KU-555-309

Shiatsu theory and practice

This book is dedicated to the memory of Brian Inglis

For Churchill Livingstone:

Commissioning editor: Mary Law/Inta Ozols
Project development editor: Valerie Bain
Project manager: Valerie Burgess
Project controller: Nicky Haig/Pat Miller
Design direction: Judith Wright
Copy editor: Holly Regan-Jones
Indexer: Tarrant Ranger Indexing Agency
Sales promotion executive: Maria O'Connor

Shiatsu theory and practice

A comprehensive text for the student and professional

Carola Beresford-Cooke
BA LicAc MRSS
Co-Principal of the Shiatsu College, London

Foreword by
Pauline Sasaki

Illustrations by
Lynn Williams

Photographs by
Nicholas Pole

CHURCHILL LIVINGSTONE

NEW YORK EDINBURGH LONDON MADRID MELBOURNE SAN FRANCISCO AND TOKYO 1996

CHURCHILL LIVINGSTONE

Medical Division of Pearson Professional Limited

Distributed in the United States of America by Churchill
Livingstone Inc., 650 Avenue of the Americas, New York,
N.Y. 10011, and by associated companies, branches and
representatives throughout the world.

© Pearson Professional Limited

All rights reserved. No part of this publication may be
reproduced, stored in a retrieval system, or transmitted in
any form or by any means, electronic, mechanical,
photocopying, recording or otherwise, without either the
prior permission of the publishers (Churchill Livingstone,
Robert Stevenson House, 1-3 Baxter's Place, Leith Walk,
Edinburgh, EH1 3AF), or a licence permitting restricted
copying in the United Kingdom issued by the Copyright
Licensing Agency Ltd, 90 Tottenham Court Road, London,
W1P 9HE.

First published 1996

ISBN 0 443 04941 6

British Library of Cataloguing in Publication Data
A catalogue record for this book is available from the British
Library.

Library of Congress Cataloging in Publication Data
A catalogue record for this book is available from the Library
of Congress.

The
publisher's
policy is to use
**paper manufactured
from sustainable forests**

Printed in the United States of America

Contents

Foreword

Although Shiatsu as a healing tool has been around since time immemorial, it has never been awarded the recognition it deserves. To the lay person, Shiatsu is something that is done in massage parlours or health spas and therefore, is a luxury for pleasure or well-being. It is thought by many to be either a sensual experience or a painful form of massage that requires little skill and offers no more than a brief period of relaxation. This misconception is so ingrained in society that many Shiatsu therapists have continually battled with a stigmatized image that does not reflect the true nature of the work. For instance, some cities in the US require Shiatsu therapists, like criminals, to be fingerprinted before they can practise. The public clearly needs to be educated in Shiatsu in order for it to be recognized as a vital therapy that can ensure the health of one's mind, body and spirit.

To the student, Shiatsu has often been regarded in the professional field of Asian therapies as a stepping stone to the study and practice of acupuncture. This logic stems from the common theoretical base which Shiatsu and acupuncture share as well as the attitude that manual therapy is inferior to the use of needles. Western medicine has trained us to think that the only effective therapies are those that are complex. This attitude has greatly influenced how Traditional Chinese Medicine (TCM) is being presented and taught throughout the world. Instead of emphasizing simplicity in nature, it has gained a reputation in the profession as being a sophisticated and intricate approach. As a result, TCM has become a complicated system to learn and practise.

Traditional Chinese Medicine is a metaphorical science designed to help us understand how we are part of nature. The key to understanding this is simplicity. This is the essence of the healing process. Preventing death or providing an instant cure is not the main purpose of TCM. The main objective is to help someone realize who he/she is as part of a universal structure and how to establish, maintain, and promote integration of all the various aspects of that structure. If we maintain the simplicity of the system, we will come to realize that by implementing the theory on a practical level, its therapeutic nature will automatically surface.

Shiatsu recaptures the true nature of Chinese medical theory. It achieves this primarily through the use of the hand. The hand is probably the most intricate instrument known to man; yet it is the least revered and most taken for granted. I do not think anyone will recall with exhilaration the times they have been pricked by a needle. However, I am sure we have all had an experience where feeling a friend's hand on our shoulder offered us a feeling of peace, love, and support that made our day much more meaningful. Research has proven the power behind simple touching. Lack of it can lead to far-reaching physical or mental results. This is a very significant finding, however students still look forward to graduating from the use of the hands in Shiatsu to the use of the needle in acupuncture. Due to our conditioning from Western medical tradition, students think that a needle gives more validity to the treatment and thus produces a more significant result.

Developing the hand as a tool for healing is not an easy task. It takes time, patience, and self-development to sensitize oneself to feeling another. Who you are, how you feel about yourself and others, and how you live your life all become a part of the quality of your touch. In this respect, Shiatsu offers more of a challenge than acupuncture. An effective quality of touch requires support and detachment at the same time. It represents the merging of the subjective and objective aspects of health. When this is achieved, a permanent healing connection takes place between the giver and the receiver.

In the Eastern medical tradition, more focus is given to the patient or receiver of the treatment. In Shiatsu, the aim is to understand an individual physically, emotionally, psychologically and spiritually. This requires a scope of knowledge that goes beyond the mere anatomical and physiological approach to the human body. The concept of energy was developed in order to be able to tap into these levels of consciousness. When we look at ourselves as an energetic structure, we translate these levels into layers of vibrations which comprise an energetic field. Because energy is constantly moving and changing, the study of these levels helps us understand the dynamics of homeostasis. Shiatsu works well with remedying physical ailments. However, a skilled Shiatsu therapist learns to incorporate all the necessary components from many different levels to establish a healthy state of balance that treats the mind, body and spirit as one entity.

Shiatsu is a very comprehensive system that can stand on its own. Not only can one work with given symptoms and circumstances, but one can also gain insight into the underlying cause of the problems which are often not apparent on a physical level. The use of the hand enables us to perceive through touch the subtle qualities of vibration that define the various levels of consciousness. Shiatsu theory helps us translate these vibrational experiences into information that assists us in our understanding of the receiver. Application of Shiatsu at this level produces a healing modality that results in a high degree of effectiveness that can match, if not exceed, that of acupuncture.

In the end, Shiatsu helps us learn to appreciate the uniqueness of each person and the value of life itself. Shiatsu allows us to treat not only others, but ourselves as well. It offers us an opportunity to discover our place in the infiniteness of the universe and to be able to participate in that continuum through transformation.

Norwalk, Connecticut 1996   Pauline E. Sasaki

Preface

Shiatsu practice is at present growing in popularity in the West, for several reasons. It is easy to learn and to practise without much theoretical knowledge, and it is enjoyable to receive. Its benefits are many, both in the maintenance of health and in the treatment of discomfort. Perhaps most appealingly, the practice of Shiatsu appears to develop the giver's mental and physical sensitivity, much as meditational or yogic techniques are said to do. Many supporters of Shiatsu feel that the intuition and healing power which the giver acquires through Shiatsu practice are themselves the only essential components of that practice, so that theoretical knowledge is not only unnecessary but also counterproductive. However, most meditative traditions have an intellectual or theoretical component; sometimes, like the *koan* of Japanese Zen, this content acts as a bone to keep the beagle of the discursive mind busy until realization dawns; sometimes, as in Hindu Vedanta, the theoretical component actively engages the conscious intellect in the support of the meditative endeavour. In Shiatsu, too, the mind, rather than being left at large to doubt and question, can be engaged in rational activity within a theoretical structure which is geared towards supporting and confirming the intuitive healing sense.

There are many different styles of Shiatsu and as many variations in theoretical content. For the student who encounters more than one approach, these variations can create doubt and confusion and therefore my endeavour in this book has been to reconcile conflicts between seemingly diverse disciplines. With apologies to the approaches which I have only mentioned in passing, such as the Namikoshi method, macrobiotic Shiatsu, barefoot Shiatsu, and others, I have concentrated on the two disciplines familiar to me from personal experience, Zen Shiatsu and Traditional Chinese Medicine (TCM). Zen Shiatsu, which has the reputation for being non-theoretical and spontaneous, in fact has a well-reasoned theoretical component. TCM, sometimes criticized as a narrow intellectual discipline, is rooted in the spacious spiritual wisdom of Taoism. Both combine theoretical structure with the spontaneity of healing practice. It is my wish that this book should encourage students of Shiatsu to find harmony between practice and theory, and to perceive the scope for originality which lies in both, so that they can develop and confirm their own individual healing power.

It is necessary for theory to harmonize with practice in Shiatsu, so that mind and body can work as one to create the potential for healing. This is the aspect of Shiatsu which cannot be written down. As W.B. Yeats wrote in a letter just before his death:

"It seems to me that I have found what I wanted. When I try to put all into a phrase, I say 'Man can embody truth, but he cannot know it'."

The heart of Shiatsu is that when we give it, with mind and body unified, we embody truth.

London 1996   C.B-C.

Acknowledgements

My profound thanks and respect go to the teachers who have given me a sense of the deeper meaning of the workings of energy in body and mind, Namkhai Norbu Rinpoche and Pauline Sasaki. I am most grateful to Giovanni Maciocia for the clarity of his teaching and of his books, and also for his support and encouragement. The work of Kiiko Matsumoto and Stephen Birch has been a constant source of inspiration and excitement, and their individual books are acknowledged constantly throughout the text.

I would also like to acknowledge the Shiatsu community, particularly my colleagues and friends in the Shiatsu College (UK), Paul Lundberg, Clifford Andrews, Elise Johnson and Nicola Pooley, for their contributions to a shared pool of knowledge from which we have all benefited.

I am most grateful to Nicholas Pole for taking the photographs from which the drawings were made. His technical expertise, dedication and presence of awareness were invaluable during several long days of work. I would also like to thank my three models, Richard Eagleton, Cheh Goh and John Rowley, for their patience and humour throughout, and our assistant, Maria Dallow, for contributing efficiency and an expensive pair of designer trousers.

I would like to acknowledge Lennie Goodings for valuable advice; Clare Maxwell-Hudson, John Rowley, Thirzie Robinson, Nicola Pooley, Claire and John Sharkey, Elise Johnson and Maria Dallow all helped by reading and commenting on the manuscript.

My thanks to Margot Gordon and Avigail Ben-Ari, who helped me through a long period of physical inactivity and mental overwork with Shiatsu and exercise respectively; to Sara Hooley, Dinah John and the Shiatsu College teachers for taking on so much work while I was writing; to my family and friends, who provided fun, support and help of all kinds; and to Sarah Flanagan for her helpful and unobtrusive presence, and for keeping my baby, Alexander, so happy and contented. My love and thanks also to John Rowley, for his help and encouragement throughout.

This book is drawn largely from my experience as a student, teacher, giver and receiver of Shiatsu. To all my teachers, students, colleagues and clients, I am deeply grateful.

Notes on the terminology used in the book

In order to emphasize the supportive nature of Shiatsu, I have used the terms "giver" and "receiver" throughout, in preference to the more clinical "practitioner" and "patient".

Avoiding the cumbersome "he or she" has been a problem, since to switch between "he" and "she" in fair proportions in the text might create much confusion as to who is doing what and to whom. Acccordingly, I have adopted the device of referring to the giver as "she" and the receiver as "he" throughout. This device has been continued in the illustrations.

Oriental medical terminology

In keeping with current practice, I have used English wherever appropriate, using capital letters to differentiate words which carry extra conceptual significance in Oriental medicine, for example Blood or Essence, and for the Oriental organ systems, for example Liver, as compared to the liver organ known to Western physiology which has no capital.

Where a concept cannot be translated adequately into English, I have used the Chinese or Japanese word. Yin and Yang have become familiar concepts in the West and need no explanation. Hara is a Japanese word which refers not only to the abdomen but also to the attributes of power, stamina, integrity and sensitivity which reside there, according to Oriental thought. Ki is the Japanese equivalent of Qi; the common translation of "energy" is non-specific and does not encompass its physical function, so I have used the Japanese term throughout. Shen is often translated as Mind or Spirit, but both English words are already too loaded with connotations; Pure Awareness comes closer but is too long, so I have stayed with Shen. Kyo and Jitsu literally mean "empty" and "full", but to translate them thus would exacerbate a basic confusion which exists between Zen Shiatsu and TCM interpretations.

Finally, in spite of the current preference for the word "channel" to denote the established pathways of Ki, I have retained the older equivalent of "meridian". While recognizing that "channel" carries a greater implication of flow, which is helpful to the acupuncture practitioner, I feel that it neglects the connotation which "meridian" conveys of a symmetrical network of lines of Ki, which is important when dealing with the whole body. When thinking of a channel, we think of one only; when thinking of a meridian, we necessarily see it as part of a pattern.

Introduction – the history and cultural context of Shiatsu

Among all the complementary therapies Shiatsu occupies a unique place. Although its pedigree is possibly one of the most ancient on the planet and although it has continued to flourish as part of the vigorous tradition of folk medicine in the Far East, it has only recently acquired a name and become a therapy in its own right.

In fact, the name Shiatsu encompasses a wide range of treatment styles and situations. One can receive Shiatsu fully clothed on a futon or naked in a Californian spa; lying with 10 other patients in a Japanese clinic or sitting on a stool at a Western health exhibition. Treatment can take the form of hard, forceful pressure with manipulation, gentler, subtle pressure with stretching of the limbs, or palm healing; one style even works entirely off the body. Diagnosis can be made from feeling the pulse, from points on the back, from pressure on the abdomen or from visual observation of face or posture.

Although Shiatsu is often thought of as deriving from acupuncture, it is likely that it predates even that venerable therapy. Since touch is the most instinctive form of healing, we may suppose that the points and meridians were rubbed and pressed long before they were stimulated with the stone needles found at Neolithic sites in China, dating back to 8000 BC. Perhaps the acupuncture meridians and points were originally discovered through touch? Some acupuncture teachers would have it that the meridians were originally perceived as lines of sensation travelling along the body after stimulation of a point with a needle, but simple pressure on a point can and does create the same lines of sensation. Some styles of Shiatsu use primarily the meridians and not the points and this method goes back to the early history of Chinese medicine – a book found in a tomb of the Han Dynasty (206 BC – 220 AD) in Hunan mentions meridians only and not points.

However, there is no doubt that stimulation of points with needles, rather than exploring the meridians with thumbs or fingers, involves less energy expenditure by the practitioner. So acupuncture gradually took over in China as the main form of "energy" manipulation, although mastery of palpation and massage techniques remained an important prerequisite of the physician's training before he was allowed to progress to needles. As time went by, however, the importance of massage in the medical repertory declined and its status is now roughly that of physiotherapy in our own medical system, while acupuncture is the dominant healing mode.

Among the people, however, massage, in the form of rubbing and pressing the meridians and points, retained tremendous popularity. Wherever the theory of Qi, or vital energy, went, there went this type of massage. Tibet, the Philippines, Indonesia and Thailand all have similar versions. Even Southern India, which adheres to its own Vedic concept of prana rather than the Chinese idea of Qi, has a form of massage employing pressure points and claims that all forms of pressure massage originated there, like the Chinese systems of martial arts, which are said to have been introduced by the Indian Bodhidharma. Although the truth is hard to come by, it is certain that some cross-cultural fertilization took place via the Spice Routes.

Japan has a close relationship with Chinese culture and took over the forms of Chinese acupuncture and massage with the least distortion of the tradition. However, after the introduction of Chinese medicine to Japan in the 6th century AD, some change was inevitable. The characteristic of Chinese culture at the height of its flowering is an irresistible outpouring of creativity; that of the Japanese is a mastery of fine detail. The Japanese did with Chinese medicine as they did with Chinese art; they refined the vigour of the Chinese creation and pursued the techniques down into the most detailed realms of form. A kind of pressure massage of the abdomen evolved, for example, called Ampuku. Ampuku practitioners would spend up to 12 years of training learning how to diagnose and treat disease exclusively via the abdomen, or Hara as it is known in Japanese. This capacity to reduce, analyse and refine is as typical of the Japanese approach as the broad sweep of creativity is of the Chinese.

The Hara or abdomen, already mentioned above, has its own unique place in the theory of Shiatsu, not only as an important area for diagnosis and treatment but also as a potent centre of energy to be developed by the Shiatsu practitioner. It is known as the Sea of Ki (the Japanese word for Qi) and all activity, when performed "from the Hara", is imbued with a vital combination of energy, relaxation and concentration. Martial arts, dance and theatre, Sumo wrestling, archery, meditation, painting and healing, even chopping wood or cooking, are done better when done from the Hara. Cultivation of a sense of the Hara is vital to Shiatsu training. To centre awareness and breath in the Hara is a practice which opens the practitioner's perceptions, so that ultimately the whole body can become a vehicle for the sensing or transmission of Ki.

The concepts of Hara and Ki are so rooted in Japanese thinking that they are enshrined in the language. "*Gen-ki des' ka?*", the Japanese equivalent of "How are you?", means literally "How is your Ki?" while the phrase for "ill" is "*byo ki*" – "bad Ki". To say that a person has a "good Hara" means that he or she has integrity, while a "bad Hara" suggests shiftiness and unreliability.

Shiatsu, a science of Ki rooted in the Hara, belongs, then, to all Japanese and not just the physicians. Small wonder that it should percolate down to the level of folk medicine and draw new energy from it. Here simple, vigorous and effective techniques evolved, among ordinary people doing traditional massage without much academic knowledge. This

uncomplicated, non-theoretical approach was to refresh and revitalize Shiatsu from the grass roots up.

By the beginning of this century, however, the original physicians' massage style had progressively become the massage of the court and then of the bath-houses, with many of the same connotations that "sauna and massage" had until recently in the West.

The more serious paramedical practitioners formed the Shiatsu Therapists' Association in 1925 to distinguish them from the "shampooers" who were giving relaxation massage and "Shi-atsu", or "finger pressure", became the official name for remedial massage in Japan.

Meanwhile, Western customs, including Western medicine, had been gaining a firm hold in Japanese culture. Aizawa Seishisai, a Confucian scholar writing in 1825, had already commented on "the weakness of some for novel gadgets and rare medicines" which led many of his countrymen "to admire foreign ways". Gradually Western techniques of manipulation, and above all Western medical terminology, were added to the Shiatsu practitioner's repertory. Points began to be known by their Western anatomical locations alone, and the concept of interconnecting meridians ceased to be emphasized.

Tokujiro Namikoshi, who founded the Clinic of Pressure Therapy in 1925, endeavoured to place Shiatsu techniques within a Western framework. His school was, and remains, the only one to receive an official licence to teach Shiatsu and as a result the Namikoshi method is the most widely studied in Japan. Namikoshi therapists characterize points by their anatomical locations rather than the meridian system and favour a Western scientific approach to treatment over classical theory.

Shiatsu continued to be practised and taught, both in the new Western style and in the traditional ways, until the American occupation in the aftermath of World War II, when General MacArthur, as part of a general repression of traditional Japanese culture, banned its practice, as well as the practice of Anma, the relaxation massage given mainly for pleasure. Anma was practised mainly by the blind, a tradition still observed in many Far Eastern countries for the preservation of modesty. Shiatsu also had its blind practitioners and the livelihood of all these was threatened by the ban. It is said that their plight was brought to the attention of Helen Keller, the celebrated writer and champion of the blind, herself blind and deaf from birth. She interceded with the American government and Anma and Shiatsu were restored to their former status.

The next chapter in the history of Shiatsu began with the work of the late Shizuto Masunaga. A professor of psychology at Tokyo University, he was deeply interested in traditional Oriental medicine and did much research into ancient Chinese texts on the subject. His mother had studied with Tamai Tempaku, who had played a major role in the renaissance of Shiatsu in the 1920s. Masunaga also studied Shiatsu, qualifying at the Namikoshi school and teaching there for 10 years. He began to blend his three areas of interest, psychology, orthodox Shiatsu practice and historical research into its roots, combining these with modern Western understanding of physiology. His style, which he named "Zen Shiatsu", thus has a comprehensive theory of its own, encompassing both Western and Eastern models of disease and healing.

Masunaga also developed further the traditional methods of diagnosing from palpation either of the patient's Hara or back, evolving a unique method of assessing the body's immediate energy pattern and of working the appropriate meridians to correct distortions within it. He also made a contribution to the meridian system, the foundation of Shiatsu. By tracing lines of Ki, apparent as lines of sensation to the receiver or palpable by himself as the giver, he extended the 12 classical acupuncture meridians throughout the body, so that almost every meridian can be treated in almost every body part. Zen Shiatsu is wonderfully flexible and geared towards the specific needs of each receiver.

Since Masunaga's death in 1981, many exponents of various forms of Zen Shiatsu have begun to teach, each with their own direction or emphasis, and the field of Shiatsu is alive with recognitions, discoveries and controversies. Most of this, however, is taking place in the West. With the increasing urbanization of Japan, the science of Ki does not appeal as much as the science of computer design. Shiatsu is still practised, as it always has been, in the clinics of traditional medicine and in village homes, and some major industries offer free Shiatsu to workers because of its role in preventing illness, but its major development and synthesis is taking place in the Western world. Shiatsu lacks Chinese acupuncture's connection with a thriving home centre, but its development in the West may in the end take it back to its homeland richer and more versatile.

Sources of Shiatsu theory and the purpose of this book

Why study Shiatsu theory?

The very multiplicity of the sources of Shiatsu theory in the West presents a difficulty for the advanced student. It is easy to learn the basics of Shiatsu technique and to apply them with minimal knowledge of theory in order to treat or manage a wide variety of conditions; the intuitive and healing quality of Shiatsu touch is extremely helpful from the beginning to both giver and receiver. But at a certain point the student may find herself at a loss, faced with a condition which fails to respond as expected. At this stage it is useful to be able to differentiate among the various models which constitute Shiatsu theory in order to select the appropriate method of treatment.

Let us take the example of a chronic and intractable sore throat. The Five Element model suggests the Lung meridian; Zen Shiatsu adds the Triple Heater and Heart Protector meridians; Traditional Chinese Medicine (or TCM) presents the possibility of Kidney Yin Deficiency, stagnation of Liver Ki or invasion of external Wind-Heat. There may be an osteopathic element such as a neck lesion or tension in the jaw area and there is also the option of a psychological cause, such as the inability to "voice emotions" or to "swallow a situation".

Truly intuitive and healing Shiatsu may remedy the problem without any need for theory but perhaps the giver is below par on that particular day and intuition is absent. Or perhaps she gives relief with her intuitive treatment but feels that the receiver needs to take steps to prevent a recurrence and is at a loss what to advise. It may be that something she does as a result of intuitive promptings works and she wants to know why, or perhaps she simply wants to know more about Shiatsu theory.

This book aims to present three important sources of Shiatsu theory to the student and to show their relevance in clinical situations. These are:

- the Five Element theory
- Traditional Chinese Medicine or TCM
- Zen Shiatsu.

Five Element theory

Although the Five Element (or Five Phase) theory (see p. 81) is only a part of the theory of TCM, it has been singled out to form the basis for most Shiatsu theory teaching in the West. It is useful for the beginner because it is at the same time simple and comprehensive. Five Element theory postulates that the Ki which constitutes and animates the universe can be subdivided into five different phases, which are like qualities or "flavours" of Ki, namely Fire, Earth, Metal, Water and Wood. The human bodymind contains all five of these qualities and each pair of meridians pertains to a separate Element and channels that Element's "flavour" of Ki. (Each Element governs a pair of meridians, except Fire, which governs two pairs.) Because Ki exists everywhere, this means that qualities of human Ki resemble similar qualities found elsewhere in the universe, for example the flexibility of plants, the coolness of water, the stability of earth and so on. These similarities have become codified in lists of "Element correspondences" which form a basic theory for the characteristics of the meridians.

For many Oriental physicians, the Five Element theory is no more than a historical relic with little practical application. Some Western schools of acupuncture, on the contrary, emphasize the Five Elements to the exclusion of all the other components of Oriental medicine. Between these two extremes, we could view the Five Element theory as a useful vehicle for the practical experience and understanding of Ki. Differentiating between the Ki of the Elements as they manifest in nature is a helpful exercise for Shiatsu practice, which itself is based on direct contact with Ki. For this reason I have included a discussion of the qualities of each Element as it is found in nature in the chapters describing the meridian characteristics.

TCM

Although the phrase "Traditional Chinese Medicine" properly refers to the entire body of Chinese medical theory accumulated throughout that vast country to the present day, with all its regional and historical variations, it is now widely used in the West to refer to the medical model currently adopted as standard by the People's Republic of China since the reinstatement of traditional methods during the Cultural Revolution. It is thus biased towards the treatment of physical conditions and does not emphasize the psychological and spiritual factors influencing health which were acknowledged in former times. Because of the research constantly in progress in China, however, TCM remains a living, changing system of medicine with immense potential for the treatment of a variety of diseases of the modern world.

The foundations of TCM are the concepts of Yin and Yang, the correspondences of the Five Elements, the Five Vital Substances (of which Ki is one) and the means by which they are produced, and the internal and external pathogenic factors of Wind, Heat, Damp and so forth. The principal methods of diagnosis are questioning, observation of the tongue and palpation of the pulse and the practitioner classifies the patient's symptoms under the Eight Conditions of Yin/Yang, Full/Empty, Hot/Cold and Interior/Exterior. TCM also includes an encyclopaedic repertoire of the functions of the acupuncture points in treatment.

A basic knowledge of TCM is useful to the Shiatsu giver for several reasons. Firstly, it enlarges the giver's view of the receiver's condition beyond the simple diagnosis of Five Element correspondences and the state of the meridians at the time of treatment. TCM allows the giver to differentiate the receiver's symptoms sufficiently to make an approximate prognosis, suggest changes in lifestyle and, if necessary, refer to another therapy. With the added perspective of TCM, the Shiatsu giver can also include in her treatment repertoire the use of specific acupuncture points, whether by pressure, moxibustion (traditional Oriental heat treatment) or the newer Japanese method of magnetic therapy. Finally, an understanding of the vocabulary and concepts of TCM offers the student an opportunity to benefit from the research findings now available in the field. In this way, and by participating in discussion with acupuncturists and herbalists, Shiatsu therapists can help to reinstate Shiatsu as one of the four main branches of traditional Oriental medicine.

There are several excellent works on TCM available in the West and an exhaustive analysis would be beyond the scope of this book, but I have approached the subject from the perspective of the Shiatsu practitioner and outlined the basics of TCM in Chapter 5. In addition, each chapter on the individual meridians contains a description of the meridian's function in terms of TCM.

Zen Shiatsu

With the publication in the West in 1977 of Shizuto Masunaga's *Zen Shiatsu*, the possibility was finally realized of a comprehensive Shiatsu theory, traditionally rooted, yet encompassing modern scientific knowledge and open to development and ongoing interpretation. Although Masunaga's ideas were as yet incompletely synthesized, Shiatsu practitioners hailed them as a great step beyond the limitations of both the popular Westernized theory and the theory of acupuncture, which was ill suited to Shiatsu in clinical practice and too complicated for the beginner.

The appeal of Zen Shiatsu theory to the student is that it is based in actual Shiatsu practice. The systems of palpatory diagnosis and the extension of the classical acupuncture meridians throughout the body mean that the Shiatsu treatment covers the whole body, providing a complete relaxation experience while at the same time focusing minutely on the receiver's current treatment needs.

Zen Shiatsu in theory and practice treats the receiver as a whole, as did the most ancient versions of Chinese medical theory. Through the meridians, the giver treats the receiver's mind, spirit and emotions as well as his physical body. Its particular attraction for the Western practitioner lies in this explicit unification of human psychology and physiology within the theory of Ki, an approach which satisfies the Western hunger to restore wholeness to the fragmented bodymind.

Though holistic, Zen Shiatsu theory is also distinguished by considerable scientific exactitude and intellectual integrity. If we can stretch our minds to the point of accepting that Ki exists and that all physical and non-physical phenomena are a manifestation of Ki, then the rest of the theory is well constructed and coherent. Indeed, it can even illuminate many aspects of the presentation of disease which continue to puzzle minds trained in the scientific reductionist model. Although Masunaga died before he could complete his theory, many of his leading students are continuing to build on his framework. The reader will find the basic outline of Zen Shiatsu theory in Chapter 6 and more detailed discussion in the chapters on the individual meridians.

SECTION ONE

Practice

1

The basics – why, when and how

Conditions which respond well to Shiatsu

In practice, there are few conditions which cannot be alleviated to some extent by Shiatsu treatment, but to what extent depends upon the ability of the giver. It depends also on the choice of pressure and techniques, a subject which is covered more fully in Chapter 14. Obviously, the greater the giver's ability and healing power, the better the results in all conditions.

However most practitioners will find that some receivers respond much better than others, even when their complaints are of a similar nature, and Chinese philosophy explains this as part of the phenomenon of *yuan*. *Yuan* is the strength of the energetic attraction between two individuals at any moment in time. *Yuan* exists between lovers and it usually exists between family members, though it can wax, wane or vanish. It links friends and it can exist between doctor and patient. The greater the *yuan* between doctor and patient, the more successful the treatment, and doctors famous for their ability have a broad spectrum of *yuan* with large numbers of patients. Western medicine used to have a similar concept. My father, a doctor trained in the 1930s, told me that a doctor who cured more patients than his colleagues was said in those days to have "clinical sense".

While the concept of *yuan* deserves consideration, there is no doubt that the element of touch is most important to the success or otherwise of Shiatsu treatment. Touch is a language which communicates with the emotions through the body, as research has

shown. In a study conducted by Harvard Medical School, when an anaesthetist held a patient's hand for the time it took to explain the surgical procedure to be undergone, the patient's postoperative stay in hospital and need for pain medication were both significantly reduced. Shiatsu is therefore very effective, either alone or in combination with another treatment mode, in conditions where emotional disturbance or stress is an underlying factor. While this could be said to include all ailments, the conditions most widely recognized as stress related are:

- insomnia
- anxiety and depression
- muscular tension
- headaches
- digestive disturbances
- menstrual dysfunction
- low resistance to infection

and all these respond well to Shiatsu treatment. From the perspective of the Shiatsu practitioner, since the body and the emotions are both different manifestations of Ki in action, the emotions are reharmonized as well as the body at the time of treatment, although the source of the stress must be eradicated if the improvement is to be maintained.

Shiatsu is also the treatment of choice for disorders of the musculoskeletal system, since it works directly on the tissues involved. It is therefore effective in the treatment of:

- backache
- synovitis
- sprains and strains
- neck and shoulder stiffness
- joint pain.

Its localized physical effects, when correct techniques are used, also relieve:

- sinus congestion
- retention of fluid in the tissues
- poor circulation.

From the standpoint of Oriental medicine, the effectiveness of Shiatsu in correcting these conditions is a direct result of re-establishing Ki flow throughout the meridians.

In practice, the effectiveness of Shiatsu extends beyond the comfort of touch and the physical manipulation of the tissues, both of which can be addressed by other forms of massage or touch therapy. The Shiatsu practitioner sees the physical body, mind and emotions as indivisibly connected by the network of Ki flow. For example, treating the Large Intestine meridian in the arms and legs can relieve symptoms of the musculoskeletal system (shoulder pain or lower back pain), the tissues (sinus congestion, skin disorders), the internal organs (many disorders of the bowel and related conditions), stress-related disorders (headaches) and the feelings (such as depression or lethargy).

Contraindications to the practice of Shiatsu

There are few disorders which the experienced practitioner cannot treat with Shiatsu, but certain conditions should be approached cautiously. In general, the Shiatsu giver should not attempt to treat any disorder which causes her any degree of nervousness and serious diseases should be avoided by the beginner.

Shiatsu is conventionally contraindicated for cancer, on the grounds that increased venous and lymphatic flow may cause the disease to spread. However, since physical exercise or deep breathing also increase venous and lymphatic flow and both these are considered beneficial, the Shiatsu giver may choose to treat nonetheless. There are many cases where appropriate Shiatsu has greatly helped the symptoms of cancer patients, but the decision on what is appropriate is best made by an advanced practitioner.

The first 3 months of pregnancy are also best treated by an experienced practitioner or not at all, in the interests of the giver as much as the receiver. A firmly rooted foetus is unlikely to be dislodged by gentle treatment but, by the same token, miscarriage in the first 3 months is an event as frequent as it is profoundly distressing and blame may subsequently attach to the Shiatsu giver.

Note: Throughout pregnancy, direct pressure on the abdomen and certain points which move the Ki strongly (LI 4, Sp 6, GB 21) are contraindicated.

Any kind of acute illness with fever is unsuitable for general Shiatsu treatment, since the fever is a sign that the body is already engaged in fighting off the infection and should not be overloaded. Judicious use of certain points, however, may help to speed recovery by eliminating the External pathogenic factor (Ch. 5, p. 71).

Shiatsu is contraindicated in osteoporosis except with the lightest pressure, for fear of damage to the bone. The same caution should be used in treating receivers who have had chemotherapy, for the same reason. High blood pressure is traditionally contraindicated, but this applies only to very hard and forceful pressure which could damage the blood vessels. If only gentle Shiatsu techniques and light pressure are used, Shiatsu can be soothing and beneficial in cases of high blood pressure.

Very weak or debilitated receivers, such as the elderly, the frail and many sufferers from myalgic encephalomyelitis (or ME, also known as chronic fatigue syndrome) should also be treated very gently, if it all, with Shiatsu. This subject is explored further in Chapter 14 (p. 252).

These are the main systemic conditions which the Shiatsu giver should approach with caution. Other contraindications refer to localized conditions, where only the affected part should be avoided during the course of treatment. These include:

- varicose veins
- wounds
- fractures
- operation scars and adhesions
- inflamed joints (showing signs of heat or redness)
- areas of inflamed, red or raw skin.

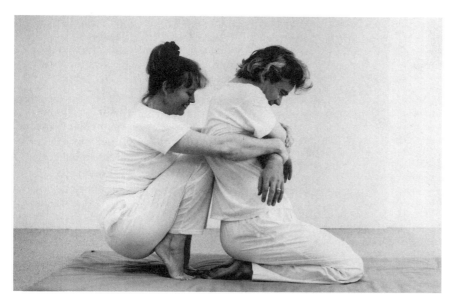

Fig. 1.1 *Working on the floor; a mid-back release using balance and leverage.*

In all these cases, general Shiatsu to the rest of the body, and in particular above and below the contraindicated area or on the opposite side if the affected part is on a limb, can be extremely beneficial.

Practical basics

Floor, bed or chair?

Shiatsu is traditionally performed on a mat on the floor, since in Japan most activities take place at floor level. For the practitioner, working on the floor permits maximum versatility, as pressure can be applied with knees and feet as well as elbows and hands and a wide variety of stretches can be used which do not require constant raising or lowering of the working surface but depend principally on the giver's choice of position and use of body weight (Fig. 1.1).

Working on the floor also encourages the giver to work from the Hara, supported by leverage from legs and feet. In the early stages of Shiatsu study, great attention is paid to the giver's posture and the relaxed application of body weight; gradually, as this becomes second nature and the giver's body flows naturally into the most effective position, then a sense of the Hara can develop and the giver begins to transmit Ki.

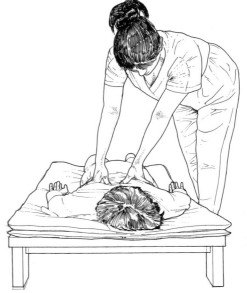

Fig. 1.2 *Using a low table.*

Shiatsu is therefore best studied at floor level to begin with, until the giver's body functions easily and powerfully in this position. However, some receivers are unable to lie on the floor and another treatment position must be chosen. For elderly receivers, the techniques traditionally performed in a kneeling or sitting position on the floor can be modified for use in

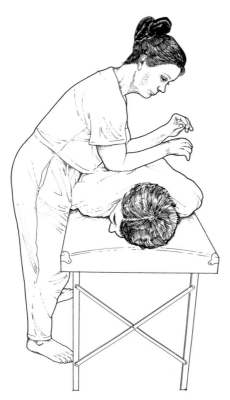

Fig. 1.3 *Working on a massage couch.*

a chair. For situations where neither floor nor chair are suitable, the solution is a treatment couch which can be lowered sufficiently to allow the giver to apply pressure through straight arms while leaning forward from the hips (Fig. 1.2). Fixed height treatment couches make it very hard to work from the Hara and unless the giver works exclusively with her elbows, it is impossible to use relaxed body weight (Fig. 1.3). The worst option is a standard domestic bed, since in addition to the above-mentioned disadvantages, the height puts a strain on the giver's back and the receiver's unsupported body sinks into the mattress with each application of pressure.

Clothed or unclothed?

One of Shiatsu's great advantages as a therapy is that it can be given through clothes. This is not only for reasons of modesty, traditional in the Far East and particularly necessary when Shiatsu techniques stretch the receiver's limbs into revealing positions; it is also relevant to Shiatsu practice. On hot days or in a warm room, giver or receiver can sweat, making the receiver's skin too slippery for stretches or pressure.

It can also feel unpleasant to receive Shiatsu from sweaty hands and for this reason many givers use a cloth when working on the face or other uncovered areas (Fig. 1.4).

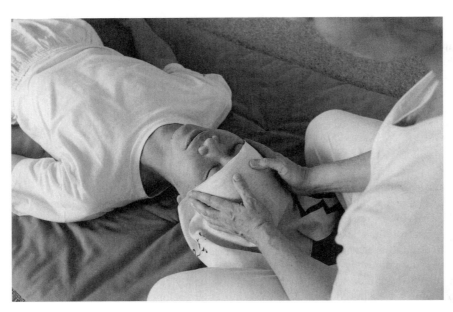

Fig. 1.4 *Using a cloth on the face.*

Note: Care should be taken not to cover the receiver's face completely with the cloth, so as to avoid possible feelings of claustrophobia.

More importantly, the focus of Shiatsu pressure is not the skin surface but the deeper body structures and above all the Ki within the body. Students are encouraged to feel through clothing for the shape and tone of the receiver's body, rather than uncovering areas "to feel them more easily", since the giver's sense of touch should not be distracted by the texture of the skin. Clothing can also be useful for observation diagnosis; to the eye of the experienced practitioner, the way clothing falls or creases can enhance rather than prevent her perception of the flow of the receiver's Ki (see p. 231).

It is thus preferable that the receiver should be clothed when receiving traditional Shiatsu; however, some practitioners prefer to work on bare skin and others use a combination of massage methods which include Shiatsu pressures and the use of oils, so that they uncover the receiver when using oils and cover him with towels when giving Shiatsu. The giver should work in the way she prefers, but a competent Shiatsu therapist should be able to work as easily through clothes as on the naked body, otherwise the Shiatsu risks being only "skin deep".

2

Recommendations for the Shiatsu practitioner

The practice of Shiatsu as a profession requires a fit and healthy body. Physical strength is not a necessity, but flexibility and the ability to relax are important since good Shiatsu is given, not with strong pressure from arms and shoulders, but with leverage and use of body weight. Stamina and energy are also required and these come with developing a strong Hara. Developing the Hara is a must for the Shiatsu giver. A strong Hara confers not only physical stamina but also the ability to sense and transmit Ki, so that powerful and effective treatments are given.

Development of the Hara

One of the best ways of increasing the energetic capacity of any body part is to bring attention to it, since awareness is a form of energy. Attention can be focused in the Hara by means of specific meditations, often combined with breathing practices. Shiatsu givers usually have their own preferred methods; for those who have none, here is a combined breathing and meditation exercise which students often find helpful.

Breathing and meditation exercise for developing the Hara

Sit comfortably with your back straight but relaxed. Close your eyes and gently draw your attention to your breathing. Observe your breathing pattern just as it is, without judging or trying to change it. Let it be slow or fast, shallow or deep, smooth or uneven; let it be. Do not focus too hard and punishingly on the breath; just observe, calmly bringing your attention back when it wanders.

Gradually, as you calmly observe your breathing and allow it to be just the way it is, it will quieten and deepen. This may take time; stay calm and patient. As it quietens, encourage your breathing to move down into your abdomen by expanding your abdomen slightly as you breathe in and contracting it slightly as you breathe out. Place your hands on your abdomen, just below the navel, if it helps.

As your breathing moves down into your abdomen, add the power of visualization to encourage it. Imagine that the lower part of your body and your pelvis are a bowl; make the bowl a beautiful one, golden or marble or porcelain, however you would like it. As you breathe steadily into your abdomen, imagine the breath as water pouring straight down the inside of your body and arriving in the bottom of the bowl; let the breath follow this image. See the bowl slowly begin to fill and imagine light illuminating both the bowl and the water pouring into it. As the bowl fills with water, watch it become more and more suffused with light.

Now let the image of the bowl gradually fade and concentrate on the sphere of light in your abdomen. As you breath in, imagine that the sphere of light becomes brighter and slightly smaller. Maintain this image through the outbreath and again imagine the sphere of light becoming brighter and smaller with the inbreath. Each time you breathe in, the sphere of light becomes brighter, smaller and more concentrated and stays that way through the outbreath. Continue until you have a tiny point of blazing white light in the centre of your lower abdomen and keep on making it smaller and brighter

15

for several breaths. Then relax your attention, let go of the visualization but remain aware of your breathing and of the place in your centre where the point of light last was.

Remain in this state of awareness for a few more breaths, then gradually bring your attention back to the present moment. Be aware of the sounds in your environment. When you are ready, open your eyes and take in the sight around you. Remain quiet for a few minutes before stretching your body and resuming activity.

Breathing and meditation exercise: advanced version

If you are already experienced in meditation techniques or Ki awareness practices – or when you have practised the above meditation for some time – you can go to the advanced version, which is quicker, simpler and more direct.

Sit comfortably with a straight back and close your eyes. Observe your breathing. Take your breath down into your abdomen and practise abdominal breathing for a few minutes. Visualize the point in the centre of your lower abdomen to which the breath is drawn. With each inbreath, halve the size of the point. Keep making the point half the size for as long as you can, then relax, release the visualization of the point but be aware of its presence, breathing gently and slowly, for a few more minutes. Gradually allow your attention to encompass your surroundings and open your eyes when you are ready. Gently stretch your body and remain quiet for a short time before resuming activity.

Do not work too hard at this meditation! If it seems like hard work or makes you feel uncomfortable in any way, relax, stretch, move around, have a soothing drink and forget about it for a while. Next time, do the first exercise.

Other ways of developing the Hara

Once you are aware of the centre of energy in the lower abdomen, it will become stronger the more you remember it. Focusing on the Hara can become a habit of attention. However, there are other ways in which you can encourage a sense of the Hara and improve your Shiatsu.

One way is to live at floor level as much as you can. A thick carpet, plenty of cushions and low-level tables can provide an attractive home environment, although some of your visitors may be more comfortable in an armchair or on a sofa. Living at floor level encourages groundedness and flexibility, as we learn to reach out for what we need or crawl towards it, rather than getting to our feet, and our centre of gravity sinks.

Consciously changing our posture can also be helpful. Many of us have the habit of keeping our knees locked straight, which cuts us off from awareness of our relationship with the ground. Unlocking the knees, keeping them slightly flexed, means that our natural balancing sensors keep us aware of our centre of gravity in the Hara. It is also important to relax the abdomen enough to feel it move slightly with the breath. Our culture encourages a "stomach-in" posture which constricts the breathing and cuts off awareness of the lower body, so let your belly out a little and relax it. Attitude of mind helps greatly here. Imagine your Hara as a powerhouse, rather than a jelly bag, and you are halfway there. It is useful to study Chinese and Japanese paintings and sculptures of warriors, sages and saints and see the power emanating from their Hara (Fig. 2.1).

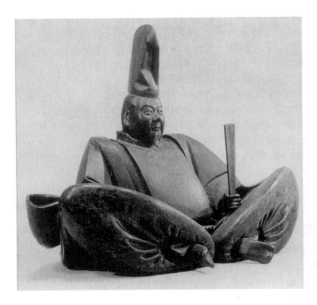

Fig. 2.1 *An example of Hara: the Shogun Minamoto Yoritomo (by kind permission of the Tokyo National Museum).*

Massaging the Hara can also help to develop energy there, as well as maintaining a healthy digestion. An easy daily exercise is to place one hand on top of the other just below the navel and rotate the whole area 50 times in a clockwise direction, not the clothes or skin only, but deeply enough to feel it in the muscular layer of your belly.

There are many exercises designed to develop the Hara within the Oriental traditions of Tai Chi and Qi Gong. One which is quick, easy and develops flexibility of the lower body as well as a strong Hara is as follows.

Stand with your feet facing straight forward and a shoulders-width apart, knees very slightly flexed, back straight, shoulders relaxed, looking straight ahead. Breathe slowly in and allow your hands to float up in front of you; breathe out and bring them slowly towards your Hara, placing them finally one on top of the other, just below your navel. Visualize a tiny pencil stub in the centre of your lower abdomen, under your hands. Imagine that the pencil is beginning to draw a clockwise spiral in a horizontal plane within your Hara and that your body is following its movements. The pencil makes 36 turns of the spiral in ever-increasing circles and your body follows it, so that you begin with movements so small and subtle as to be imperceptible to the eye. Then gradually your hips begin to rotate clockwise and towards the end of the 36 turns the pencil is drawing such large circles that your whole body is compensating for the wide movements of your hips. Try to keep the circles as even in shape as possible. After the thirty-sixth circle, pause, then rotate in the opposite direction while you visualize the pencil drawing a decreasing spiral of 36 circles, so that the large movements become smaller and eventually almost imperceptible. When you reach the point at the centre of your spiral, relax, gently lower your hands to your sides and stand, still with knees slightly flexed, aware of the point in the centre of your Hara.

Achieving flexibility – exercise

The Shiatsu giver needs to develop the Hara in order to transmit Ki effortlessly for sustained periods of time. She also needs to be physically flexible in order to increase her repertory of techniques. In the long term this saves energy, since using exactly the appropriate technique for a particular receiver in a particular position ensures maximum treatment effect.

Yoga, Tai Chi and Qi Gong

These are all taught increasingly widely in the West and the Shiatsu student is advised to gain some experience of at least one of these systems of exercise in addition to Western exercises or activities, since all of them are based on principles of energy flow as well as stretching and developing the physical body. Tai Chi and Qi Gong are tailormade for the Shiatsu giver, since they are rooted in the science of Ki, while Yoga stretches, though based on a different concept of energy, that of prana, also encourage the flow of Ki through the meridians.

The Makko-Ho

A series of exercises called the Makko-Ho (translated as Mr Makko's Method) was made available to the Shiatsu world in the 1970s. It remains the most basic form of exercise taught in Shiatsu schools, since it involves a specific stretch for each pair of meridians. The yoga-based stretches are easy to master and express the psychological quality of the meridian pairs, as well as stretching them physically. In sequence, they provide a simple, short but comprehensive workout for the meridian system; singly, they can be taught to receivers with a bias towards problems in a particular meridian pair as a way of improving their own health between treatments. A detailed account of the Makko-Ho is given in Chapter 15.

Hand and foot exercises

Hands need to be strong and feet flexible for giving Shiatsu and specific attention may need to be paid to them.

A simple hand exercise taught by Pauline Sasaki (one of the most highly regarded teachers and exponents of Zen Shiatsu in the West) is to kneel down in a crawling position with the tips of the fingers and thumbs resting on the floor in front of you. Shift your weight forward into the fingers of the left hand, then across to the right hand, then back to the right knee, then to the left knee, completing a circle. Repeat the circle four more times, then reverse your direction and complete five more circles the opposite way. This encourages a sense of the Hara as well as strengthening your hands, if you imagine your Hara making the circles.

A sequence of foot exercises taught to me by the healer Annie McCaffry has proved very helpful to Shiatsu students.

Start by standing relaxed, with your feet shoulders width apart, arms by your sides, making sure your knees are not locked, and put your awareness in your feet. See how you experience your contact with the ground. Now slowly shift your weight completely on to one foot, so that you can take your other foot off the floor without altering your balance. Then slowly and evenly shift your weight on to the other foot in the same way. Usually one feels more comfortable to stand on than the other. Start the exercises standing on the more comfortable foot.

1. Place the ball of the other foot on the floor and stretch the toes back as far as you can against the resistance of the floor. Stretch three or four times (Fig. 2.2).
2. Curl the toes of the same foot underneath your sole and stretch the foot in this position three or four times. Try to keep the top of your foot in line with your lower leg, not bending at the ankle (Fig. 2.3).
3. Shift your weight on to the other foot and repeat 1 and 2 on the other side.
4. Stand on both feet again and raise both your big toes from the floor (Fig. 2.4).

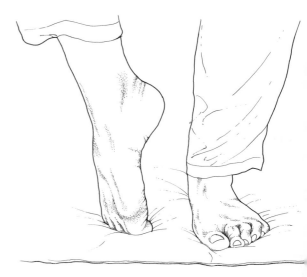

Fig. 2.3 *Foot exercise 2.*

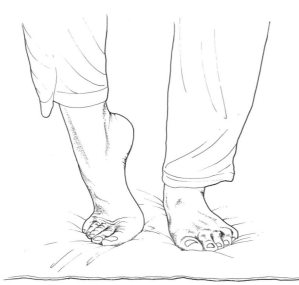

Fig. 2.2 *Foot exercise 1.*

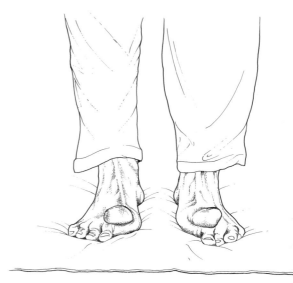

Fig. 2.4 *Foot exercise 4.*

5. Put your big toes down flat again and try to raise all your other toes from the floor. Try not to let your feet roll inwards (Fig. 2.5).
6. Repeat 4 and 5 several times.
7. Bring both feet together and stand on the outer edge of both feet, with your soles touching as much as you can (Fig. 2.6).

Now stand on both feet again and see how you experience your contact with the ground. Shift your weight slowly from one foot to the other. If there was a difference between your feet when you first started, you may feel that the difference has lessened or disappeared.

These exercises not only increase the flexibility of your feet so that when giving Shiatsu you can move easily around the receiver; they also increase your awareness of your feet, so that you can use them as Shiatsu "tools" and also generally increase your groundedness.

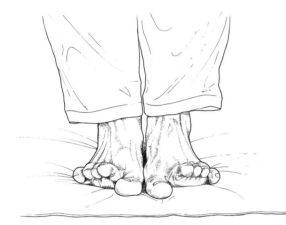

Fig. 2.5 *Foot exercise 5.*

Maintaining health

There is a saying among Shiatsu practitioners that the Ki of the giver should be greater than that of the receiver if the treatment is to be beneficial. In fact, the study and practice of Shiatsu should increase the giver's Ki and general well-being. However, there are a few guidelines which should be at least considered by anyone thinking of Shiatsu practice as a career.

Conserve your energy

1. Moderation in all things was advocated by the great Oriental physicians of the past. Too much work, including self-development such as meditation or exercise, is as detrimental to health as too many late night parties.
2. Try to observe your own energy; do not push yourself. When giving Shiatsu, keep your treatment time to the minimum required to create a positive effect (Ch. 14) and keep your own body movements to a minimum, relying on comfortable use of your weight.
3. If you become ill, even with a cold, rest. According to TCM, many diseases can develop if the body is not allowed to heal itself fully. Observe the condition of your Ki and pace yourself accordingly.

Take care of your diet

Many of us who study Shiatsu come to adopt Oriental principles of diet. These may be macrobiotic principles or the more eclectic Chinese way of eating.

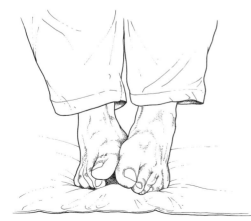

Fig. 2.6 *Foot exercise 7.*

Some of us may prefer the Western naturopathic model of raw food vegetarianism and some may be vegans. Food combining is also an increasingly popular option. Within this varied spectrum of eating habits, there are certain commonsense principles which all can follow.

1. Firstly, try to eat foods which retain the maximum of their original Ki; fresh foods, if possible organic, which have undergone the minimum of chemical, mechanical or radioactive interference. Foods are best when they are local and in season and have not travelled far or been kept in storage. If you eat meat of chicken, try to find free range or organic sources so as to avoid taking in extra hormones or antibiotics from intensive farming. The same applies to salmon and trout.
2. It is also a good idea to maintain balance between the different aspects of your diet. Even if you are food combining, make sure that your diet overall is balanced, with more carbohydrate than vegetables, more vegetables than protein and more protein than fat.
3. To ensure the best use of food by your body, keep your food intake moderate and regular. Do not skip breakfast. Make sure mealtimes are unhurried and devoted to eating only, not work, discussion or argument. Neither give nor receive Shiatsu immediately after a meal and try to rest for a short time afterwards.
4. Within the limits of whichever dietary principles you are following, try to eat as much as possible according to inclination rather than principle. Ask your body what it needs and follow its promptings, without indulging habitual cravings. And finally, while endeavouring to eat wisely, try not to allow correct diet to become an obsessive concern. While nutrition is an important factor in health, so is enjoyment.

Avoid over-reliance on stimulants, alcohol or recreational drugs

The Oriental concept of balance, as well as the Western principle of homoeostasis, has it that the body must compensate for the effect on it of any stimulant or sedative substance. In Oriental terms, this means that any substance-induced change of mood or behaviour depletes or alters the vital source of Ki which must last our lifetime. This does not mean that occasional or moderate enjoyment of mood-alterers such as coffee or wine will have disastrous consequences. On the contrary, the ancient texts tell us that, in the tradition of moderation, occasional indulgence is preferable to punishing self-restraint. It is the *habitual* abuse of any substance, which we often begin in an unconscious attempt to heal an imbalance in our energy patterns, which eventually fosters and intensifies that imbalance, thus compromising our health.

Receive Shiatsu

Once introduced to the principles of Oriental medicine, we can take our habitual behaviour or cravings as a sign of imbalance and take steps to correct it. Receiving Shiatsu is important for the Shiatsu giver. It maintains health and restores depleted energies. It is also a valuable teaching aid, since as much can be learned about Shiatsu by experiencing it as by giving it. Most importantly, it restores the balance between giving and receiving, a problem area for many therapists.

Attitude

Most of us choose to practise Shiatsu as a profession out of a desire to help others. However, Shiatsu is a situation of mutual support and the desire to help is often interwoven with our own needs for approval or recognition. Some of us may give of ourselves because we find it difficult to receive and some may find that only when in the role of the therapist can we safely make contact with others.

Even the greatest practitioners are not immune from this meshing of personal agenda with the compassion of the healer but it will often take its toll, if not from the quality of the Shiatsu then from the well-being of the practitioner. Shiatsu is best given from the clarity of an objective standpoint, while maintaining the basis of compassionate motivation, and while it would be unrealistic to think we could discard our personal motivations completely, we can at least acknowledge them objectively, without condemnation, and let them be.

We should also remember that our interaction with the receiver extends far beyond the Shiatsu treatment itself. It begins at the moment of making the first appointment and does not end until the receiver leaves at the end of the final session. Often, over a long period of receiving Shiatsu, the receiver will come to expect the fulfilment of dependency needs from the giver and it is vital that from the start the giver both acknowledges to herself her own needs from the therapeutic relationship and makes the limits of that relationship clear to the receiver.

This situation can become confusing for both when it takes place in the context of an existing relationship, when giving Shiatsu to family, friends or partners for example. In these cases the underlying emotional issues may affect the outcome of the Shiatsu treatment and where possible it is often advisable for long term Shiatsu treatment to be given by a practitioner who is not involved with the receiver.

If the relationship between giver and receiver begins to involve the giver emotionally beyond her normal extension of compassion, it is part of the Shiatsu Code of Ethics for her to transfer the responsibility for the Shiatsu treatment to another practitioner. It is advisable, when entering into professional practice, to obtain a copy of the Code of Ethics from the Shiatsu Society of the country where you live. If there is no association or society there, one can be obtained from the British Shiatsu Society (see p. 283 for address).

3

Shiatsu tools and techniques

When giving Shiatsu, it is helpful to envisage the experience as a dance between two people, rather than a process in which an active therapist applies thumb pressure to a passive recipient. The Shiatsu giver uses her whole body for leverage, support and pressure and the receiver, far from being permanently prone and inert, is a source of subtle movement, to which the giver attunes herself, as well as providing counter-balance and support for the movement of the giver.

The basic movement – crawling

For most Shiatsu students at their first class, expecting to learn the use of thumbs on pressure points at once, it is a surprise to spend an hour crawling on the floor and on each other. But many of them are giving the best Shiatsu they will give for a long time in this way. Even after many years of professional practice, at the end of a tiring day they may find, as I do, that their best results are achieved by relaxing into the crawling technique.

Crawling is the transmission of body weight through straight but relaxed arms and relaxed hands, aided by support from legs, hips and Hara. If you practise crawling on the floor with full awareness of your body posture and how it changes, you can recognize some of the most basic principles of good Shiatsu technique – controlled use of body weight and relaxation. You can then apply a modified version of the technique and "crawl" around the receiver with your hands only, not your knees, on the

receiver's back, shoulders and hips. Keep your arms at right angles to the body surface, your hands relaxed and only lean on areas which feel that they will support your weight comfortably.

Controlled use of body weight occurs naturally in crawling, as we shift our body weight gradually on to each limb in turn, while allowing the other three limbs to support us. In giving Shiatsu, this is the correct way to modify pressure; not by using muscular strength to apply or withhold it but by continuing to "crawl" and use body weight, only keeping more weight invested in the supporting limbs when we need to use a lighter touch.

Relaxation is what we experience by abandoning our body to the floor's support. Tension disappears from our shoulders and hips as we crawl – our body weight is naturally supported by the floor. This depends largely on the vertical position of our arms and thighs; they are at right angles to the floor. When applying the crawling principle to the giving of Shiatsu, we should remember this and keep our body at a correct distance from the receiver, so that our body weight can be applied at right angles to the receiver's body surface (Figs 3.1A and B).

Another aspect of relaxation is the moulding of our hands to the surface which supports us. If, as we crawl on the floor, a hand lands on a cushion or a pencil or the edge of a thick rug, it automatically moulds itself around the new surface. The more relaxed our hands are, the more they contribute to our support, and the less we think about our hands, the more relaxed and accommodating they are.

This relaxation can bring great depth and sensitivity to our Shiatsu. Instead of concentrating on

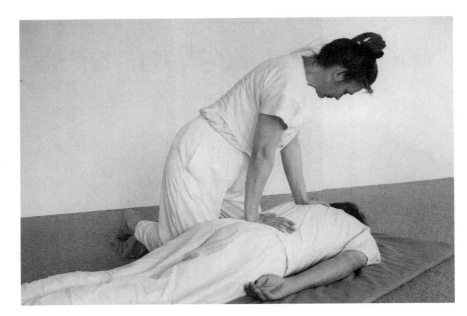

Fig. 3.1A *Using body weight correctly.*

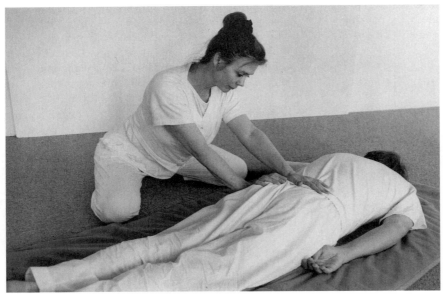

Fig. 3.1B *Using body weight correctly.*

the surface on which our hands rest, which would involve the hand–brain connection and analytical effort, we are relaxing into the support which the receiver's body gives us, which involves the deeper sensing and balancing mechanisms of our own whole body. This means that we are not "doing something to" the receiver; we are involved in the process on a deeper level. As we relax into the support of the receiver's body, we are also automatically aware of whether that contact is comfortable, so that we can stay there for a long time, or whether the receiver's body is tense and uneasy in any particular area and seems to want to throw us off. This is the central sensation in "feeling" diagnosis, the sensing of parts of the receiver's body which are empty of Ki or overfull.

From crawling to use of the Hara: guidelines

Once the student has been "crawling" on the body of the receiver long enough to relax and to be able to control the application of her body weight without diminishing her relaxation, she is beginning to understand the use of the Hara. New techniques and working positions can then come into use, but there are still certain basic "crawling" guidelines which should be checked through constantly.

Are you feeling comfortable in what you are doing?

Good Shiatsu has to feel comfortable to the giver. If the giver is uncomfortable, the receiver will also be uncomfortable. The giver should at all times make use of the support of the receiver's body, rather than expending effort in awkward positions. Only use techniques with which you feel comfortable. Only apply pressure to areas which you can reach comfortably.

Are your arms, hands, neck and shoulders relaxed?

If they are not, you are expending unnecessary effort. Take a deep abdominal breath and focus your attention in your Hara for a while or go into a basic crawling technique until you feel more relaxed.

Do you feel your connection with the ground?

Even if you are doing a modified Shiatsu on a treatment couch, be aware of the ground and your own and your receiver's connection with it.

Is your base as wide as you can make it?

You should be making full use of the ground's support. Keep your knees apart and your groin area open as much as you can, to ensure maximum stability, support and Ki flow.

Is your Hara facing the area on which you are working?

If it is not, you will not be making use of your body weight. As you progress in Ki awareness, it can help to imagine your Hara as giving out a spotlight beam which illuminates the part of the receiver's body you are working on. The Hara can also direct Ki, so that you can position yourself with your Hara pointing in the direction in which you wish the receiver's Ki to go.

Once the use of the Hara and the art of crawling have been mastered, it is easier to understand the Five Principles of Zen Shiatsu, which were first formulated by Shizuto Masunaga, although they are common to many Shiatsu styles.

The Five Principles of Zen Shiatsu

Relax!

This has been discussed above.

Penetration, not pressure

This refers to the quality of Shiatsu touch. When we "press", we are aware of a resistant surface against which we act with physical effort. Conscious "pressing" originates from the muscles of hands and arms; contact is limited to the physical manipulation of tissues and the giver is a "doer", while the receiver is an object.

When Shiatsu is given from the Hara in a state of relaxation, as when crawling, the surface becomes less important and the receiver becomes a source of support to the giver, who senses the quality of that support throughout her body. In this way, the receiver also becomes aware of the quality of the support which his own body provides and thus of his own strong areas, weak areas and centres of greater or lesser concentrations of Ki. A connection takes place in which both giver's and receiver's whole-body awareness is involved. This is when pressure becomes penetration (Fig. 3.2). This form of penetration is not active but receptive; the giver penetrates into the

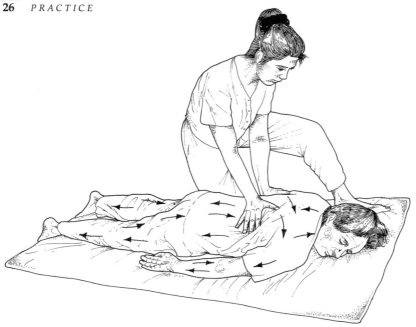

Fig. 3.2 *Penetration, not pressure, leads to whole-body awareness.*

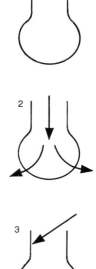

Fig. 3.3 *Perpendicular penetration into a tsubo.*

awareness space of the receiver's body in order to form a connection and to "listen".

However, penetration can be active. Active penetration is most useful in Shiatsu when working deeply into a particular point or tsubo and can be greatly increased by the giver's intention. In the martial arts, students are taught not to aim their blow at the presenting body surface of their opponent, but through the body to a point on the other side. This principle also works in Shiatsu to increase the power of penetration; when applying pressure with the thumb, elbow or knee, imagine that your pressure is going through, like a knife through butter, to the receiver's other side. When you penetrate in this way, your work will be doubly deep and effective without causing discomfort to the receiver.

Stationary, perpendicular penetration

This principle follows on from the preceding one. Penetration must be stationary to be effective; that is, the movement is only inwards, not from side to side or round and round. Beginners are often tempted to rock rhythmically into their pressure, as in massage, but this process only affects the surface tissues, as their pressure does not have a chance to penetrate. It is only by being still when leaning into a point that penetration occurs.

Perpendicular penetration means the application of pressure in towards the centre of the receiver's body, at right angles to the body surface. In order to achieve this, you will need to alter your own posture in order to lean your weight into different areas of the receiver's body.

The reason for perpendicular penetration lies in the structure of the points or tsubos (Fig. 3.3). In the ancient Taoist script, the character for tsubo is similar to a jar with a narrow neck (1). When the point is penetrated perpendicularly, the way is clear and open into the larger space of the receiver's whole body energy (2). If it is not, you pressure will encounter the sides of the neck of the vessel, in the surface tissues of the body, and penetration will not occur (3).

There are exceptions to the general rule of perpendicular penetration. Sometimes, if a meridian is distorted, you may find that you have to change your angle in order to contact the Ki. There are also certain areas where the meridian can only be reached by penetrating at a certain angle and these are discussed in detail in the chapters on the individual meridians in Section Two.

Two-hand connectedness

One of the characteristics of Zen Shiatsu which differentiates it from most other styles is that both the giver's hands are always in contact with the body. Sometimes, as when giving symmetrical pressure down the meridians of the trunk, both hands work together but very often one hand is still, supporting one part of the meridian, while the other hand works down another part of it. Masunaga called the stationary, or Yin, hand the "mother hand" so that by inference the working, or Yang, hand is the "child hand". The mother hand, although it does not appear to be doing anything, is the more important of the two; it provides a reassuring touch for the receiver and support where it is needed. More importantly, it provides stillness to counterbalance the movement of the child hand, not only from the standpoint of the receiver but from that of the giver as well. When calm attention and awareness is invested in the mother hand, a vital source of stability and meditative calm remains open in the giver's state of being, which

informs and guides the Shiatsu given by the child hand. The mother hand does not always have to be the same one; in fact, in some techniques (see p. 42) the hands swiftly alternate their roles.

Two-hand connectedness means that the mother and child hands are always equally in the giver's awareness and thus connected in the giver's state of being. This connection plays an important part in working with the meridians, since the child hand as it works "draws a line" of awareness in the receiver from the mother hand outwards along the meridian. For this reason, it is always preferable to have the mother hand resting closer to the centre of the body than the child hand, or above the child hand when it is working down the body (Fig. 3.4).

Masunaga emphasized the "two hands as one" sensation derived from the experience of two-hand connectedness by both giver and receiver. When the giver experiences the connection between Yin and Yang, stillness and movement, from maintaining awareness of both hands together, the receiver experiences the same thing. In Oriental philosophy, Yin and Yang are both derived from the One, the ultimate source of being. When both giver and receiver feel the "two as one" sensation, both experience a sense of unification, not only with each other for the duration of the Shiatsu but with the One source, which allows profound healing to take place.

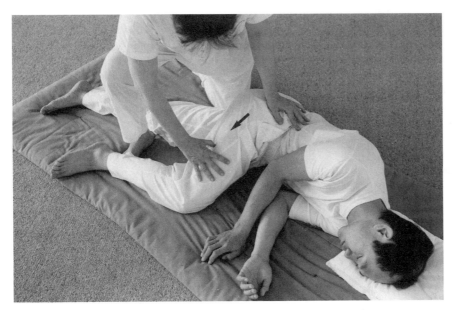

Fig. 3.4 *Two-hand connectedness.*

Meridian continuity

This refers to the practice in Zen Shiatsu of working with the Ki in the whole meridian, as if it were a pipeline, rather than concentrating on points, as many styles of Shiatsu do. In true Zen Shiatsu, the giver follows her perception of the Ki's condition and movement, with appropriate techniques. In treating a meridian, therefore, a standard procedure is to rest the mother hand as high as possible on the meridian and to work down the meridian with the child hand, with fairly continuous running pressures, in order to detect any changes in the Ki flow along it. This means that palm and thumb pressures must be close enough together for both giver and receiver to experience a sense of continuity along the meridian path. Contact should never be completely broken. Your palm, thumb, elbow or knee should slide along the meridian in between pressures.

The tools of Shiatsu

Once the Five Principles have been understood, the hands, knees, elbows and other Shiatsu "tools" can come into play, with their appropriate techniques.

The palms

The most basic beginner's technique, and at the same time one of the most powerful, is palming. When we begin our "crawling" Shiatsu, the palms are relaxed and moulded to the body part which is supporting us. As we progress to the intentional use of palming, the hands remain relaxed but with experience comes an awareness which informs us of the quality of Ki in the receiver's body.

We therefore often use palming on a meridian before thumbing or more focused work, both to open and prepare the meridian and also as a "read-out" to inform us of the areas which need further work. It can also be used as a technique on its own, for body parts or meridians which do not need more specific attention but which need to be acknowledged as part of a full-body treatment.

The palms can also be used with hardly any pressure simply to hold a weak or deficient area and transmit Ki to it (Fig. 3.5).

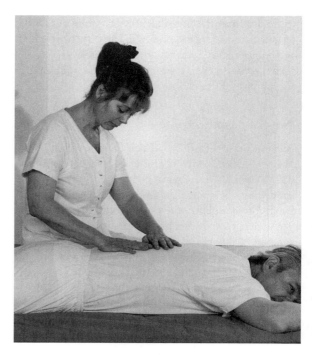

Fig. 3.5 *Transmitting Ki through the palms.*

The thumb

Thumbing is one of the most useful and characteristic Shiatsu techniques, suitable for applying strong and focused pressure. The thumb is robust enough to penetrate deeply into the tissues when required and sensitive enough to receive Ki messages as to when to lighten up or to stop. Care should be taken when using the thumb not to poke or press and the use of gradual pressure is especially advisable. Only the ball of the thumb should be used, not the tip, and the thumb should not be flexed, unless you have double-jointed thumbs, when it may be necessary.

It is advisable when using your thumb to allow another part of your hand to contact the receiver's body as well, in order to stabilize both the thumb and the area being worked on and also to counteract the tendency to "poke". For example, when both thumbs are working down the Bladder or Kidney meridians on the back, your fingertips can rest on the back to support the thumbs (Fig. 3.6). Keep your intention focused in your thumbs, however, and try to keep your palms above the receiver's body surface while thumbing or else the technique becomes another kind of palming.

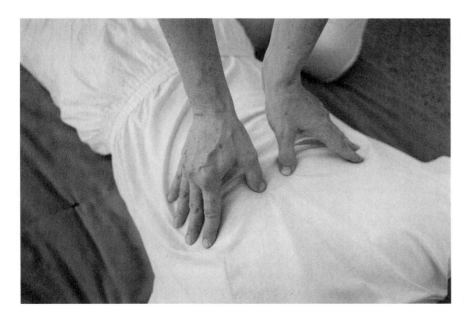

Fig. 3.6 *Supporting the thumbs.*

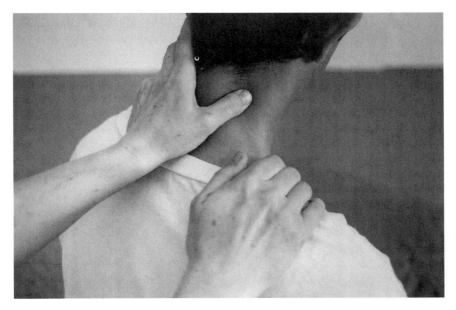

Fig. 3.7 *Support for both giver's thumb and receiver's neck.*

Another example is when working the neck meridians in the sitting position. Rather than pressing with your thumb alone, lightly hold and support the receiver's neck in such a way that your thumb rests on the chosen meridian (Fig. 3.7).

Supporting the working thumb is important for keeping it aligned with your arm as much as possible and thus maintaining a free flow of Ki. Any part of the body used for giving Shiatsu should not be bent or cramped in such a way that the flow of Ki from your Hara is obstructed.

The fingertips

The fingertips, while they can be strengthened by the hand exercises in Chapter 2, tend to be too weak for strong, deep pressure. They are, however, ideally suited for delicate areas where accurate rather than strong pressure is required, such as the face.

For work on the face, your fingertips should be curled inwards to reach into the crevices of the facial bones, such as under the cheekbone or eye socket. Rather than applying pressure with all your fingertips at once, use them in running sequence, one after the other, as if playing the piano (Fig. 3.8).

The fingertips can also be used when Ki penetration, rather than vigorous technique, is required. They can be very useful in working the back meridians with the receiver in the side position, if there is not a great deal of muscle tension (Fig. 3.9). For this technique, the fingertips of one hand penetrate the tsubos on the meridian at the top of the back, while your other hand works down the meridian in the same way, concentrating on the areas where penetration is deepest. All the fingertips work together and usually the middle finger and sometimes the ring finger will have to bend in order to keep level with the index. It is important to keep your fingertips aligned with your hand and arm and to penetrate perpendicularly to maintain maximum Ki flow.

Fingertip pressure is also useful on the meridians of the upper torso, where it is necessary to work between the ribs. Your fingers should be aligned in a gentle curve with your hands and arms. This technique is illustrated in the chapters dealing with the treatment of the different meridians.

One fingertip at a time can be used to penetrate the points between the vertebrae, connected to a mother hand on the shoulder. Depth of penetration must be monitored to make sure that the pressure is enough to be felt by the receiver, yet not so forceful as to damage spinal ligaments. This is where Ki penetration, rather than surface pressure, is important.

One technique which allows maximum penetration by the fingertips is the occipital balancing technique (see p. 50). It is important that the hands and arms support the fingers for this technique. Kneel behind the receiver's head with your elbows and forearms on the ground and your fingertips in the groove under the base of the receiver's skull (Fig. 3.10). With the backs of your hands on the ground for leverage, push upwards with fingertips curled back slightly towards you, so that the weight

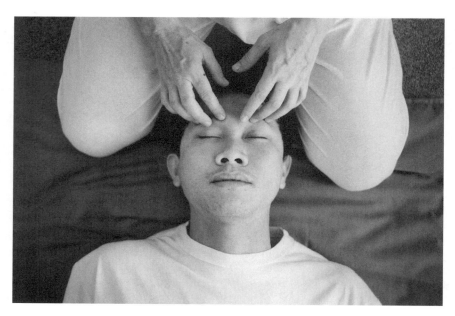

Fig. 3.8 *Fingertips on the face.*

of the receiver's head rests entirely on your fingertips, causing them to penetrate deeply into the groove. You can then explore for areas of deep penetration, by tilting the receiver's head to one side and moving your fingertips to different places under the occipital ridge, then leaning the weight of the receiver's head on to them once more and continuing until the whole occipital groove has been treated. When not actively penetrating with your fingertips (which is done by allowing the whole weight of the receiver's head to do the work), you can support part of the weight of the head on your palms.

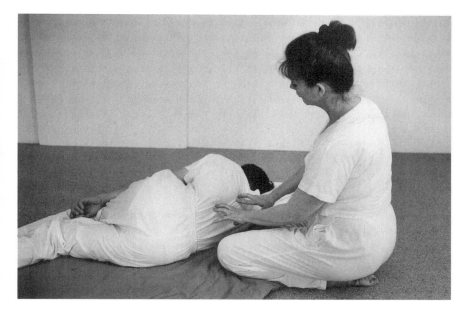

Fig. 3.9 *Working the back meridians with the fingertips.*

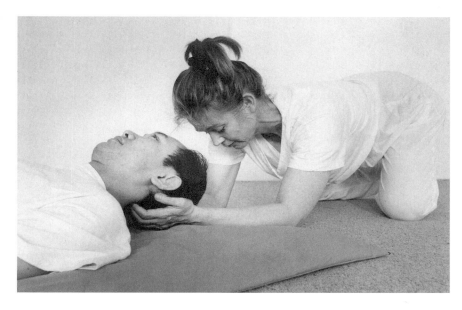

Fig. 3.10 *Occipital balancing.*

The Dragon's Mouth

The Dragon's Mouth is the exotic name for a technique in which the giver's hand grasps the receiver's limb, to stabilize and support it, while positioned in such a way that the knuckle of the first joint of the index finger applies pressure to a meridian or point (Fig. 3.11). This technique is particularly useful when working on the arms, which are inclined to roll out of position if unsupported.

A variation of the Dragon's Mouth is the technique in which pressure is applied with the thumb and the knuckle of the second joint of the index finger at the same time (Fig. 3.12). This technique is mostly used for working down both sides of the spine at once, particularly in the sitting or side positions.

The elbows

The elbow is a powerful tool, capable of applying deeper and more sustained pressure than the thumb. It should therefore be used judiciously, since inappropriate elbow work can cause pain or physical damage to the receiver. It is most important to remember the two basics of the crawling technique when applying the elbow, i.e. relaxation and controlled use of body weight. When these principles are put into practice, the elbow can apply pressure which is deep yet comforting and surprisingly accurate. When working from the Hara, using your deeper body sensing mechanisms to find working postures which are comfortable and supportive for both yourself and the receiver, you will find your elbows are as sensitive and receptive as your hands.

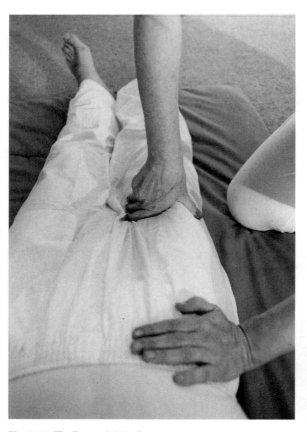

Fig. 3.11 *The Dragon's Mouth.*

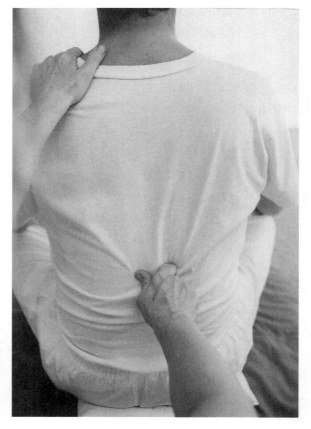

Fig. 3.12 *Index finger and knuckle used together.*

When beginning to learn elbow techniques, many students, afraid of causing pain, use only their forearms and thereby lose the accuracy which is the result of using the elbow point. The key to good elbow technique is to rest the point of your elbow on a specific tsubo or meridian but to relax your forearm and hand; then to lean your body weight gradually on to the elbow, as if leaning comfortably on the back of a sofa. In this way, just enough of your forearm will relax on to the body surface to soften the impact of your elbow point, which nonetheless carries the emphasis of the pressure (Fig. 3.13).

Elbow work is best applied to areas of dense, compacted muscle in robust receivers, until the giver has acquired real proficiency in the technique. This is more of a dispersing method (see p. 255). Later it can be used with more delicacy for tonifying specific areas which would otherwise be hard to reach, such as the deep crevices which some receivers have alongside the spine. *The elbow must never be used directly on a bony surface.*

The elbow can also be used simply to save your thumbs, when the receiver's physique is strong enough to take it.

The elbows can also be used both at once, as in leaning on the area between the shoulderblades. Be

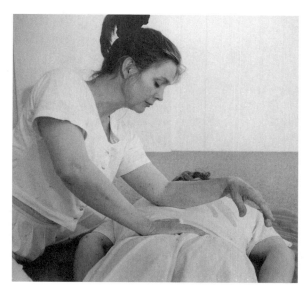

Fig. 3.13 *Applying focused but comfortable pressure with the elbow.*

careful not to lean too much weight on this area; relaxing your upper body on to it is sufficient (Fig. 3.14).

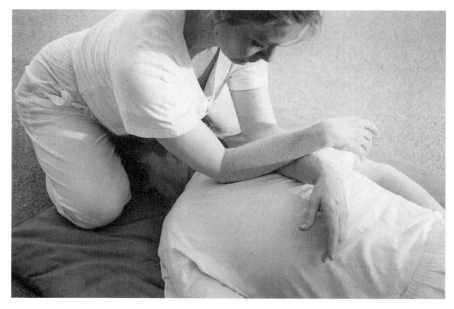

Fig. 3.14 *Double elbow technique.*

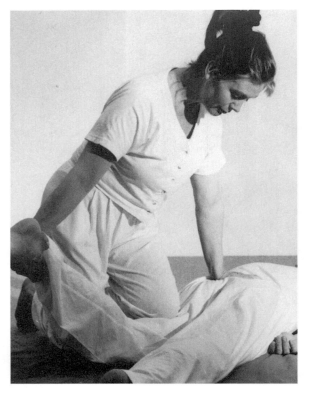

Fig. 3.15A   *Knee pressure on the thigh.*

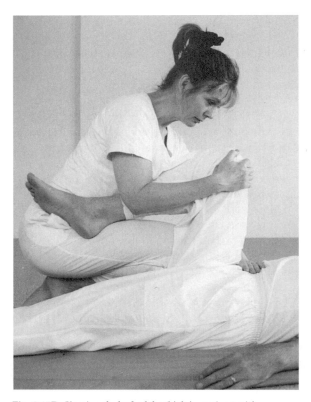

Fig. 3.15B   *Kneeing the back of the thigh in supine position.*

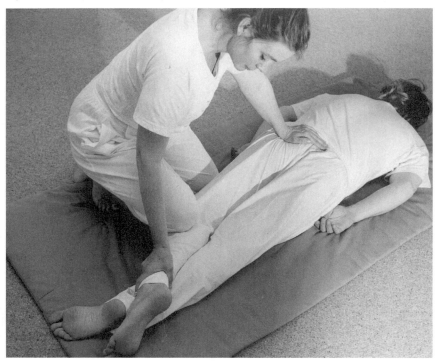

Fig. 3.15C   *General work with the knee.*

The knees

The knee, like the elbow, is capable of applying powerful and sustained pressure but because of its greater surface area it is not used for deep penetration. This limits the scope of its application and you will usually use your knee for supporting a limb in a specific position or for general work which does not require much focus. Only on the heavy muscles of the backs of the thighs is the knee used at anything like its full pressure potential and you should proceed gently even here.

When using your knee to apply pressure to the backs of the thighs, you should be well supported by a mother hand on the receiver's sacrum. The other hand holds the receiver's foot, bent back towards the torso to release and open the thigh muscles. Your weight should be well invested in the other leg and foot, so that your position is stable, before you lower your knee to apply gradual, controlled pressure to the back of the receiver's thigh (Fig. 3.15A).

The knee can also be used to work the same area when the receiver is in the supine position. With your mother hand on the receiver's Hara, bend the receiver's leg towards his opposite shoulder and position yourself close to his flexed hip, with your knee resting on the chosen meridian on the back of his thigh. While maintaining awareness in your mother hand, encircle his knee with your other hand and bring his leg back on to your knee in the correct direction so that your knee applies pressure to the meridian. Stretch his leg back towards his shoulder again and move your knee slightly higher up the meridian before repeating the procedure (Fig. 3.15B). It is important to maintain a grounded position close to the receiver and to keep the receiver's hip well flexed during this technique, so that your knee remains fixed while applying pressure.

One or both knees can be used to apply light or normal pressure along accessible meridians, though the knee is not suitable for detailed, penetrative work and is best for general work or to spare your hands. Suitable areas are the side of the torso and the side of the leg when it is supported in the correct position (see p. 42). For this method of working with the knee, you should be sitting on your haunches and well supported by both hands in contact with the receiver's body (Fig. 3.15C).

The feet

The feet can be used by a skilled practitioner almost in the same way as the hands, for deep softening and relaxing of the tissues. For an illustration of this kind of work the reader is referred to *Barefoot Shiatsu* by Shizuko Yamamoto. However, these techniques are unsuited to focused work with Ki and can be dangerous unless the giver is highly experienced. Walking on the back is a technique often associated with Shiatsu in the lay person's mind, but in fact more properly belongs to the practice of Anma and, once again, it can be dangerous.

One foot technique which is both safe and useful is that of standing on the soles of the receiver's feet, if they are capable of lying flat and inverted, as shown. Your heel should not rest on the receiver's instep, but in the hollow just below the ball of the foot. If the receiver's ankles are stiff, so that there is a space between the dorsum of the foot and the floor, the feet can be laid on a cushion for comfort (Fig. 3.16).

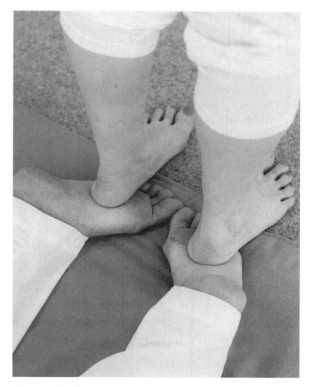

Fig. 3.16 *'Walking' on the feet.*

Other techniques

To a great extent, the tools of Shiatsu and its techniques are synonymous, since much of Shiatsu technique consists of working down the meridians with the different parts of the giver's body described above. However, there are two additional techniques which form an important part of the Shiatsu repertory.

Stretches

There are many varieties of stretches and manipulations associated with Shiatsu; some have been acquired from Western osteopathic methods, but others are traditional to many of the Oriental massage therapies. There are two types of stretch; the first type aims to open up and adjust the receiver's physical framework, the second type, more a position than a stretch, aims to bring a meridian to the surface of the body in order to work it better.

The first type of stretch, like an osteopathic technique, can be complicated to perform and almost impossible to describe in writing. I have confined myself to describing the simplest of the useful stretches in this category in the next chapter.

These stretches should be used sparingly and performed as a conclusion, either to the Shiatsu on a particular area or to the treatment as a whole. They should not be used until the area to be stretched has been strengthened and balanced by appropriate work on the meridians. When used in this context, they can be highly relaxing, as the receiver's physical structure is encouraged to accommodate the energetic changes produced by the Shiatsu.

They should only be used, however, on receivers who enjoy them and cooperate with them; any resistance will negate the benefits of the technique. The receiver can be encouraged to cooperate with the stretches by the giver's own relaxation and confidence, by constant reassurance and mutual feedback – "Is this all right? Can you go a bit further? Tell me when it's as far as you would like to go" – and by performing the stretch slowly enough to allow the receiver to relax into it.

The second type of stretch is used to place a limb in position so that the meridian concerned is activated. A famous Shiatsu master, Yoshio Manaka, has demonstrated that stretching a meridian causes increased reactivity in the Bo diagnostic points related to that meridian (see p. 239) and it is suggested that the increased tension in the fasciae encourages conductivity, or Ki flow, in the meridian concerned (*Hara Diagnosis: Reflections on the Sea*, p. 147). The meridian stretches in this book are those devised by Shizuto Masunaga and are dealt with individually in the chapters on the meridians.

Rotations

Rotations, like stretches, can be performed simply as physical manipulations to increase mobility. When they are done sensitively and with attention, on a joint supported by the mother hand, the effect is very different. Not only is the receiver encouraged to release tensions in the small muscles surrounding the joint, but the giver becomes aware of areas of restriction and stiffness in that joint and the meridian imbalances which they indicate. Rotations, like all Shiatsu techniques, can be an aid to "listening in" to the receiver's body (Fig. 3.17).

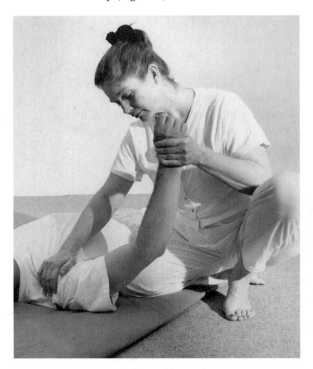

Fig. 3.17 *'Listening' to the joint while rotating.*

The first requirement for rotations is a position which provides potential for easy rotation of the limb or joint concerned. The prone position, for example, offers scope only for ankle rotations, the side position is good for shoulder and arm rotations, the supine for hip, ankle, wrist and limited arm rotations, and the sitting position for arm, wrist and neck.

The second requirement is adequate two-handed support for joint and limb. Your mother hand should be placed as close as possible to the joint to be rotated and the working hand should support the rotating limb in such a way that the receiver can relax it completely. Specific instructions on the rotation of the limbs are given in the following chapter.

It is important that the receiver relaxes completely into the rotation, otherwise both the diagnostic effect and the treatment value are diminished. Many receivers, however, have difficulty in relaxing, to the point of being unaware that they are doing the rotation for you. They need to be made aware of this and encouraged to make their limb heavy and relaxed, by whatever visualizations or methods are at your disposal. You can also try firmer support from the mother hand and a much slower rotation technique, to encourage the receiver to "listen in" himself to his own patterns of holding.

4

Shiatsu treatment routines in the four positions

Most Western forms of massage are performed in two basic positions, prone and supine. Shiatsu makes use of two additional positions, side and sitting. Although it is not often necessary to adopt all four positions in one treatment session, each position has its own special advantages and the Shiatsu practitioner should feel equally at home working in any one of them.

The student will usually begin to learn Shiatsu techniques with the receiver in prone position (face down). This is the best position in which to experiment with the "crawling technique" and the controlled use of body weight, since for most receivers the back of the body is the strongest, most protected area. Once the correct techniques for the back have been mastered, the giver progresses to work with the receiver in the supine position (face up). Here subtler techniques which require accuracy and sensitivity, rather than strong pressure, can be learned. The side and sitting positions follow, so that the giver can begin to change her own working position to meet the needs of the receiver.

In practice, any sequence of positions can be chosen; the choice of positions is discussed in Chapter 14. In this chapter, a basic outline of the commonest treatment procedures in each position is given, together with a discussion of the general advantages and disadvantages of the position. Only standard techniques are shown; the giver can adapt any of the techniques and add her own, according to preference. The location of the meridians and specific techniques for working them are given in the chapters on the individual meridians in Section Two and the giver can incorporate these into the general treatment routines below.

Prone position

Advantages

The prone position is one in which most receivers are used to receiving bodywork and in which they feel less exposed, so they can relax. It is the best position for deep, penetrative work on the back meridians and points, on the sacrum in particular, and for emphasizing the relevant postural connections with the backs of the legs.

Disadvantages

Correct penetration of the meridians and points in the upper back is only possible if the receiver's arms are by his side and this can be uncomfortable for some. The position generally places a strain on the receiver's neck and is unsuitable for receivers with stiff necks. It can also exacerbate lower back pain and receivers with weak lower backs should have a pillow under their abdomen. Pillows may also be needed to support the upper chest, if a woman has large or tender breasts, and under the shins if the receiver has stiff ankles or painful knees. This position is unsuitable for women after the third month of pregnancy and for receivers with breathing problems. The side position is a useful alternative.

Most accessible meridians

Bladder, Kidney, all hip meridians.

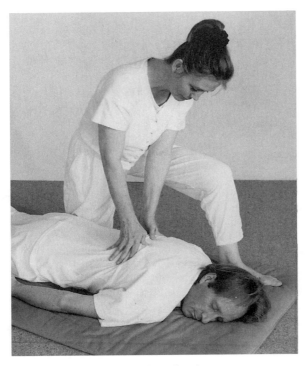

Fig. 4.1A *Bilateral thumbing down the spine.*

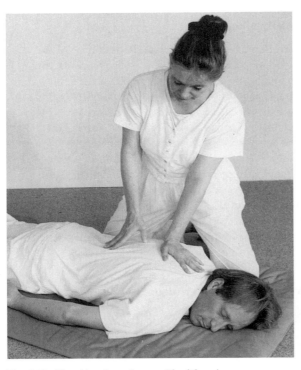

Fig. 4.1B *Thumbing down the nearside of the spine.*

Treatment procedure

Palming and thumbing down both sides of the spine

From a "lunge" or kneeling position, the meridians of the back can be worked both sides at the same time, with palms or thumbs (as shown). This technique is particularly suitable for working on the Yu points (see p. 239). Pressures should be applied to the full length of the meridian, all down the back (Fig. 4.1A).

Palming and thumbing down one side of the spine

The mother hand remains at the top of the meridian, on the side of the back nearest to the giver. The working hand palms and thumbs down the rest of the meridian to its full length (Fig. 4.1B). With this one-sided technique, work on the leg nearest the giver follows and the giver changes sides to work on the other side of the back and the other leg.

The giver is kneeling, facing in towards the receiver's side.

Palms, thumbs or elbows on the hips and buttocks

The giver moves down to face the side of the receiver's hip. The mother hand gives support to the lumbar area while the working hand palms and thumbs the meridians of the hips and buttocks. Alternatively, the elbow can be used, as shown (Fig. 4.2).

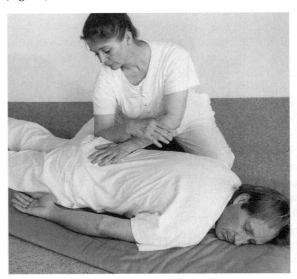

Fig. 4.2 *Elbowing the hips.*

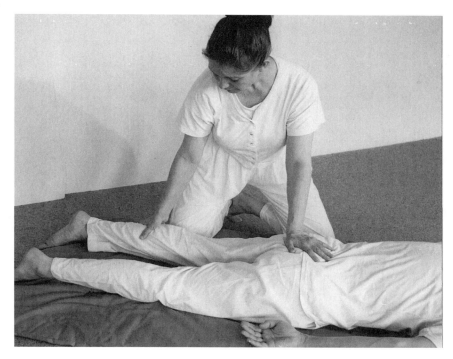

Fig. 4.3 *Working the lower leg.*

Palm, thumb, elbow, Dragon's Mouth or knee down the back of the leg

The giver moves down to face the side of the leg and her mother hand moves down to the sacrum. The working hand palms and thumbs the meridians of the back of the leg. For some meridians, the hand position may need to change on the lower leg, as shown (Fig. 4.3). The elbow or Dragon's Mouth can be used instead of the thumb and knee pressure can be used on the upper leg, as described on p. 35.

Three-way stretch for the Stomach and Spleen

Without changing position, the giver slightly increases the pressure invested in the mother hand to stop the receiver's hips flexing and picks up the receiver's foot with the working hand. She gently and slowly stretches the toes back towards the buttocks, first straight, then towards the opposite buttock, then towards the nearside hip, as shown, releasing the leg to an open angle in between each stretch (Fig. 4.4). This stretches the muscles and meridians in the front of the leg. It should not be used if the receiver has knee problems.

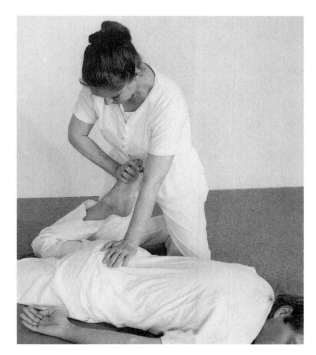

Fig. 4.4 *The three-way stretch.*

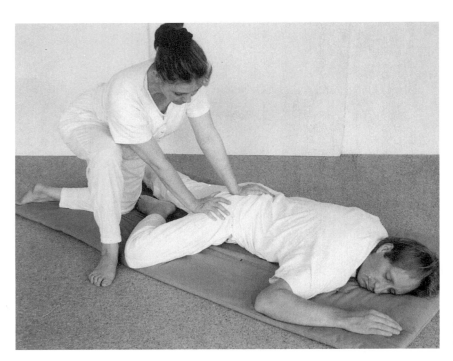

Fig. 4.5 *A meridian stretch for specific work.*

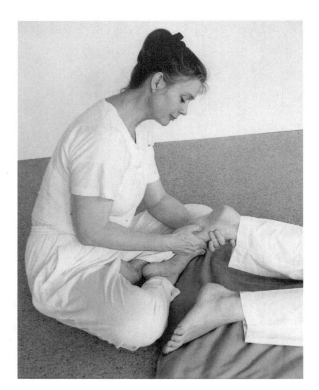

Fig. 4.6 *Thumbing the feet.*

Stretches for the meridians of the back of the leg

When the Large Intestine or Gall Bladder meridians are worked in the prone position, the leg must be moved into one of the meridian stretches discussed in the previous chapter before being palmed and thumbed, elbowed or kneed. Here the position for the Gall Bladder is shown (Fig. 4.5).

Work on the feet

Walking on the soles of the feet is a technique illustrated in the preceding chapter (see p. 35) and which can be used here. More detailed foot work with the thumbs can be done with the giver in a sitting or kneeling position (Fig. 4.6).

The top of the shoulders

The giver kneels behind the receiver's head to work on the meridians at the top of the shoulders; she may use a stationary mother hand at the top of the spine while the working hand palms and thumbs each meridian outwards toward the shoulder joint (Fig. 4.7). Alternatively, the hands may palm and thumb out across both shoulders simultaneously, alternating pressure and release; in this case, they alternate their roles as mother hand and working hand. The upper part of the back meridians, between the shoulderblades, can also be treated from this angle with palms, thumbs or elbows.

Supine position

Advantages

The supine position is restful for the receiver and requires a minimum of padding with pillows. The giver can observe the receiver's facial expression for feedback on her pressure. The position's main advantage is its extreme versatility; because the limbs can be rotated and moved into many positions, almost every meridian can be treated and the only areas which are difficult to access are the back, hips and buttocks. It is also the easiest position in which to perform stretches and rotations.

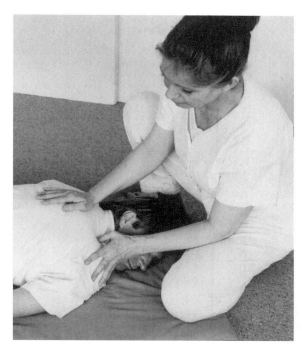

Fig. 4.7 *Working the top of the shoulders.*

Disadvantages

Because the face and the front of the body are exposed, the receiver may feel emotionally vulnerable and find it hard to relax. The lower back and sacrum can begin to ache after a while in this position.

Most accessible meridians

Stomach, Spleen, all arm and chest meridians.

Treatment procedure

Hara work

The experienced practitioner will often begin a session with the receiver in this position, in order to diagnose from the Hara.

Hara diagnosis or treatment is traditionally performed with the giver kneeling hip to hip beside the receiver, facing the receiver's head. If penetration is required, the giver leans her body weight in towards the receiver, to give controlled, gradual pressure (Fig. 4.8). Both hands remain on the Hara at all times, for support and feedback.

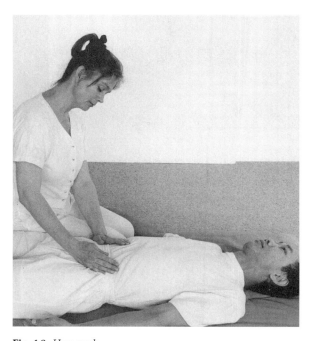

Fig. 4.8 *Hara work.*

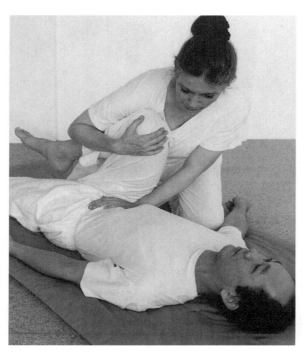

Fig. 4.9 *Leg rotation.*

Leg rotation

This is a good preliminary to work on the legs. With a mother hand on the Hara, the giver places a hand under the knee of the leg nearest her and raises it to a flexed position. Facing the receiver's head, she then moves her body so as to support the receiver's bent knee with the front of her shoulder, lightly encircling it with her arm, and moves the leg with a circling movement of her own whole body, first towards the opposite shoulder, then the shoulder on the same side and so on (Fig. 4.9). Awareness is in the mother hand on the Hara and the giver is tuning in to the smoothness or otherwise of the joint rotation. Care should be taken not to over- or understretch.

Front of the legs

The giver keeps her mother hand on the Hara in order to palm and thumb the meridians on the front of the leg. If this becomes too wide a stretch, she can move her mother hand down on to the thigh. If the leg needs supporting, the giver can use her knee or foot (Fig. 4.10). The working hand should not avoid

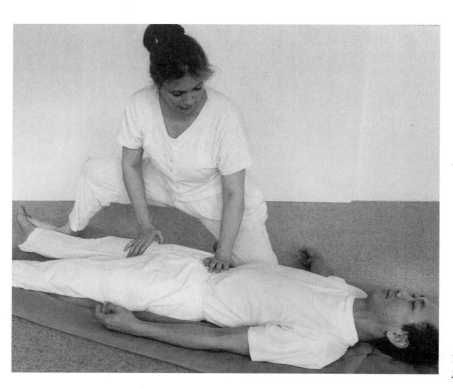

Fig. 4.10 *Working the front of the leg.*

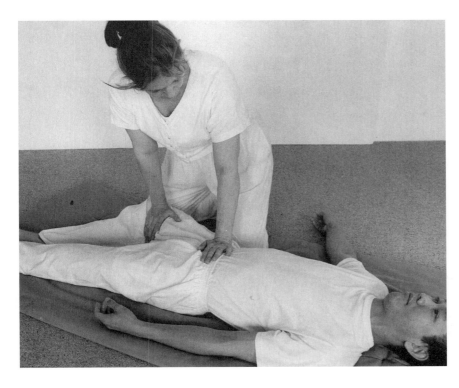

Fig. 4. 11 *A meridian stretch for specific work.*

the knee joint, but should work the edges of the kneecap with fingers and thumb, while applying light pressure over the kneecap with the palm.

Stretches for the leg meridians

Most of the leg meridians will need to be worked in a specific position in order to stretch and expose the meridian. These stretches are all illustrated in the chapters on the individual meridians. The mother hand remains on the Hara throughout and the working hand palms and thumbs down the relevant meridian to the foot, while the leg is in the appropriate stretch. Here work on the Spleen meridian is shown (Fig. 4.11).

Foot work

For both general and specific work on the foot, it can be useful to balance the back of the receiver's heel on top of your thigh. In this position, ankle rotations can be performed using the thigh's support as a pivot point, the meridians of the top of the foot can be worked and the toes can be stretched (Fig. 4.12).

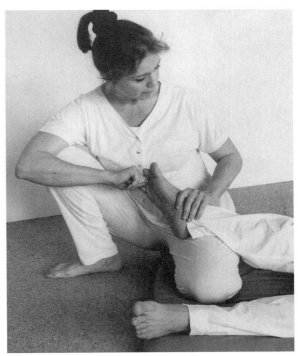

Fig. 4.12 *Foot work.*

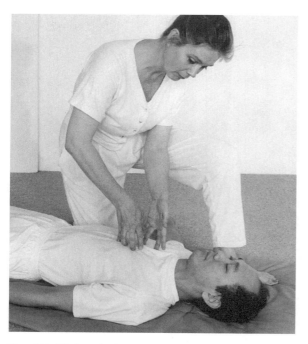

Fig. 4.13 *Work on the chest meridians.*

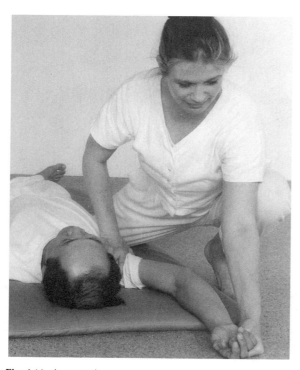

Fig. 4.14 *Arm rotation.*

Work on the chest

The giver repositions herself at the side of the receiver, either kneeling or in the lunge position, as shown, for work on the individual meridians of the chest. Here fingertip work on the Kidney meridian is shown. The locations of the individual meridians are described in the chapters of Section Two (Fig. 4.13).

Arm rotation

Kneeling in the lunge position, the giver rests her mother hand on the receiver's shoulder joint to stabilize it and picks up the receiver's hand with her thumb resting in the hollow of his palm. Encouraging the receiver to relax his elbow joint if necessary, she takes his arm above his head to the floor, then draws it in a wide circle back towards herself, moving her own body speedily to allow space for the arm to rotate as fully as the receiver's flexibility will permit (Fig. 4.14).

Stretches for the arm meridians

The 12 meridians in the arm are all worked in their own stretch positions and these are given in detail in the chapters in Section Two. The basic techniques for working in these stretches are as follows.

Horizontal and upwards stretches – Heart Protector, Liver, Heart. The arm is laid in the appropriate stretch and the giver's mother hand stabilizes the shoulder joint while the working hand palms and thumbs the meridian. Here the Heart meridian is shown (Fig. 4.15).

Downwards stretches – Large Intestine, Bladder, Lung, Spleen. The procedure is the same as that given above, but the Dragon's Mouth may be more suitable for some meridians than the thumb and the giver may feel more comfortable taking her weight further forward, in the lunge position. Here the Large Intestine meridian is shown (Fig. 4.16).

Transverse stretches – Kidney, Small Intestine, Stomach, Triple Heater, Gall Bladder. The giver lays the receiver's arm across his body in the appropriate stretch. She can use her mother hand to support the

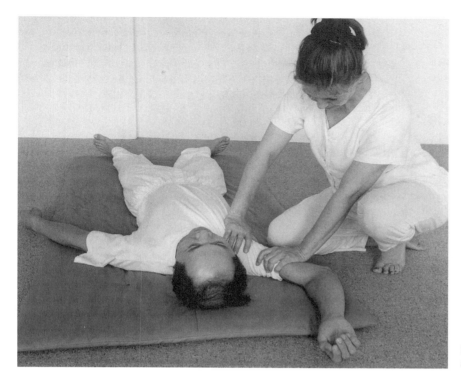

Fig. 4.15 *Arm stretches: an upwards stretch.*

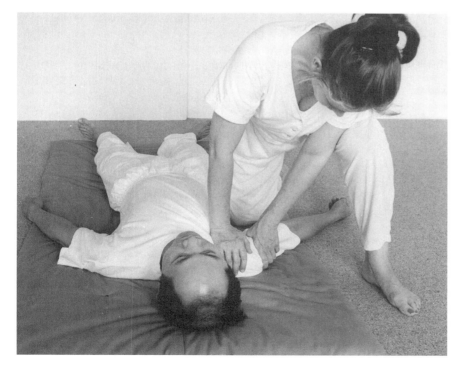

Fig. 4.16 *Arm stretches: a downwards stretch.*

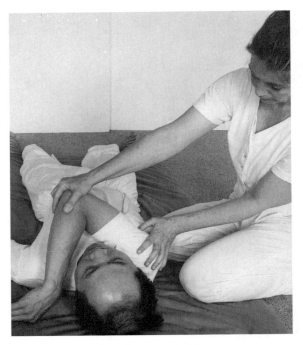

Fig. 4.17 *Arm stretches: a transverse stretch.*

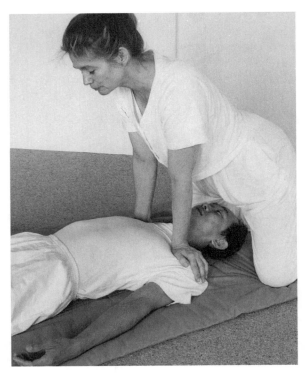

Fig. 4.18 *Opening the shoulders.*

shoulder while using palm, thumb or knee on the chosen meridian, but it is more effective to secure the receiver's arm at the elbow while working the meridian with the palm or thumb of the other hand, changing hands when reaching the elbow. Here the Kidney meridian is shown (Fig. 4.17).

Opening the shoulders

The giver moves behind the receiver's head and lightly grasps the rounded part of his shoulder joints with both hands, the heels of her hands resting in the natural hollow between chest and shoulders. Bringing her weight forward, she leans in to open his shoulders and chest (Fig. 4.18).

Neck stretches and work on the neck meridians

Many practitioners prefer to use a cloth when working on the face and neck, in traditional Japanese style. For clarity of illustration, the neck techniques have been shown without a cloth, but it is shown in the section on the face on p. 50.

Still kneeling behind the receiver's head, the giver stretches his neck in four different directions.

Straight back, by interlacing her fingertips under the occipital ridge, moulding her palms to the sides of his neck and drawing his head firmly back towards her Hara (Fig. 4.19A).

Diagonally at the front, by rotating his head slightly to one side, *gently* stretching the exposed side of the head diagonally back towards herself, while stretching the front of the opposite shoulder more firmly downwards in the opposite direction (Fig. 4.19B).

Sideways, by turning the receiver's head to face straight up again and gently moving it sideways, as if taking his ear down towards his shoulder-tip, while maintaining support on the opposite shoulder (Fig. 4.19C).

Diagonally at the back, by rotating the receiver's head so that his nose faces his shoulder-tip and stretching his head gently down towards the shoulder, while maintaining support on the opposite shoulder. This position is also suitable for working on the meridians of the back of the neck. Here the giver's thumb works the Triple Heater meridian while the neck is held at a stretch (Fig. 4.19D).

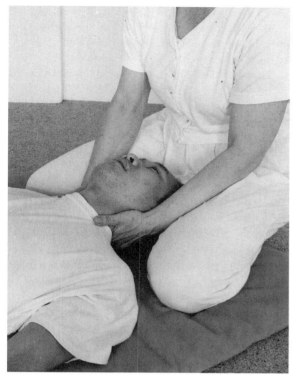

Fig. 4.19A   *Backwards neck stretch.*

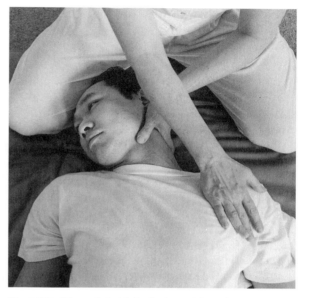

Fig. 4.19B   *Diagonal stretch for the front of the neck.*

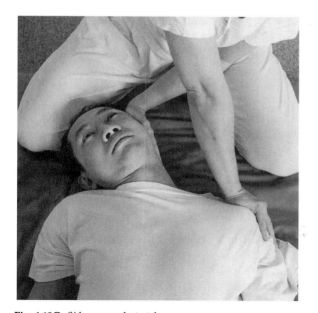

Fig. 4.19C   *Sideways neck stretch.*

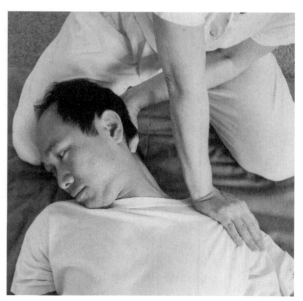

Fig. 4.19D   *Diagonal stretch for the back of the neck.*

Fingertip work under the occipital ridge

This technique, illustrated in Chapter 3 (see p. 30), is used for rebalancing uneven tensions in the neck muscles. The giver stretches the receiver's head back towards her with the fingers of each hand in turn, to discover which side of the neck is weaker and stiffer. She works on the weaker side first, finding the points of deepest penetration with her fingertips and leaning the weight of the receiver's head on to each in turn to increase penetration, then repeats the process on the more robust and resilient side.

Face work

When using a cloth on the face , cover only the part you are working on and at no time allow the cloth to cover the nose. Although very light pressure is used on the face, the giver should continue to work from the Hara and with whole-body awareness, with an upright posture.

Work on the face has more fluency if a general treatment following the shape of the bones is adopted and the face points and meridians incorporated into it.

First work outwards across the forehead with both thumbs. Curl the fingertips to work under the upper

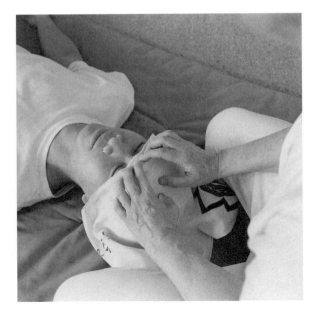

Fig. 4.20 *Face work.*

part of the eye socket (see p. 30 and Fig. 4.20) and work in the same way on the cheeks and under the cheekbones. Use both thumbs to press along the edges of the jawbone. Gently massage the ears.

The head can be tilted if necessary for work on the meridians; these are illustrated in Section Two.

Side position

Advantages

This is the most comfortable position for the receiver, especially if he has neck or lower back problems. It allows the giver plenty of scope for working on the shoulder joint, since the arm can be rotated fully into all positions. It also permits deep work into the side of the hip joint.

Disadvantages

The accessibility of the receiver's shoulder can be compromised if his upper torso is permitted to slump forward and this can require some effort for support from the giver. The position generally requires the giver to move around and change her working posture frequently, which can be distracting for the less experienced Shiatsu giver. It is also difficult to give the deep pressure into the back meridians which some receivers require and the position does not give much scope for work on the front and back of the legs.

Most accessible meridians

Gall Bladder, Liver, Triple Heater, Large Intestine, Small Intestine.

Treatment procedure

Head work

From the lunge position behind the receiver, the giver palms and thumbs the meridians of the side of the head, while supporting the forehead with the mother hand. A cloth can be used for thumbing the side of the face and jaw. The receiver's head should be comfortably supported on a pillow (Fig. 4.21).

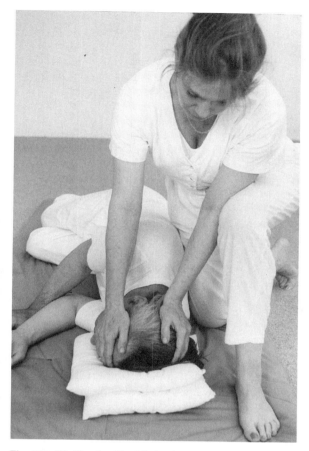

Fig. 4.21 *Working the side of the head.*

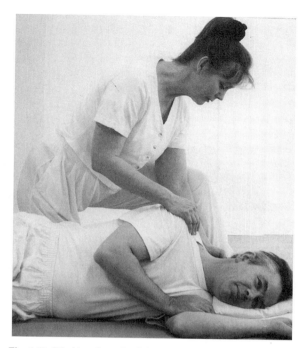

Fig. 4.22 *Working the neck while stretching the shoulder down.*

Neck work

The giver thumbs under the occipital ridge and the meridians of the side of the neck from a lunge or kneeling position, with her mother hand encircling and slightly drawing down the receiver's shoulder, to give a slight stretch to the neck meridians. The working hand should lightly grasp the neck while thumbing, for added support (Fig. 4.22).

The top of the shoulder

The giver moves behind the receiver's head. Her mother hand stabilizes the shoulder joint and stretches it slightly downwards, while she thumbs the meridians of the top of the shoulder outwards from the base of the neck (Fig. 4.23).

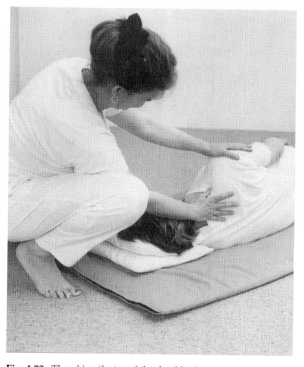

Fig. 4.23 *Thumbing the top of the shoulder from behind the head.*

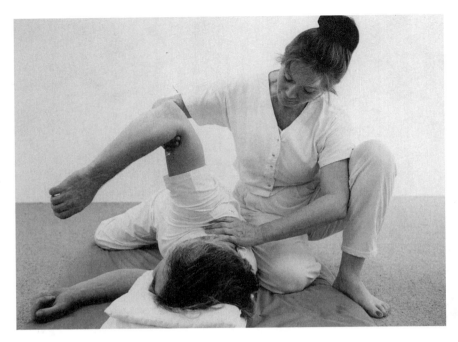

Fig. 4.24 *Shoulder and arm rotation.*

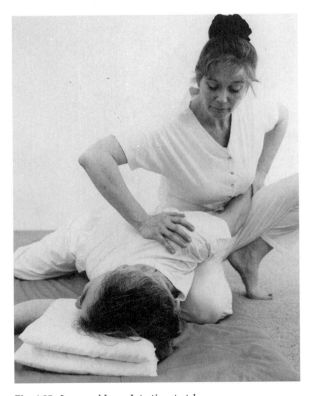

Fig. 4.25 *Lung and Large Intestine stretch.*

Shoulder and arm rotation

The giver moves to a position behind the receiver's back and kneels with her nearest leg contacting and supporting it. Her mother hand holds the shoulder for support with her thumb under the shoulderblade, while her other hand supports the receiver's arm by loosely grasping under the elbow and takes it in a wide, slow circle, forward, up, back and down (Fig. 4.24). The arm can then be laid in one of the following meridian stretches.

Lung and Large Intestine stretch

Still kneeling in close contact with the receiver's back, the giver draws his arm downwards and backwards to lie across her thighs. Holding his wrist, she leans her body weight backwards to stretch the arm, while her mother hand leans into the front of his shoulder to open the chest (Fig. 4.25). The meridians can be palmed, thumbed or elbowed with the arm in the stretch position.

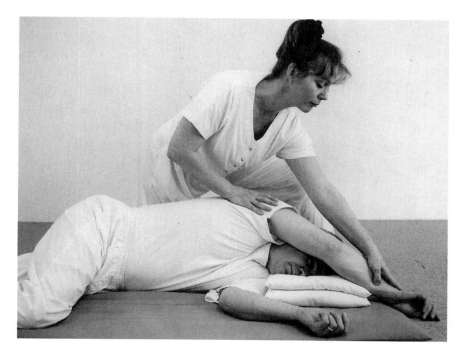

Fig. 4.26 *Heart and Small Intestine stretch.*

Heart and Small Intestine stretch

The receiver's arm is laid over his ear and the giver moves into the lunge position. Her mother hand leans on the opened shoulder to stabilize it, while she thumbs the accessible meridians in the arm (Fig. 4.26).

Working under the shoulderblade

Kneeling close in to the receiver's back, with her outside knee raised, the giver clasps the front of the shoulder joint with her mother hand and uses it to lift the shoulder towards the pressure of her working hand, which works under the edge of the shoulderblade with fingertips or thumb, supported by the leverage of the raised knee (Fig. 4.27). Even more support is provided if the arm of the mother hand is slipped under the receiver's arm while supporting the shoulder joint.

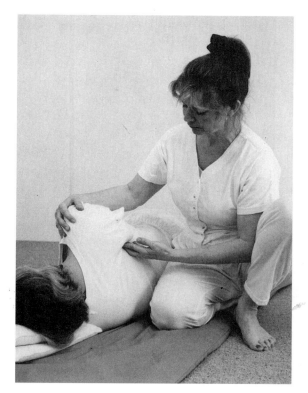

Fig. 4.27 *Working under the shoulderblade.*

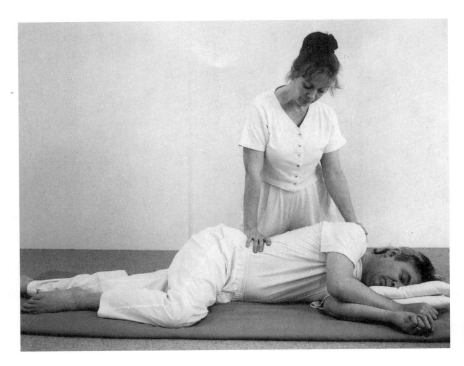

Fig. 4.28 *Working the side of the torso.*

Working the side

The giver turns to face the receiver's torso and supports the shoulder with her mother hand, while she palms, thumbs or elbows the meridians of the side, down to the hip (Fig. 4.28). The top of the arm can be worked in the same way, if it is laid on top of the torso.

The spine and back

From the working position shown above, the giver can kneel down and work the accessible back meridians, either with the fingertip technique shown in Chapter 3 (see p. 31) or by thumbing down them while supporting the shoulder with the mother hand. Penetration rather than pressure is necessary to avoid pushing the receiver's body forwards. A more supportive technique is to adopt the working position shown in the shoulderblade section above and to work down both sides of the receiver's spine with the thumb and knuckle (see p. 32) (Fig. 4.29). All of these techniques can be continued on to the sacrum.

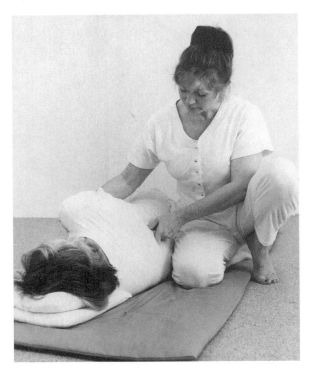

Fig. 4.29 *Thumb and knuckle down the sides of the spine.*

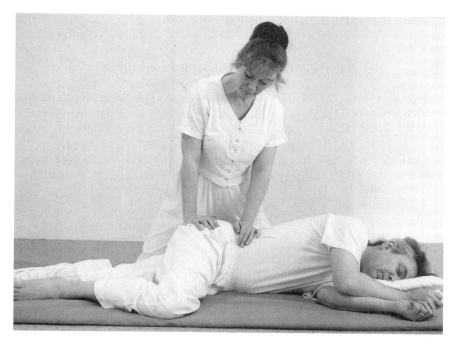

Fig. 4.30 *Working the hips.*

Hips

The giver kneels facing the receiver's torso and rests her mother hand on the side of the waist while she palms, thumbs or elbows the meridians of the side of the hip (Fig. 4.30).

Legs

Moving her mother hand down to the hip, the giver palms and thumbs the meridians of both the upper and lower leg. The knee can also be used on the lower leg (Fig. 4.31).

Sitting position

Advantages

There is great scope for work on the neck and shoulders in this position, since arms, shoulders and head can be supported, rotated and stretched. The receiver can be made aware of the natural potential for uprightness and movement in his torso and remains alert and energized. Shiatsu in this position

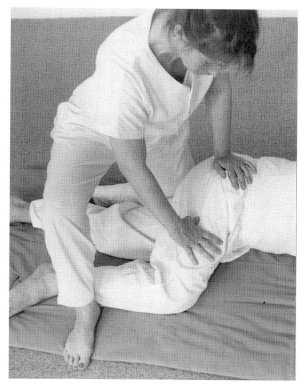

Fig. 4.31 *Thumbing the legs.*

does not require a large treatment space and can be adapted for use in a chair.

Disadvantages

Very few Westerners can sit comfortably for any length of time in the Japanese kneeling position, which is the best for sitting Shiatsu. The cross-legged position encourages the receiver to slump and he may need to sit on cushions or a low stool. The position makes considerable demands on the giver, who must pay constant attention to supporting the receiver and to maintaining her own relaxation and sense of the Hara (although this is wonderful for her practice!). It is difficult to work the lower torso effectively in this position.

Most accessible meridians

All neck, shoulder and arm meridians and meridians of the upper back.

Treatment procedure

Palming down the back

The giver kneels an arm's length away from the receiver, with a mother hand on his shoulder. (N.B. If the giver maintains the correct distance and a straight arm, this position provides excellent support for the receiver.) With her other hand she palms and thumbs the back meridians (Fig. 4.32). The thumb and knuckle technique (see p. 32) can also be used down the spine.

Elbows on shoulders

Kneeling in contact with the receiver's back and thus supporting him, the giver rests her elbows on the tops of his shoulders (Fig. 4.33).

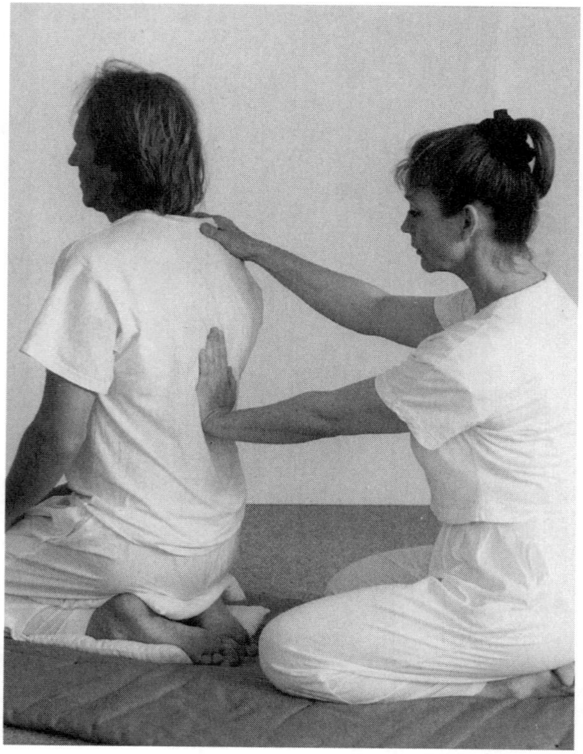

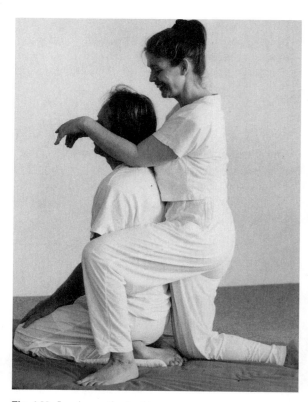

Fig. 4.32 *Palming down the back.*

Fig. 4.33 *Leaning on the shoulders.*

Arm rotation

Supporting the receiver's elbow and with a mother hand on the shoulder, thumb pressing next to the edge of the shoulderblade, the giver rotates the arm forward and up, back and down (Fig. 4.34).

Shoulder slash

Grasping and supporting the shoulder joint at the upper arm with the mother hand, the giver moves the joint backwards to meet the pressure of the thumb of the other hand, which presses around and slightly under the edge of the shoulder blade (Fig. 4.35). It may be helpful to put the receiver's arm in a half-nelson for this technique .

Arms

Two techniques for working the arm meridians are possible in the sitting position. The first is effective for a few of the Yang meridians only, the second for all the meridians.

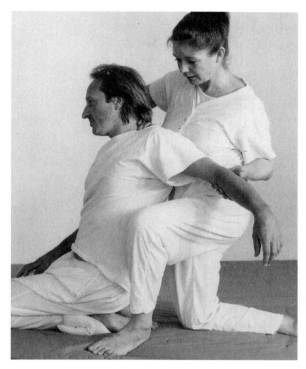

Fig. 4.34 *Arm rotation.*

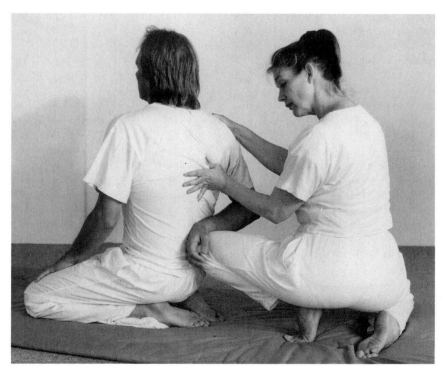

Fig. 4.35 *'Slashing' the shoulder.*

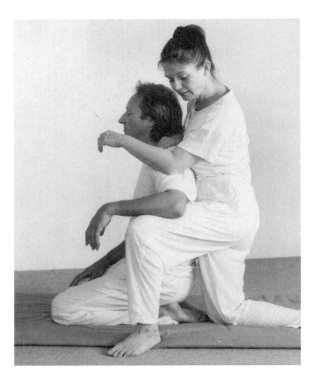

Fig. 4.36A *Elbowing the meridians of the top of the arm.*

Elbow technique. Kneeling close to the receiver, so as to support his body with her own, the giver lays the receiver's arm over her raised knee, elbow bent for complete support. With a mother hand on his shoulder, she then works the meridians of the top of the arm with her elbow (Fig. 4.36A).

Fingertip technique. Kneeling behind the receiver, the giver stretches his arm backwards in such a way as to stabilize him in an upright position. One hand holds his hand to maintain the position, while the other grasps the arm as close to the shoulder as possible. The fingertips or thumb of the working hand can then penetrate into any chosen meridian of the arm. The working hand continues to grasp down the arm, working the length of the chosen meridian (Fig. 4.36B).

Hand and wrist work

This technique is performed from the same position as the fingertip technique above. Supporting the wrist joint firmly with fingers and thumb, the giver holds the receiver's hand as if shaking hands and rotates the wrist (Fig. 4.37). Without releasing the wrist, she then stretches each finger in turn.

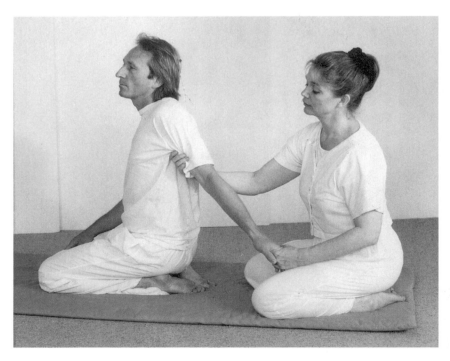

Fig. 4.36B *Working the arm meridians with thumb or fingertips.*

Thumbing the neck meridians

Kneeling behind the receiver at arm's length and with a mother hand on his shoulder for support, the giver holds his neck with her thumb on the chosen meridian on the opposite side of the neck to her palm and works down it to the shoulder on both sides (Fig. 4.38).

Neck rotation

The giver kneels close to the receiver, supporting his body with her own and with her raised thigh across his back for support. Her mother hand rests on his forehead and the other firmly holds the groove below his occiput, if possible with the thumb penetrating into one of the points there. Slightly lifting his head upwards for a stretch to the neck, she uses her mother hand to take the head slowly round in a circle, avoiding force and waiting at points of stiffness for the natural flexibility of the neck to reassert itself. This technique should be performed slowly and with sensitivity. Repeat it on the other side, reversing your position (Fig. 4.39).

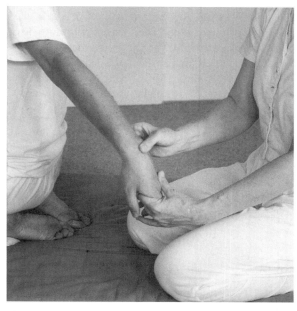

Fig. 4.37 *Hand and wrist work.*

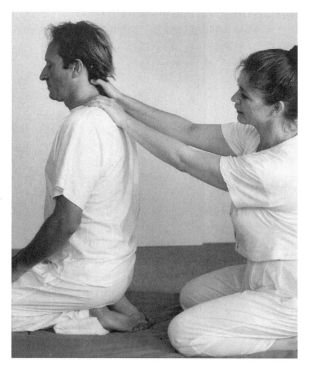

Fig. 4.38 *Thumbing the neck meridians.*

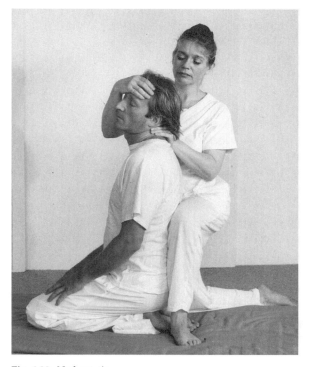

Fig. 4.39 *Neck rotation.*

Whole body stretch

The giver stands behind the receiver, with the side of one leg supporting his back and the other leg stretched behind her for stability. She picks up his hands or wrists and holds the back of his hands to her upper chest. She stretches the receiver upwards and backwards by lifting her own torso in the same direction (Fig. 4.40).

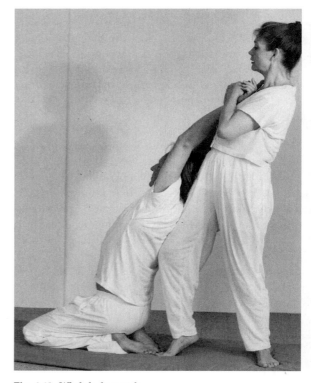

Fig. 4.40 *Whole body stretch.*

Theory

5

Traditional Chinese Medicine for the Shiatsu practitioner

What is TCM?

As mentioned in the Introduction, the acronym TCM is now widely taken to mean the model of Traditional Chinese Medicine re-established by Chairman Mao during the Cultural Revolution and currently practised and taught throughout the People's Republic of China. This model serves as a basis for the treatment of disease by acupuncture, herbal medicine, moxa, diet, exercise and medical massage, which includes Shiatsu.

It is not based, as a purely Shiatsu-oriented model would be, on the movement of Ki in the meridian network. Rather, it includes Ki among the Vital Substances which form and animate the human organism and sets forth the processes by which these substances are produced, maintained and distributed. It also classifies the disharmonies which can impede these processes as a result of the failure of any internal organ functions, whether from internal causes or external pathogenic factors (resulting from such influences as climate or diet).

Since much practical research on the efficacy of traditional medicine is taking place in China, and since large numbers of Western practitioners visit China for training, the concepts of TCM tend to take on the colouration of modern Chinese culture; TCM is taught as a pragmatic system, dealing primarily with the physical symptoms of acute disease. As a result, many Shiatsu practitioners in the West, many of whose clients come for help with emotional or psychological stress, feel that TCM has little relevance to the work they do. However, the history of Chinese medicine spans thousands of years and many eras in which values and philosophies were different from those of modern China and these are preserved in the ancient writings which are still medical classics. In fact, the roots of TCM are interwoven with those of Taoism and this connection can be valuable to the modern Western Shiatsu practitioner, who finds herself dealing with many psychological difficulties which in previous times would heve been prevented or remedied by the support of a spiritual tradition.

Practical uses of TCM

Although Shiatsu students do not need to learn TCM theory in order to give effective Shiatsu, it can enhance their practice in many ways.

Prognosis

One vital benefit which some knowledge of TCM confers is the ability to make a prognosis. An experienced Shiatsu practitioner can make a prognosis for a receiver's condition based purely on the information which the receiver's Ki supplies to her fingers. Less experienced or gifted practitioners need the support of a theoretical system to allow them to assess the seriousness and probable duration of the condition under treatment.

Points, moxa and magnets

The practitioner can decide with the help of TCM differentiation what points would be particularly helpful for the receiver and can treat them herself, with pressure, moxibustion (see p. 260) or magnets (see p. 260). She can also suggest that the receiver treats himself with them.

Referrals

If the prognosis indicates that the receiver's condition requires a treatment mode for which the giver is not qualified, such as herbs, the giver can refer the receiver to another practitioner.

Recommendations

TCM allows the giver to establish the cause of the receiver's condition and this in turn empowers her to suggest to him possible changes in lifestyle which may remove the cause and thus alleviate the condition.

Many Shiatsu practitioners are deterred from the study of TCM by the large number of lists of symptoms classified under "syndromes" which appear in the TCM reference books and which seem complex, dry and unrelated to Shiatsu. However, with a thorough understanding of some of the essential principles of TCM, together with some idea of tongue diagnosis, there is no need to learn all the details of the various syndromes by heart – the practitioner can put her own picture together. An explanation of the basic principles follows.

The root concept of TCM – Yin and Yang

In Taoist cosmology, Yin and Yang are the two archetypal principles produced by the movement and stillness of the Void* and which by their interaction together create Ki and the world of phenomena. On the philosophical level, movement and stillness, activity and receptivity are the key words for the understanding of Yin and Yang.

The Shiatsu student, when studying Yin and

Yang, may be confronted with lists of opposites such as night and day, male and female, which do little to further her understanding of the relevance of Yin and Yang to Shiatsu. First of all, it should be understood that the two principles do not indicate static and opposed states, but rather a continuum of relative relationship. Thus the muscles are Yin compared to the skin, but Yang in relationship to the bones. If this is understood, Tables 5.1 and 5.2 may be helpful.

Table 5.1 *Yin and Yang relationships of body parts and substances*

Yin	Yang
Lower part (e.g. Hara)	Upper part (e.g. head)
Front (e.g. throat)	Back (e.g. nape)
Interior (e.g. bones)	Exterior (e.g. skin)
Substance (e.g. Blood)	Energy (e.g. Ki)

Table 5.2 *Yin and Yang relationships of bodily and metabolic functions*

Yin	Yang
Cooling	Warming
Relaxing	Activating
Downward movement	Upward movement
Centreing	Expanding
Anchoring	Transporting
Nourishing	Consuming
Moistening	Drying
Storing	Protecting

All living things ideally possess Yin and Yang in equal balance. Human beings are born with a full and equal quota of each, not only as part of our form (front/back, bones/skin, etc.) but as reserves of the vital Yin and Yang principles stored in the Kidneys as Kidney Yin and Kidney Yang (see p. 102). Each organ possesses Yin functions, such as the capacity to cool, relax or moisten in the appropriate sphere of influence, and Yang functions such as the ability to transform, warm, move or protect. Excess Yin and Yang can only enter the body in the form of external influences such as cold, heat, etc. (see p. 70); any other disharmony of Yin and Yang is in the form of deficiency of either principle which leads to an apparent Excess of its counterpart (see p. 77).

---

*"It is the ultimate of nothing which is the Supreme Ultimate. The Supreme Ultimate moving produces the Yang, and at the ultimate of movement becomes still. Becoming still, it produces the Yin; and at the ultimate of stillness again moves. Movement and stillness alternate, each the root of the other". Chou Tun-Yi, quoted on p. 32 of *Two Chinese Philosophers* by A.C. Graham, Lund Humphries.

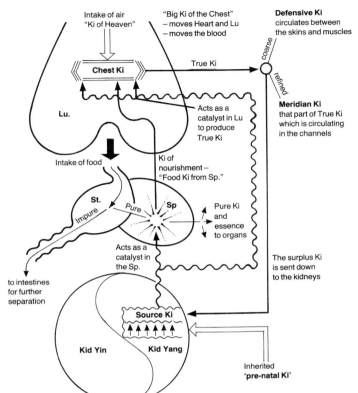

Fig. 5.1 *The production of Ki (by kind permission of Paul Lundberg).*

The Vital Substances

In TCM terms, the Vital Substances are responsible for all aspects of human form and function. Essence, Blood and Body Fluids perform the Yin functions of nourishing, moistening and satisfying our substance. Ki and Spirit are the Yang, non-substantial factors which animate and move it; Ki in particular governs our metabolism.

Ki

Ki is at first taken by the Shiatsu student to mean the movement of energy in the meridian network. Although this is indeed one aspect of Ki, the word "energy" is a Western approximation of an Oriental concept which has the sense of something physically palpable, a kind of rarefied fluid which can condense into substance. The Chinese character for Ki contains the radicals for both "steam" and "rice". In its refined forms Ki moves and flows almost invisibly, like steam.

In its denser aspects it slows or coalesces into form, such as rice. Ki is the product of the interaction of Yin and Yang and is itself the basis of the world of phenomena. In the human body, Ki is the principle which moves, warms and protects us from outside influences. Since on the physical plane Ki is the agent for movement and transformation, similarly on the psychological level free-flowing Ki gives an ability to change our state, to alternate between different emotions, between work and pleasure, activity and rest.

Production of Ki (Fig. 5.1)

We have three sources of Ki: our genetic inheritance, our food and the air we breathe. Each of these is stored or processed in a different area of the body, corresponding to the "three burning spaces" of the Triple Heater.

1. In the Lower Burning Space is stored our Source, or Original Ki. Part of this is present from

conception. This Ki which we inherit from our parents, what we might understand as the energy of our genes, remains within us, fuelling the activity of all our systems and organs and thus we gradually deplete it throughout our lives. The other part is formed from the purest of the Ki produced by the processes of breathing and digestion, which is sent down to the Lower Burning Space to replenish the source. Source Ki is pure and concentrated, like rocket fuel; a little goes a long way. It acts as a catalyst for all bodily processes and for each meridian, via internal connections governed by the Triple Heater, the "messenger of the Source Ki". Every meridian has a Source Point, from which it takes its feed of Source Ki. Source Ki forms the basis for Kidney Yang, which powers all the Yang energy of the body.

2. The Middle Burning Space is the area in which we process food in order to obtain its Ki, which has different characteristics from those of human Ki, and change it into our own. This is done by the Stomach and Spleen which , with the help of Source Ki, break down the food into the Food Ki (Gu Qi, or "Grain Ki" in Chinese) and send it up to the chest to unite with the third type of Ki.

3. The Ki of air ; this is already in a pure state, requiring no processing, and is taken in by the Upper Burning Space to combine in the chest with Food Ki. Source Ki also acts as a catalyst for this process. Thus all three forms of Ki unite to form the individual's True Ki, which flows in the meridians. A by-product of this transformation is Defensive Ki which is highly active, "strong and bold", and is sent by the Lungs to defend the surface of the body and protect it from outside influences.

Each of the three transformational areas, or Burning Spaces, of the Triple Heater contributes its own measure of Source Ki to facilitate the processes described above and to combine with the Ki of the organs in that area to provide energy for transformation. Thus the Fire of the Lower Burner contributes to Kidney Yang, the Fire of the Middle Burner is allied with Spleen Yang and the Fire of the Upper Burner combines with the Ki of the Heart and Lungs to contribute to the transformational power of the Zong Ki, the "Big Ki of the Chest".

I am grateful to my colleague Paul Lundberg,

co-founder of the Shiatsu College in London and author of *The Book of Shiatsu*, for permission to reproduce his chart, illustrating these processes in a direct and simple form (Fig. 5.1).

Disharmonies of Ki

In health, Ki flows freely, imperceptible except as a sense of well-being. In disharmony, four things can happen to Ki: it can become deficient; it can go in the wrong direction; it can be in relative Excess; and it can be obstructed.

Ki Deficiency. Ki can become deficient in one particular organ or in the whole body. This systemic condition, known as Ki Deficiency, usually arises from a problem in the process of Ki production by the Spleen or the Lungs. Symptoms of Ki Deficiency are therefore those of Spleen or Lung Deficiency* (see Chs 8 and 9):

- fatigue
- pale face
- breathlessness
- loose stools
- weak voice
- daytime sweating with little or no exertion.

Shiatsu can be helpful in cases of Ki Deficiency, especially with attention to some of the following tsubos. Moxa may be useful if there are no signs of Heat and dietary advice and breathing exercises are good recommendations.

■ *Points for Ki Deficiency* – LI 4, 10; St 36; BL 17, 43; CV 6, 17; GB 30

Ki Sinking or Rising. Ki can also go in the wrong direction. The natural direction of the Ki of the Spleen is upwards, that of the Stomach and Lungs downwards. When the Spleen Ki fails to go up, the condition is known as Ki Sinking (see p. 187) and leads to symptoms such as prolapse. If the Stomach or Lung Ki fails to go downwards it is known as

---

*Any syndrome in TCM, such as Ki Deficiency, will manifest a variety of symptoms. Not all the symptoms will necessarily appear every time, but at least three must be observed in order to confirm the diagnosis.

Rebellious Ki. In the case of the Stomach, this leads to hiccups, vomiting or reflux of stomach acids; in the case of the Lungs it can lead to fullness in the chest, coughs, sneezes or asthma (see p. 269).

- *Points for Ki Sinking* – GV 20 (especially with moxa)

- *Points for Rebellious Ki* – Stomach – HP 6; CV 13; St 21; BL 17, 19, 21. Lungs – Lu 1, 2, 5, 7; BL 13

Ki in relative Excess. Ki can also be in relative Excess, when some organs, body parts or meridians have more Ki than others. In itself, this is not a condition of disease, since it is a normal part of the movement and flow of Ki in the course of human activity. It is when the flow stops and the relative Excess of Ki becomes lodged in one particular organ or body part that disharmony and thence disease occur. Shiatsu deals with this condition by dispersing the Ki from the Excess areas (sedation) and bringing it to the deficient ones (tonification). This is discussed in detail in Chapter 14.

Ki Stagnation. Ki can also become obstructed or stagnant. This can occur as a local problem, resulting from physical injury or an invasion of one body part or meridian by cold, wind or damp. It can also occur as a more generalized whole body condition in which the internal processes are affected and this is generally as a result of repression of emotion (see p. 125). The symptoms of Ki stagnation include:

- sense of fullness, discomfort or pain (which comes and goes)
- swellings which come and go, e.g. swollen breasts
- sense of blockage in the throat
- irritability
- slightly purple tongue (not always the case).

- *Points for Ki Stagnation* – Liv 3; GB 34; LI 4; Sp 6; BL 18

Shiatsu is a good treatment for disharmonies of Ki, especially the last two, since it re-establishes the balanced flow of Ki throughout the body, even though ingrained patterns of Ki distribution are often linked to the receiver's personality and lifestyle and may need some time to shift.

Local treatment with moxa can be helpful for Ki stagnation, if there are no signs of Heat.

Essence

The second of the Vital Substances, Jing, is often translated as Essence. Essence is the Yin or substantial form of Source Ki, part of which we inherit from our parents. In the same way that Source Ki, being Yang, is the motive force for all our body processes for our lifetime, Essence, being Yin, is the basis for our body substance, the seed of our physical form. One cannot exist without the other.

On the philosophical level, Essence represents the historical continuity of living form as generation succeeds generation, whereas Source Ki is the force which activates and motivates each individual. On the practical level, the quality and quantity of our Essence determines our physical constitution for our lifetime and the quality of the constitution we hand on to our children. This is discussed further in the chapter on the Kidneys (see p. 100).

Essence, like Source Ki, comes in two forms. The first, Prenatal Essence, cannot be supplemented or replenished and gradually decreases with age. Sexual activity in men and childbearing in women deplete our Prenatal Essence the most, since its ultimate function is to provide physical form for our descendants. Postnatal Essence is produced by the processes of breathing and digestion and can be replenished by a healthy diet, breathing exercises and a moderate lifestyle.

Prenatal Essence is stored "between the Kidneys", which some authorities maintain is the Hara*. Postnatal Essence is produced by the Stomach and the Spleen, which transports it to all the organs and body parts, and what is left is stored in the Kidneys. It is considered to belong to the Kidneys more than to the Spleen. Both forms of Essence form the basis for Kidney Yin, the underlying Yin reserve which supports the Yin of the whole body.

Disharmonies of Essence

Essence can only be deficient, never in Excess. Shiatsu, though it can do little to augment the quantity of Prenatal Essence, can help to increase the

---

*"In the dantian (lower abdomen) is jing qi; the jing qi disperses (to the whole body)" from the Huan Ting Wai Jing Jing: quoted in *Hara Diagnosis: Reflections on the Sea*, p. 81.

activity of the organ systems which produce Postnatal Essence. Qi Gong exercises and treatment with Chinese herbal medicine are helpful. The symptoms of Deficiency of Essence include:

- retarded growth
- impotence or infertility
- weak constitution
- brittle bones
- poor memory
- prematurely grey or thinning hair
- red tongue with no coating.

■ *Points to tonify Essence* – BL 23, 43; GB 39; GV 4; Ki 3

Blood

"Blood" with a capital 'B', the third Vital Substance, represents more than the actual analysable substance which flows in the veins; to the Chinese it is the Yin complement to Ki. Where Ki goes, Blood goes and Ki also follows Blood. Whereas Ki performs the Yang functions of moving, warming and transporting, Blood's role is to moisten, nourish and relax. Without Blood, all body tissues, substances as diverse as those of the eyes, skin, nails, brain and tendons, lose their moisture, elasticity and nourishment, and thus part of their function.

Blood also has an effect on the emotions. It nourishes and satisfies on the psychological as well as the physical level. According to Ted Kaptchuk: "Ki represents the tension of change from one state into another. Blood represents the completion and acknowledgement of that change, resting in the change, the change made substance...Blood is more than a gynaecological issue. It has to do with how kind we can be to ourselves, how much space we can give ourselves to be comfortable" (Lecture in Oxford , UK, November 1991)

Particularly in the Heart, Blood stabilizes and provides a resting place for the Spirit, or Shen, which otherwise becomes agitated, leading to symptoms such as anxiety and insomnia.

Blood is produced from the Food Ki sent up by the Stomach and Spleen to the chest. In TCM the Heart is ultimately responsible for the making of Blood but it cannot do this unless the Spleen is providing enough Food Ki, so that Deficiency of Blood is frequently caused by a deficient Spleen. Excessive loss of blood, for example in menstruation or childbirth, can also lead to Blood Deficiency and this can also be due to a deficient Spleen failing to keep the Blood in the Vessels (see p. 187).

Another organ whose function is vital for the quantity and quality of the Blood is the Liver, which stores the Blood when we are at rest and sends it out when we need it for action (see p. 125). Since inefficient storage and distribution can lead to the unavailability of Blood when we need it, the Liver may be a key factor in creating a Deficiency of Blood; and as the healthy functioning of the Liver is connected with emotional balance, Blood Deficiency can result from emotional causes.

Disharmonies of Blood

Deficiency of Blood. Blood can be deficient from loss of blood or because the Spleen is failing to hold it in the Vessels or is not making enough Food Ki to create it or because the Liver is not making it readily available from storage. The symptoms of Blood Deficiency include:

- dull pale face
- dry skin and hair
- brittle nails
- weak tendons
- weak eyesight or "floaters" in the eyes
- insomnia (difficulty getting to sleep, but then sleeps well)
- depression or anxiety, poor memory
- dizziness
- numbness
- scanty periods
- pale, thin tongue, or slightly pale or orange sides to the tongue.

Deficiency of Blood, like that of Ki, does not present severe pathological symptoms but can lead to many syndromes which do. Shiatsu is helpful for Blood Deficiency because of its comforting and relaxing effect, but in severe or chronic cases dietary advice or herbal treatment will usually be needed.

Moxa can be helpful for Blood Deficiency on the following points, as long as there are no signs of Heat.

■ *Points for Blood Deficiency* – Sp 6; St 36; BL 17, 20; CV 4; GB 30; Liv 8

Heat in the Blood. If the Liver becomes too Yang and hot, which it is inclined to do, either from Interior emotional causes or from Exterior factors such as food or alcohol or from insufficient cooling by Liver Yin, the Blood which it stores also becomes hot. Heat in the Blood may manifest as red and itchy skin rashes or as a tendency of the Blood to "move wildly", causing sudden, heavy or profuse bleeding. The symptoms of Heat in the Blood include:

- feeling of heat
- itchy red rashes
- profuse bleeding (e.g. heavy nosebleeds, menstrual flooding)
- red tongue body.

■ *Points for Heat in the Blood* – Sp 6, 10: LI 11; BL 40; Ki 6; Liv 2, 14

DO NOT USE MOXA!

Blood Stagnation. The Blood can stagnate as a result or either Blood Deficiency, where the flow is slowed through weakness, or stagnation of Ki (see above), since the Ki moves the Blood. It can also be caused by physical injury or by invasion of Heat or Cold. It can be a fairly serious condition, when it affects the internal organs such as the Heart; many receivers who present with these symptoms will be on Western medication and herbal treatment may be advisable as a complement to Shiatsu. The symptoms of Blood stagnation include:

- pain which is severe, fixed, drilling or stabbing
- congestion or swelling which does not come and go
- bleeding which is dark with clots
- purple tongue.

■ *Points for Blood Stagnation* – Sp 1, 10; HP 6 (for stagnation in the chest); St 30 (for stagnation in the lower abdomen)

Shen

The Shen is the most rarefied and pure of the Vital Substances. It is only by courtesy a Substance at all, since it is most commonly translated as "Spirit" or "Mind". However, it is linked to the physical body by Essence and Ki and cannot manifest without them. Shen gives us our capacity to be present in the moment, aware and able to respond appropriately to our circumstances. Shen is considered to reside in the Heart.

Disharmonies of Shen

Although Shen is not itself a Substance but a presence of awareness, its condition depends upon other Vital Substances. Essence invites its presence in the body and nourishes it, so that Deficiency of Essence can cause Deficiency of Shen, with the additional symptoms of:

- low spirits
- dull, unresponsive behaviour.

The other Vital Substance which is important for the condition of the Shen is the Blood, specifically Heart Blood. Shen resides in the Heart and Heart Blood provides it with a tranquil, nurturing environment. Being Yin, the Blood calms and rests the Shen and if Blood is deficient the Shen becomes restless, leading to:

- anxiety
- insomnia.

The Shen can also be affected by the presence of Heat or Phlegm (see p. 74) which heat or obstruct the Blood in the Heart, so that the Shen loses its resting place, becoming scattered or disturbed. This manifests as:

- manic or depressive behaviour
- confusion
- delirium.

Shiatsu is an excellent short term treatment for disharmonies of Shen, because of its calming and balancing effects. However, in order to have a long term effect, the conditions which caused the Shen to become deficient, restless or scattered must also be addressed.

■ *Points to calm the Shen* – Ht 3, 7, 8; HP 6; CV 15

Body Fluids

The last of the Vital Substances, the Body Fluids, encompass all the liquid substances of the body, from the viscous lubricants of joints and marrow to the more watery fluids such as sweat and lymph. The Blood is the most important Body Fluid and is in a category of its own. All the Body Fluids, including the Blood, are supported by the basic Yin of the body, Kidney Yin. They are derived from our drink and the fluid content of our food by a complex process involving many of the organs.

This process begins with the action of the Spleen, assisted by Source Ki from the Kidneys, in obtaining the fluids from our food. These are separated into pure and impure. The pure fluids are sent up to moisten the Lungs, which descend them to the Kidneys and disperse them throughout the body to the skin and muscles. The Kidneys, having sent further vaporized fluids to the Lungs to moisten them, send the rest of what they have received down the Bladder. The Bladder further separates and refines them, sending the pure around the body and excreting the impure as urine. The impure part of the fluids which are extracted from food and drink by the Spleen go to the Small Intestine for further refining; the resulting pure fluids are sent to the Bladder for distribution around the body, the impure to the Large Intestine, which, having reabsorbed some fluid, excretes the rest in the faeces.

The transformation and distribution of Body Fluids, like that of Ki, is mediated by the action of the three Burning Spaces of the Triple Heater.

Disharmonies of Body Fluids

It is not vital for the Shiatsu giver to know all the details of the above process. The main points to remember are that the principal organs involved in the transformation and distribution of fluids of the Lungs, Spleen and Kidneys and that fluids cannot be transformed and distributed by any of these without the help of the Triple Heater. If the Lungs or Upper Burning Space are obstructed in their functions, there will be fluid accumulation in the upper part of the body. If the Spleen or the Middle Burning Space are in disharmony, there will be fluid accumulation in the middle of the body and if the Kidneys or Lower Burning Space are dysfunctional, fluid oedema will occur in the lower part of the body.

■ *Points for accumulation of Body Fluids* – BL 22; Lu 1; Sp 6, 9; CV 6, 9

MOXA MAY BE HELPFUL IF THERE ARE NO SIGNS OF HEAT.

If Body Fluids are not transformed, transported or excreted by any of these three organs (but primarily the Spleen) and are allowed to accumulate over a long period of time, they can condense to form Phlegm (see p. 74).

■ *Points for Phlegm* – St 40; CV 9, 17

Deficiency of Body Fluids can be caused by Deficiency of Blood or of the Yin moistening principle and has the same symptoms as those of Dryness (see p. 75).

■ *Points for Deficiency of Body Fluids* – Sp 6; Ki 3, 6; CV 4

DO NOT USE MOXA!

The causes of disease

We have examined Yin and Yang and the Vital Substances as being the components of the mind and body in TCM and how their disharmonies can manifest as disease; but what causes those disharmonies? The causes can be internal or external. Just as TCM sees no separation between body and mind, matter and energy, so it sees the internal environment of the body as corresponding to the external. In many texts the body is likened to a territory, with a ruler and government officials; this territory has its own climates and seasons, the natural conditions of the Vital Substances. Thus during the Yang phase of daytime activity, the body is warmed and moved by Ki; during the Yin rest period of night, it is nourished and relaxed by Blood. The climate of this territory can be influenced by changes in the condition of the Vital Substances; it can also be influenced by the conditions of the surrounding environment.

It is relatively easy for the Western mind to understand how internal emotional states can cause disease in the form of heat, cold or obstruction. Our language preserves these concepts from former times; we say, for example, "frozen with terror" or "blazing with anger". These are the same connections that TCM makes between temperature and emotion. We also have the metaphors to describe the movement of energy; "a knot in the stomach" describes the effect of worry upon the flow of our Ki and the phrases "I jumped out of my skin" or "I was beside myself" vividly describe the effect of shock in momentarily dislodging the Shen. It is harder, perhaps, to envisage external climatic influences actually penetrating the body's territory to lodge there in the form of wind, cold, heat or damp. This, however, is how TCM views the influence of the environment on the body's Ki.

There are three categories of the causes of disease (see Table 5.3). These can be resisted according to the strength of the individual's heredity and constitution when balanced against the strength of the cause of the disease. Thus a short exposure to cold or a brief episode of worry will cause few problems to someone with a strong constitution, but may cause much greater damage to a person who is frail and weak.

The "Gateways of Change"

There are certain transitional periods in every individual's life when he or she is particularly susceptible to the causes of disease, but conversely when a great change for the better may take place in his or her health. These are times when the whole constitution can be either strengthened or weakened and obviously, during these periods, extra care should be given to protection from external pernicious influences and maintaining a balanced and healthy lifestyle. The Gateways of Change are:

- birth and the perinatal period (for the baby)
- puberty
- onset of full sexual activity ("marriage" in the texts)
- pregnancy, labour and the postnatal period (for the mother)
- the menopause.

These periods can lead to better health if proper care is taken to avoid emotional tension, overwork or exposure to extremes of climate. An extremely common effect of the Gateways of Change is seen in

Table 5.3 *The causes of disease*

Internal	External	Other
Fear	Wind	Diet
Anger	Cold	Overwork
Grief	Heat	Too much sex
Joy	Damp	Trauma
Thinking too much	Dryness	Poisoning
Worry	Summer Heat	Parasites
Shock		Wrong treatment

women who develop problems after a pregnancy but regain health after a subsequent one (or vice versa).

The internal causes of disease (the emotions)

The internal causes of disease are mental and emotional. Five of them, namely joy, anger, grief, fear and thinking too much, are linked with a specific Element and organ function. These emotions cause disease by exhausting or obstructing the Ki of the organ linked with them, so that the organ is weakened in the performance of its physical function. The emotional links with the organs are discussed individually in Section Three.

Two of the internal causes, shock and worry, are not ascribed to any one organ or meridian. Shock, however, is particularly associated with the Heart in TCM, since it disturbs the Shen. It can also deplete the Kidneys, which must release a large measure of Source Ki to restore normal balance after severe shock. Worry is said to "knot" the Ki in general. Since the Lungs disperse the Ki to all parts of the body, this has a backlash effect on the Lungs and since worry is a form of "thinking too much" it also affects the Spleen.

All the emotions can have a specific effect on bodily functioning, depending upon the organ – emotion link in question. However, a general, non-specific effect of any emotion in the long term is to create Heat because the Ki, instead of flowing freely, is concentrated and internalized.

The external causes of disease (and "internal climates")

In a state of health, when our internal climate is adjusted to the external one, the Ki of our bodies is in harmony with that of the environment. Our

Defensive Ki protects us, forming a shield so that external influences cannot penetrate, but only stimulate a healthy response. (In cold weather, for instance, we feel braced and energetic, in hot weather, relaxed and expansive.)

If our internal climate is out of balance, however, or if our Defensive Ki is weak, we become susceptible to external influences. Wind, cold, dampness or heat can penetrate and lodge within the body, causing symptoms of disease which resemble the effects of the external climatic influence.

For example, if someone lives in a damp environment, dampness can penetrate his body, causing stiffness and swelling in his joints. The same symptoms can be created by a Deficiency of the Spleen, which causes internal fluids to collect and create internal Dampness, since they are not being transformed or transported.

If internal Dampness is already present as a result of Spleen Deficiency, the external dampness will penetrate more easily. By the same token, external dampness penetrating the body will obstruct the function of the Spleen, preventing it from transforming fluids, thus creating more Dampness.

To summarize: external climates can penetrate the body to become internal climates. Internal climates can also arise as a result of Deficiency of one of the organs. If an internal climate already exists, the same external climate establishes itself more easily in the interior. If the external climate establishes itself, it creates imbalance in the related organ function, increasing the production of the internal climate.

Wind

Wind is the most powerful, most penetrating of the external causes of disease. It is considered very important to protect the body from Wind for this reason. Since Wind can be encountered in many forms, such as air-conditioning, the stream of air from a fan, travelling on a motorbike or in an open car, or even as draughts in the home, people with weak Defensive Ki or who are susceptible to exterior influences should avoid these situations or wrap themselves up well if exposed to them.

Wind causes symptoms which are like wind in nature:

- sudden and acute in onset

- affecting mostly the upper part of the body
- causing shivering and fear of draughts.

The most usual manifestation of Wind is the common cold, which affects the Lungs, the uppermost organ, and the upper part of the body, but it often signifies the beginning of some other disease. There is a TCM saying that "every disease begins with the symptoms of a cold". Wind can carry other external influences, such as Heat or Cold, into the body with it and Wind-Heat or Wind-Cold are much more common than Wind on its own (Table 5.4).

Table 5.4 *The symptoms of Wind-Cold and Wind-Heat*

Wind-Cold	Wind-Heat
Headache	Headache
Shivering and fear of draughts	Shivering and fear of draughts
Sneezing	Sneezing
Cough	Cough
Aching muscles	Sore throat
Runny nose, clear or white mucus	Stuffed-up nose, yellow mucus
No fever or sweating	Fever and sweating

Exterior Wind can easily affect the eyes, causing the symptoms of acute or chronic conjunctivitis (swelling and watering of the eyes). Hayfever is another common manifestation of external Wind.

When Wind is created by a disharmony of the internal organs, it has different symptoms from the Exterior Wind described above. (This is the only case in which the symptoms of an external climate invading are different from those of the same climate internally.) Internal Wind is usually associated with some syndrome of the Liver, the commonest of which include severe Blood Deficiency, rising out of Liver Yang or extreme Heat. The symptoms include:

- tics
- tremors
- convulsions (in extreme Heat cases)
- a moving or deviated tongue (when extended).

Internal Wind is discussed further in Chapter 8 on the Liver.

■ *Points for External Wind* – GB 20; BL 12; LI 4; St 36; GV 14

■ *Points for Internal Wind* – Liv 3; GV 20: BL 18; LI 4 (for facial tics)

■ *Points for Heat* – LI 11; TH 6; Liv 2; BL 40; HP 3

DO NOT USE MOXA!

Heat

The characteristic effects of heat on substances in the external environment are to:

- concentrate fluids
- intensify colour and smell
- speed up movement
- cause a burning sensation
- cause thirst and sweating

and these are also the symptoms of invasion of the body by Heat. They will shortly be compared with the effects of Cold for easy reference (Tables 5.5 and 5.6 overleaf).

External causes of Heat are: exposure to hot climates, central heating and hot working conditions, such as boiler rooms or kitchens. Heat can also develop within the body as a result of heating food or drink such as spices, coffee and alcohol or from emotional causes. Heat symptoms can also arise from a lack of the cooling principle of Yin and this is discussed further in the section on the Eight Principles.

Summer Heat

Summer Heat is a strong form of climatic external Heat which produces the symptoms of sunstroke and fever. Points used are the same as for Heat.

DO NOT USE MOXA!

Cold

The characteristic effects of cold in the external environment are to:

- maintain fluids
- reduce intensity of colour and smell
- slow down movement
- cause biting or cramping pain
- reduce thirst and sweating

and Cold invading the body produces the same symptoms. External causes of Cold are exposure to a cold climate or cold working conditions. Cold can also develop internally from an intake of cold food such as ice cream or Cold energy foods such as yoghourt or

Table 5.5 *The manifestations of Heat*

Action	Effect on body
Concentrates fluids	Dry stools (constipation) Scanty urine Thirst
Intensifies colour	Red face and lips Red tongue Yellow tongue coating Dark urine Yellow mucus or discharge
Intensifies smell	Smelly stools and secretions Strong sweat
Increases movement	Explosive diarrhoea Restlessness/agitation
Characteristic hot sensations	Itching Burning pain Dislike of heat Pain or symptoms better for cold (e.g. ice pack)

Table 5.6 *The manifestations of Cold*

Action	Effect on body
Maintains fluids	Loose stools Copious urine Lack of thirst
Reduces intensity of colour	Pale face and lips Pale tongue White tongue coating Clear urine White or clear mucus or discharge
Reduces intensity of smell	Little smell from stools or secretions No sweat or odourless sweat
Reduces movement	Stools not so urgent Slowness and stagnation
Characteristic cold sensations	Cramping Sharp or biting pain Dislike of cold Pain or symptoms better for heat (e.g. hot water bottle)

salad or it may manifest from a lack of the warming principle, Yang, usually the Yang of the Kidneys and Spleen. This is discussed further in the section on the Eight Principles.

■ *Points for Cold* – GV 4; St 36

MOXA IS AN IMPORTANT TREATMENT FOR COLD CONDITIONS, BOTH LOCALLY AND ON THE POINTS ABOVE.

Dampness

This, like Wind, combines readily with Heat and Cold. Dampness in the external environment causes stickiness, moisture oozing forth, swelling, obstruction and turbidity, and affects structures near the ground. It is slow to arise and difficult to eliminate.

Dampness in the internal environment is similar; it causes sticky, turbid discharges, oozing skin diseases, swellings (e.g. stiff and swollen joints in arthritis), obstruction such as difficult urination (Damp obstructing the Bladder) or nausea (Damp obstructing the Spleen). It gives sensations of heaviness in the limbs and stuffiness in the chest or head (although it

tends to affect the lower part of the body). It often manifests as a thick, sticky coating on the tongue, which may be white or yellow depending on whether the condition is Damp-Cold or Damp-Heat.

Dampness can invade the body from the outside as a result of climatic humidity, damp living conditions, remaining in damp clothes for too long and occupational causes such as gardening or working in a laundry. Dampness can also build up as a result of too much sweet food, dairy products or alcohol. Spleen Deficiency causes internal Dampness, since the Spleen does not transform and transport fluids, which then accumulate.

■ *Points for Dampness* – BL 20, 22; Sp 6, 9; St 36, 40; CV6, 9, 12

MOXA MAY BE HELPFUL IF THERE ARE NO SIGNS OF HEAT.

If Dampness is present for some time, it may condense to form Phlegm. Phlegm may manifest as substantial Phlegm, in the form of mucus or fatty lumps and swellings, or insubstantial Phlegm, which obstructs the flow of Ki in the meridians causing numbness and paralysis, or clouds the Mind causing symptoms of mental illness. Phlegm, being derived

---

EXAMPLES

To show the usefulness of differentiating between the internal climates, let us take three hypothetical women presenting with cystitis.

Ms A is feverish. Her urine is dark and scanty with blood in it and smells strong. it is frequent, urgent and burning. Her face is flushed and her tongue is red, with a yellow coating. Her symptoms are much worse if she drinks coffee or alcohol. She has Heat in the Bladder. The Shiatsu treatment incorporates pressure on BL 40 and Ki 6. She is told to avoid heating foods and drinks (see Fig. 5.2, p. 76), to drink plenty of water and is sent to a herbalist for cooling herbs.

Ms B looks pale. She is shivering and bundled up in lots of clothes. Her pain is sharp and biting and feels better for a hot water bottle. Her urination is

frequent, in reasonable amounts; the urine is clear and has no smell. She craves hot drinks. Her tongue is pale, with a white coating. She has Cold in the Bladder. She is given moxa treatment on the lower abdomen and back, in addition to the Shiatsu, and is advised to use it at home.

Ms C has had chronic cystitis for some time; it seems to flare up whenever she goes camping with her boyfriend, which she enjoys. Her urine is cloudy; she has a heavy, dragging sensation in her lower abdomen and although she feels a frequent need to urinate, the flow is slow, difficult and obstructed. She has a vaginal discharge most of the time. Her tongue has a thick white coating on the root. She has Damp in the Bladder. She is advised to avoid sweet foods and dairy products and is given moxa treatment on St 36 and Sp 9.

from Dampness, is often rooted in a Deficiency of Stomach and Spleen, although substantial Phlegm is most often present in the Lungs. There is a TCM saying that "The Spleen is the generator of Phlegm, the Lungs are the container of Phlegm".

■ *Points for Phlegm* – St 40; CV 9, 17

Dryness

This condition manifests as dry skin, mouth, throat and eyes, a dry cough and dry stools. It may arise from dryness in the environment, such as a desert climate, or excessive central heating and air-conditioning. Internally, it can arise as a result of Blood Deficiency or Yin Deficiency (see p. 79).

■ *Points for Dryness* – Sp 6; Ki 3, 6; CV 4

The examples on page 74 show the usefulness of differentiating between the internal climates.

Other causes of disease

Overwork

Physical overwork includes overexercising and its effects can be general or local. In general it depletes the Spleen and Kidneys and commonly leads to backache and other Kidney-related symptoms. Local problems occur in specific areas through wear and tear; a runner may develop painful knees or shin splints; a writer may suffer from wrist or finger pain. Often the meridian which is most affected locally is one which is already out of balance for other reasons.

Mental overwork can affect the Stomach or Spleen if only the intellect is involved, but there are often other factors related to our working lives, such as decision-making or fear of failure, which are rooted in other causes and stem from other meridians.

Too much sex

It is always controversial in the West to teach that there can be too much sex, let alone that it can be a cause of disease. However , in TCM terms, excessive sexual activity leading to climax, with or without a partner, depletes the Essence and thus the Yin principle. Since Essence is responsible for the general health of our constitution and decreases with age, sexual activity should be rationed according to our age and state of health.

Diet

It is extremely common to find problems caused by poor diet, even if the receiver is diet-conscious and thinks he is eating healthily. A common problem is the excessive consumption of cold or raw food, such as salad and fruit, which use up the warming and transforming power of the spleen Yang.

According to its warming or cooling properties, food or drink may produce internal Heat or Cold if taken in excess; greasy or fatty food, dairy products, sugar and alcohol can produce Dampness. The Stomach and Spleen are particularly vulnerable to disharmony from dietary causes.

Diet in TCM is a vast and complex subject, and every Chinese receives at his or her mother's knee a fund of information on foods which can be helpful for various health problems. It is suggested that the reader refers to one of the specialized books on diet (such as *Prince Wen Hui's Cook* by Bob Flaws and Honora Lee Wolfe, Paradigm Publications, 1983) for more detailed information. However, since Heat and Cold are among the simpler principles of Chinese dietary therapy, I include overleaf a chart (redrawn in Fig. 5.2 and reproduced by permission of Christina McCausland, who created it) showing the Hot and Cold energies of food.

As important as the quality of the food itself are the circumstances in which it is eaten. Food should be taken at regular intervals, in tranquillity. Irregular eating, eating "on the run" or while working, or family rows at mealtimes all injure the Spleen and Stomach, particularly the Stomach Yin.

Since this chapter is specifically on TCM, it is the TCM view on diet which is given here. For more general dietary recommendations, see Chapter 2, p. 19.

Trauma

Physical trauma means injury to the tissues from outside causes, such as blows, wounds, chemical damage or burns. Trauma can result in local stagnation of Ki or Blood, which may cause problems, either immediately or in the long term. Shiatsu can be very effective in minimizing the effects of trauma. In the case of recent injury, the giver should work above and below the traumatized area, on the meridians

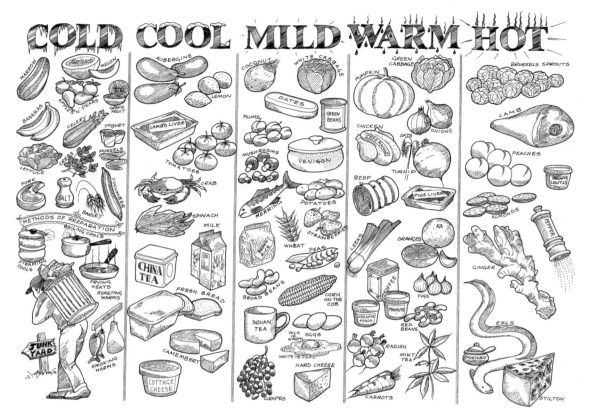

Fig. 5.2 *Hot and Cold energies of food.*

indicated in the Hara diagnosis and also on any other meridians which feel imbalanced in any way. If the trauma is to a limb, Shiatsu can be given to the same area on the opposite limb. If the trauma was not recent but has left a damaged area such as a scar, the same treatment principles can be observed, avoiding the scar tissue but paying particular attention to holding the meridians involved on points above and below the scar, to encourage the Ki to flow through it.

Poisoning

In the modern world the category of poisoning is enlarging all the time. Poisoning may be sudden and violent, as when a person ingests a harmful quantity of a poisonous substance, or it can be slow and insidious. The diseases caused by pollution, such as reactions to air pollutants, chemical substances or radiation, are a modern form of poisoning and the list is likely to grow.

Once the cause of poisoning is eliminated, Shiatsu can be effective in minimizing the symptoms remaining and increasing the emotional well-being of the sufferer.

Parasites

Examples of visible parasites which cause disease are worms and lice. Shiatsu has little effect on these and they must be eliminated by other means before treatment can progress.

Fungi such as tinea (athlete's foot) or yeasts such as candida (thrush) could be said to be "invisible" parasites but since their presence is inseparable from the symptoms of Dampness coming from the damp environments in which they thrive, they are usually considered a manifestation of Dampness. Shiatsu can help greatly here, but needs to be combined with dietary changes and herbs or other treatment.

Wrong treatment

It is unusual for a wrong diagnosis in Shiatsu to result in lasting ill effects, if the cautions in Chapter 1 are observed, since Ki has a natural tendency to balance itself out. Wrong treatment by Shiatsu would be treatment which is too vigorous for the receiver's constitution or violent techniques of manipulation, which would cause damage.

The "wrong treatment" mentioned in the TCM texts mainly refers to herbal medicine, which has a slow but lasting effect. Occasionally, it is possible to identify a problem as the result of wrong self-treatment, since many receivers will take strong herbs, such as ginseng, with little knowledge of their effects. Apart from cases such as this, the Shiatsu practitioner may not be able to identify wrong treatment by herbs, but she can familiarize herself with the side-effects of the main prescribed Western drugs. These are unlikely to respond significantly to Shiatsu treatment until the medication has been reduced, although Shiatsu can prevent further deterioration.

The Eight Principles

The Eight principles are ways of differentiating a multitude of symptoms into recognizable patterns. The receiver's symptoms are examined and classified under the categories shown in Table 5.7.

The purpose of this classification is to determine:

- the extent and seriousness of the condition
- how to treat it, in terms of approach and points
- whether to use moxa or not
- what recommendations to make concerning lifestyle.

Yin and Yang

The differentiation of symptoms in terms of Yin and Yang is a prerequisite for classifying them further according to the remaining six Principles. As well as looking at the Hot or Cold, Deficient or Excess, Interior or Exterior nature of the symptoms, the giver needs to look whether they are in the upper or lower part of the body and whether they indicate a failure

Table 5.7 *The Eight Principles*

Yin	Yang
Cold	Hot
Deficient	Excess
Interior	Exterior

of the receiver's Yin functions of moistening, nourishing and storing, or the Yang functions of moving, transforming and protecting.

Hot and Cold

The differentiation of symptoms according to Hot and Cold has been discussed above under the causes of disease. Since one receiver may present symptoms of both Heat and Cold at once, it is important not to make a diagnosis based on only one or two symptoms or signs of either, but on a clear predominance of several symptoms of either Heat or Cold. It is then necessary to decide whether the Heat or Cold is of a Deficient or Excess nature and whether it is in the interior or exterior of the body.

The main purpose of Hot and Cold differentiation for Shiatsu purposes is in order to decide on possible lifestyle changes (diet, occupation, relaxation, living environment) and whether or not to use moxa.

Deficient and Excess

This classification in TCM goes far beyond the vague description terms of "he is a very Excess type" or "she is really Deficient", even though such descriptions can be useful in determining whether the receiver should receive vigorous or gentle treatment. Obviously a receiver with an Excess (robust and vigorous) constitution needs stronger treatment than a Deficient (depleted) one but, in order to be more specific, it is important to find out *what* is Deficient or Excess in the receiver.

We can be Deficient in:

- any of the Vital Substances (Ki, Blood, Essence, Shen, Body Fluids), either generally or in one particular organ, e.g. Lung Ki, Liver Blood, Kidney Essence
- the Yin principle
- the Yang principle.

We can have an Excess of:

- any of the external causes of disease (Heat, Cold, Wind, Damp) or Phlegm, produced by Dampness
- Fire, which is not the Element of Fire but the natural activity of an organ gone wild and combining with Heat to produce extreme Heat symptoms going upwards
- Ki, Blood or Body Fluids, in relative Excess because they are stagnating in one particular area.

Note: For the practitioner of Zen Shiatsu, there can be considerable problems in confusing Excess and Deficiency with Kyo and Jitsu. They are not the same and the difference between them is discussed further in Chapter 6 on Zen Shiatsu.

Conditions tend not to be completely Excess or completely Deficient. If we are Deficient in one of our vital principles or substances, we invite the invasion of external pathogenic factors and by the same token, if an Excess condition exists, there must have been a Deficiency which allowed in to establish itself. Thus a Spleen Ki Deficiency allows Excess to build up in the form of Dampness, and Liver Fire (Excess) presupposes a lack of the cooling principle of Yin. In practice, however, some conditions, such as Blood Deficiency, can exist without Excess.

When an Excess factor is present it often masks the underlying Deficiency, so that when it has been removed during the curative process, the receiver may seem more Deficient than before. It is, however, important in TCM terms to remove the Excess before tonifying the Deficient organ since otherwise the Excess pathogenic factor will be tonified. For the practitioner of Zen Shiatsu this does not have much bearing on the actual Shiatsu treatment procedure, but it can be important for the recommendations and when choosing any extra points for treatment. For example, a receiver should not take large amounts of a tonifying herb such as ginseng if he or she has significant amounts of Excess Heat, Damp, Phlegm, etc. In the choice of points recommended for self-treatment, the clearing of Excess should be considered as well as the tonification of Deficiency; for example in a case of Phlegm or Damp in the Lungs causing symptoms of bronchitis, points to remove the Dampness and Phlegm should be chosen before points to tonify the Ki of the Lungs.

All of the above conditions of Excess and Deficiency have been discussed elsewhere, except the Deficiencies of the Yin and Yang principles.

If the Yang principle of moving, warming , transporting and protecting is Deficient, there are symptoms of Yang Deficiency:

- feeling cold
- cold limbs
- tiredness
- low motivation or depression
- bright pale face
- copious pale urination
- loose stools
- frequent colds or infections
- tendency to put on weight (not always an indication)
- pale, wet, swollen tongue, perhaps with teethmarks.

Many of these symptoms are those of Cold, since the Yang function of warming is Deficient; and in fact, Yang Deficiency invites invasion of Cold rather than Heat, so that Excess Cold often accompanies this condition.

Yang Deficiency is usually rooted in a Deficiency of the Yang of the Kidneys or the Spleen and sometimes both. Kidney Yang is injured by overwork, although a Deficiency may be present for constitutional reasons. Spleen Yang is most often affected by dietary factors, especially an intake of cold, raw food. Kidney Yang Deficiency will lead to Spleen Yang Deficiency over time and vice versa, since the Kidneys store and the Spleen replenishes the Source Ki. Shiatsu can be an effective treatment for Yang Deficiency, but there must be a gentle approach and care not to exhaust the receiver.

■ *Points for Yang Deficiency* – GV 3, 14; St 36; CV 6

MOXA (ON THE ABOVE POINTS) IS AN EFFECTIVE TREATMENT FOR YANG DEFICIENCY. (SINCE HEAT, FOR EXAMPLE IN THE HEART, CAN COEXIST WITH YANG DEFICIENCY, THE GIVER SHOULD CHECK THAT THERE ARE NO SIGNIFICANT SIGNS OF HEAT BEFORE PROCEEDING.)

If the Yin principle of nourishing, cooling , moistening and relaxing is Deficient, there are symptoms of Yin deficiency:

- anxiety
- dry mouth, especially at night
- insomnia (hard to get to sleep and frequent waking)
- tendency to be thin (not always)
- night sweats
- hot feet, hands, chest ("five-palm heat")
- feeling hot, or low fever, in the afternoon
- scanty dark urine (not always)
- flush on cheekbones only
- red tongue with no coating (peeled) or peeled patches on tongue.

These general symptoms are usually combined with other symptoms, depending on the organs affected.

Yin Deficiency is sometimes called Empty Heat in TCM and it can be seen that there are symptoms which indicate Heat, but that they have a Deficient quality. For example, a person with Full Heat will feel generally hot, whereas a person with Yin Deficiency (or Empty Heat) will just have hot feet or a sensation of heat in the chest; someone with Full Heat has a generally red face, whereas someone with Yin Deficiency has a flush only over the cheekbones.

The support for all the Yin of the body is the Kidneys (see p. 100) and if Kidney Yin is Deficient, the Yin of the other organs is unsupported and vulnerable. Yin in general can be depleted by constitutional factors or by an injudicious lifestyle which exhausts the Essence or emotional stress which generates Heat. Stomach Yin is particularly affected by irregular eating habits. Chronic illness can also deplete the Yin.

Yin Deficiency, since it affects the most essential aspects of the body's substance, is a deep disharmony and difficult to rectify completely, although it may never produce pathological symptoms if care is taken in matters of health and lifestyle. It is usually linked with deep patterns of emotional sensitivity and an inability to relax; and relaxation, rest and emotional rebalancing are essential in treating Yin Deficiency. Shiatsu can be an aid to relaxation, but herbal treatment is usually needed to replenish the body's substance. Royal Jelly can be helpful, if taken for no more than a couple of months.

■ *Points for Yin Deficiency* – Ki 3, 6; CV 4, 15; BL 23; Sp 6

DO NOT USE MOXA!

Interior and Exterior

The terms Interior and Exterior refer primarily to the location of symptoms of disease in the body rather than to the cause of the disease, although Exterior conditions almost always have an Exterior cause.

The Exterior part of the body consists of the skin, the muscles and the meridians; the Interior part encompasses the internal organs and all other internal structures and the Vital Substances. (Fig. 5.3)

An Exterior condition may be only a short stage in the penetration of an external pathogenic factor into the body territory, after which it penetrates into the Interior portion and becomes an Interior condition, affecting the internal organs and thus producing changes in the body processes, with signs such as cough, diarrhoea, etc. An Interior condition may thus have had an Interior or Exterior cause. Even if an Interior condition manifests on the exterior in the form of skin eruptions or pain in the muscles, it

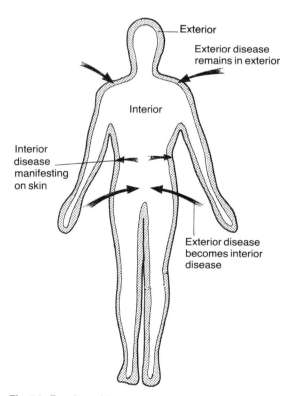

Fig. 5.3 *Exterior and Interior conditions.*

remains an Interior condition as long as it affects the Interior organs in any way.

Most of the conditions which the Shiatsu practitioner can expect to treat are Interior conditions. However, it is important to be able to recognize an Exterior condition, for reasons outlined shortly.

Exterior conditions can be of two kinds:

1. The invasion of the muscles and meridians by an external pathogenic factor such as wind, cold or damp which causes symptoms such as pain, swelling, stiffness or numbness but does not produce any other symptoms. This condition responds well to local Shiatsu treatment and to the use of moxa if there are no signs of Heat; also to cupping and skin scraping (see below).
2. The initial stage of an acute illness, while the body's Defensive Ki is still keeping it at bay, but the outcome of the battle is not decided. The symptoms are:

    *   shivering or "fever with chills" (skin)
    *   body aches (muscles and meridians)
    *   stiff neck or headache (muscles and meridians).

The Exterior phase of an illness, before it penetrates into the Interior, may last only a matter of hours. However, appropriate treatment at this stage of the illness may result in complete elimination of the external pathogenic factor and thus cure, before the disease develops. A whole body Exterior condition of this kind does not respond well to normal Shiatsu treatment since the Exterior, which includes the meridians, is obstructed by the pathogenic factor; the Defensive Ki is doing battle with it on the surface and the normal Ki responses are difficult to obtain. However, there are other options available:

1. *Cupping* A process in which a vacuum is created in a cup placed on the skin, so that the flesh rises up into the cup, increasing local circulation and, in TCM terms, drawing out the external pathogenic factor. Traditionally, the vacuum is created by heating the inside of the cup, a technique which requires some training, but there are now vacuum suction kits available of which there are good reports and which are easier to use. This folk medicine method is commonly used over tsubos to draw out the external pathogenic factor and the point of choice is BL 12; though GB 20 or GV 14 are possibilities, they are technically harder to cup.
2. *Causing sweating* This is another folk medicine method of releasing the pathogenic factor through the pores and is effective in receivers who are not particularly Deficient in Ki or Body Fluids, which are also lost to some extent through this method. The commonest way of causing sweating is to drink some hot (or heating) drink such as a herbal tea (a Western favourite is peppermint, elderflower and yarrow) or hot toddy and then to wrap up warmly and lie down.
3. *Skin scraping* This technique is extensively used in China, where it is called Gua Sha. The skin surface is lubricated and then scraped with a coin or the edge of the spoon down the affected area; for example, the upper back and neck for a cold, the hips for sciatica. Red marks are created as stagnation is released and fade in a couple of days.
4. *Points to release the Exterior* – BL 12; GV 14; Lu 7; LI 4; GB 20 plus points for Wind, Cold, Heat or Damp if signs of these are developing. These can be used with pressure alone or with moxa if it is absolutely certain that there are no signs of Heat developing.

Interior conditions can be treated by normal Shiatsu methods, either through the meridians alone, as in Zen Shiatsu, or with the addition of the relevant points to tonify Deficiency or disperse Excess.

In conclusion to this chapter on TCM, it can be seen that:

1. TCM is not meridian-orientated, like Shiatsu, but uses various different methods of treatment, of which the most easily available to the Shiatsu giver is the use of points;
2. TCM also recognizes general conditions such as Blood Deficiency or Dampness, which are not linked to one specific meridian, although they may be related to some organs or meridians more than others;
3. TCM relies on different methods of diagnosis from the primarily palpatory methods of Shiatsu, such as pulse diagnosis (not covered in this book) and inspection of the tongue. "Asking diagnosis", or questioning, is also specifically geared to the TCM differentiation of syndromes.

It is important when using TCM, therefore, to use it in parallel with the Shiatsu treatment and not to amalgamate the two. In other words, if a receiver complains of a cough with profuse mucus, indicating Damp-Phlegm in the Lungs, it would not be appropriate to give Shiatsu to the Lung meridian on the basis of the symptoms alone; it might make the condition worse. It would, however, be appropriate to press points such as CV 17 or Lu 5 to resolve Phlegm during the course of Shiatsu treatment based on the current diagnosis from the Hara, which may or may not include the Lung meridian.

Even if the Shiatsu giver does not use the points in her treatments, it can be very useful to have some knowledge of TCM in order to make recommendations (see case history below).

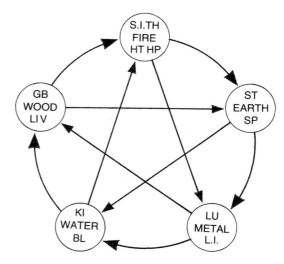

Fig. 5.4 *The Five Elements.*

CASE HISTORY

A third-year Shiatsu student was treating a receiver with irritable bowel syndrome. Her symptoms were loose stools, bloating and discomfort after eating and dull abdominal pain. The student diagnosed Spleen Yang Deficiency with consequent internal Empty Cold, but treated the receiver with Zen Shiatsu methods, according to the Hara diagnoses. These were very helpful in treating most of the symptoms, but the bloating remained until the receiver took the student's advice and ate only warm, cooked food which tonified the Spleen Yang.

Five Element theory

The theory of the Five Elements is included here as a part of the body of TCM theory, although the individual Elements are discussed at length in Section Two. Five Element theory refers to a differentiation between the different vibrational qualities of Ki which manifest in the universe, sometimes called Elements, sometimes Phases. The literal translation of the Chinese expression is "the Five Walkings", which indicates the connection with the characteristic *movement* of different qualities of Ki. As such it has particular appeal to the Shiatsu giver and forms the basis for much Shiatsu theory taught in the West, as explained in the Introduction.

The Five Elements are Fire, Earth, Metal, Water and Wood and the principal constituents of Five Element theory deal with the relationships between the Elements themselves (the Creative and Control Cycles) and the relationship between the Elements and the cosmos, represented by the Element correspondences. A popular model for the relationships between the Elements is represented in Fig 5.4.

The arrows forming the outer circumference of the circle show the Creative Cycle, in which each Element fosters and nourishes the succeeding Element. It can be memorized by a simple list of analogies:

- Fire creates Earth – think of ashes
- Earth creates Metal – think of goldmines
- Metal creates Water – think of condensation
- Water creates Wood – think of watering the garden
- Wood creates Fire – think of logs in a grate.

In clinical practice, this means that disharmony in an Element is passed on to the next Element in the cycle. This phenomenon is known as the Law of Mother–Child and relates to a TCM saying: "If the child screams, treat the mother". If an Element is weakened and symptoms develop in the "child" Element because the "mother" is not nourishing it, then the root cause of the problem is in the "mother", which should be treated as well as the "child". For example, if the Spleen is Deficient it encourages the formation of Phlegm which lodges in the Lungs, the Spleen's "child"; in this case the Spleen should be treated as well as the Lungs. The Law of Mother–Child is very commonly seen in practice.

The Control Cycle refers to the crossing arrows within the circle of Elements, which represent the counterbalancing forces which hold the Creative Cycle in check. It too can be memorized by simple analogies:

- Fire controls Metal – it makes it malleable
- Metal controls Wood – it cuts it down
- Wood controls Earth – its roots bind it together
- Earth controls Water – as banks contain a river
- Water controls Fire – it extinguishes it

Although sometimes mistranslated as the Destructive Cycle, the Control Cycle is an agent of harmony and balance which fails to function only when one of the Elements becomes weakened and fails to control its opposed Element, which then becomes relatively in Excess, or vice versa. Thus, if the Kidneys become weak, they cannot control Fire and circulatory problems such as high blood pressure can develop.

The Element correspondences are a formulation of the manifestations of the Ki of the Elements in the physical universe. They are discussed in detail in the chapters of Section Two, but are listed in Table 5.8.

The Six Divisions

The Six Divisions is a method of grouping the 12 meridians into alternative pairings. It has most relevance for treatment in the domain of herbal medicine, where the Six Divisions describe six different levels of disease, and its significance for the Shiatsu giver is mainly meridian-related and largely academic. It is, however, helpful to be able to understand the terminology of the Six Divisions when reading TCM texts and the relationship of the Zen Shiatsu meridians to the classical pathways makes more sense when the Six Divisions are considered, hence a brief explanation.

In ancient times, the meridians were not named by organ, such as the Large Intestine meridian; this is a Western innovation. They were labelled according to the Six Divisions which paired a meridian from the

Table 5.8 *Element correspondences*

Element	fire	earth	metal	water	wood
Colour	red	yellow	white	blue/black	green
Sound	laughing	singing	weeping	groaning	shouting
Odour	scorched	fragrant	rotten	putrid	rancid
Emotion	joy	empathy/ reflective thought	grief	fear	anger
Power	to flourish	to mature	to decline	to store	to give birth
Spiritual capacity	Shen	intellect	corporeal soul	will	ethereal soul
Sense Organ	tongue	mouth	nose	ears	eyes
Body tissue	blood vessels	flesh	skin	bones	tendons
Season	summer	end of each season	autumn	winter	spring
Time of day	11 am–3 pm 7–11 pm	7–11 am	3–7 am	3–7 pm	11 am–3 am
Taste	bitter	sweet	pungent	salty	sour
Climate	heat	dampness	dryness	cold	wind
Meridians	HT SI HP TH	Stomach Spleen	Lungs LI	Kidneys Bladder	Liver Gall Bladder

top half of the body with one from the bottom half, according to certain classifications of Yin and Yang.

The Six Division pairings are:

- Tai Yang (Lesser Yang) – Bladder, Small Intestine
- Yang Ming (Bright or Sunlight Yang) – Stomach, Large Intestine
- Shao Yang (Greater Yang) – Gall Bladder, Triple Heater

- Tai Yin (Lesser Yin) – Spleen, Lungs
- Shao Yin (Greater Yin) – Kidneys, Heart
- Jue Yin (Terminal or Utmost Yin) – Liver, Heart, Protector

Each meridian of a pair would occupy a similar position on the limb and the body posture to reveal these similarities is sitting like a teddy bear, with arms and legs straight out in front (Fig. 5.5). Thus the Large Intestine meridian, Arm Yang Ming, is in the same relative position on the arm that the Stomach meridian, Leg Yang Ming, occupies on the leg. It confirms the holistic approach of Chinese medicine that the meridians refer to an energetic zone of the body which happens to include an internal organ, rather than the other way around.

The organs of each division are linked and influence each other and the meridians can substitute for each other to some extent in treatment. The meridian pairings are particularly interesting to the student of Zen Shiatsu theory since the Masunaga extensions to the classical meridians are often next to the placement of the meridian's Six Division partner.

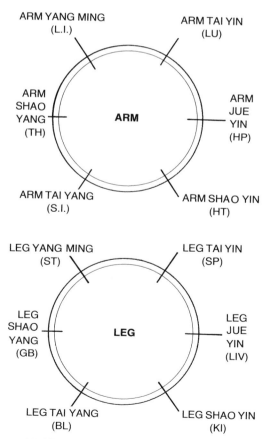

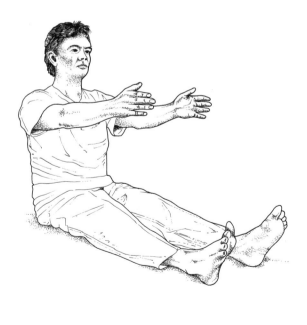

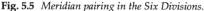

Fig. 5.5 *Meridian pairing in the Six Divisions.*

6

Zen Shiatsu theory

Zen Shiatsu, the system created by Shizuto Masunaga in the 1970s, is the first Shiatsu model with its own theory, entirely integrated with the practice of Shiatsu. Masunaga's sources were:

- the ancient Taoist roots of TCM theory
- the traditional use of Shiatsu as folk remedy
- modern knowledge of physiology
- the Western psychological model
- the philosophical approach of Zen Buddhism
- his own clinical experience over thousands of Shiatsu treatments.

Zen Shiatsu theory is a cohesive whole; diagnosis, theory and treatment are inseparable and all have as their source the meridian network and the movement of Ki within it. Zen Shiatsu deals with the direct experience of Ki in a fresh and immediate way and before examining its theoretical content, this is a good opportunity to look again at the Five Principles of Zen Shiatsu to see how the *practice* of Zen Shiatsu permits this direct experience of Ki.

The Five Principles – a reminder

Relax!

This allows the giver to sense the receiver's Ki without interference from distracting tension or thoughts.

Penetration, not pressure

The giver does not press on the surface tissues of the receiver's body but, with the aid of relaxation, penetrates into the receiver's Ki dimension.

Stationary, perpendicular penetration

Stationary penetration allows time to "listen" to and sense the receiver's Ki. Perpendicular penetration ensures direct access to the receiver's Ki dimension without hitting the sides of the narrow neck of the tsubo.

Two-hand connectedness

The use of a stationary Yin mother hand to support the active Yang child hand, keeping both equally in the giver's awareness, establishes a connection between the active and receptive sides of the giver's consciousness and thus allows a continuous following of the receiver's Ki flow.

Meridian continuity

The receiver's Ki is followed throughout the course of the meridian, not contacted at specific points only.

It was the direct experience of Ki which led Masunaga to extend the pathways of the classical meridians of acupuncture throughout the body. Although some purists may doubt the authenticity of these extended meridians, discovered through one man's subjective experience, the fact that many of them follow the deep pathways of the traditional meridians, subsidiary branches or connections within the Six Divisions tends to endorse them.

There are a few instances in which Masunaga's version of the classical meridians appear to deviate from the accepted pathways. In some cases, this is a result of inaccurate annotation on the Masunaga charts. In some cases the TCM version may be the inaccurate one, since in modern acupuncture charts it is the position of the points, not of the pathways between them, which is accurately located. The traditional Japanese approach to the location of meridians and points tends, in any case, to be empirical, based to a great extent on the sensations of both giver and receiver when the point is contacted. This was also the case in ancient China and Japan, in the era when palpation was an integral part of acupuncture practice. It is written in the Ling Shu "...ask above and below the point, because each person's meridians are not the same" (Ling Shu 10.145, quoted in *Hara Diagnosis: Reflections on the Sea*, p. 24) Where there has been any controversy regarding the difference between the meridians of Zen Shiatsu and those of acupuncture, it is discussed in the chapter on the location of the relevant meridian in Section Three.

Zen Shiatsu is meridian-orientated. Masunaga's theory structure arose from his interest in the meridian locations and their relevance to the specific effects of the meridians on the body, mind and emotions. He reasoned that if the meridian system was a valid expression of our energy structure and not an arbitrary, academic arrangement, then there would be a relationship between the energetic functions of the meridians and their place on the body. Working on this hypothesis, he took as his starting point the sequence of the meridians known in the West as the Chinese Clock (Table 6.1). By following this sequence, the entire meridian network

can be traced continuously over the body; the end of one meridian, for example, let us say on the chest, is near the beginning of the next in sequence, also on the chest.

There is a symmetry in the arrangement of the meridians on the body and their alternation between Yin and Yang but the meaning of the symmetrical sequence has always been linked mainly to the successive times of day in which the meridians were said to be most active. Masunaga took the sequence to refer not to a day but to a lifespan or to the cycles of activity, from initiation to completion, which occur within a lifespan. To explain his theory in the simplest possible terms, he took as his model the life cycle of one of the simplest beings known, the one-celled animal, so that his seminal theory is often taught as "the life cycle of the amoeba".

The life cycle of the amoeba

■ *"So...the primordial soup. Now...we'll set out to shock. Tell it from the point of view of the soup, maybe? Have one of those drifting, floating, feathery crustaceans narrate. Or an ammonite? An ammonite with a sense of destiny. A spokesperson for the streaming Jurassic seas, to tell it how it was."*
PENELOPE LIVELY, 'MOONTIGER', PENGUIN, 1988

Stage One – making a border and initiating exchange

If we imagine the beginnings of life on this earth as it is still conventionally taught, we must envisage what used to be called the primordial soup. In this rich brew of amino acids and life-supporting nutrients, life appeared, we are told, perhaps through an electrical impulse from lightning. The simplest life form came into being, one cell, more or less primordial soup with a skin around it. This is the first stage of existence, the establishing of an individual

Table 6.1 *The Chinese Clock*

Meridian	Quality	Time of day	Beginning	End
Lung	Yin	3–5 am	Chest	Hand
LI	Yang	5–7 am	Hand	Head
Stomach	Yang	7–9 am	Head	Foot
Spleen	Yin	9–11 am	Foot	Chest
Heart	Yin	11 am–1 pm	Chest	Hand
SI	Yang	1–3 pm	Hand	Head
Bladder	Yang	3–5 pm	Head	Foot
Kidney	Yin	5–7 pm	Foot	Chest
HP	Yin	7–9 pm	Chest	Hand
TH	Yang	9–11 pm	Hand	Head
GB	Yang	11 pm–1 am	Head	Foot
Liver	Yin	1–3 am	Foot	Chest

identity, separate from the rest of the universe yet coexisting with it. Masunaga called this energetic action "making a border"; we could also call it the establishment of an identity structure. The border is what separates the amoeba from the universe and yet it must be a permeable border, allowing exchange of Ki with the universe; the amoeba will die if it is a sealed unit (Fig. 6.1).

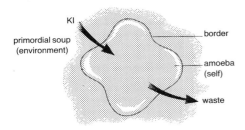

Fig. 6.1 *The outside.*

In the human organism according to TCM, the Lungs rule the skin, which is our permeable border. The Lung and Large Intestine meridians are on our anatomical border, forming the "outside" of our outline if we stand with palms facing forward in the anatomical position. The Lungs and Large Intestine represent the functions of intake and elimination through that border, both equally necessary for the replenishing of our supplies of Ki; we cannot take in if we do not let go. The catch phrase summing up this phase in the cycle is "vitality through exchange"*.

Stage Two – satisfying needs

In the first stage of the cycle, the amoeba is unaware of any particular needs. The functions involved are so vital that we do not feel a craving to perform them; we simply cease to be, as a separate entity, if they stop. In the second stage, once an individual identity has been established, needs necessarily arise. The most basic need of any life form is for nourishment. In the case of the amoeba, let us imagine that it espies some particularly tasty food molecule before it in the primordial soup. Its actions then are to bulge itself forward (in biological terms, to put out a pseudopodium) to reach what it desires, then to enfold it and begin to break it down into a digestible form (Fig. 6.2).

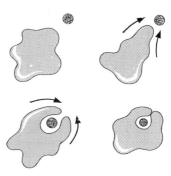

Fig. 6.2 *The front.*

The two parts of this phase of the cycle represent the activity of the Stomach and Spleen meridians. The Yang or active energy of the Stomach embodies the appetite factor, the perception of a need and the movement towards satisfying it. The Spleen performs the Yin function of drawing in and enfolding the object of our need; it also breaks it down into usable form. The object can be anything which we perceive as being necessary for our well-being, even our survival; anything, in other words for which we hunger. It may be information, love, approval, possessions or status that we crave, as well as food. The Stomach hungers and pursues; the Spleen establishes possession and knowledge of attainment. The activity in this phase of energy is all at the front; the perception of an object of desire outside ourselves, which attracts us to move forward till we have grasped and enfolded it, is acted out by the Spleen and Stomach meridians which are at the front of the body. The catch phrase for the meridian activity in this phase is "hunger and satisfaction".

Stage Three – assimilating and integrating nourishment

At the end of Stage Two, the desired object has been drawn in and broken down into usable form, but it has not yet been assimilated. Stage Three is the absorption into our own identity of the desired

---

* For this and the Stomach and Spleen catch phrase which follows, I wish to acknowledge the class of 1991 at the Shiatsu College, London, who worked them out in a class discussion.

object; it is the process by which a cheese sandwich, say, becomes Joe Everyman or, in this case, Joe Amoeba (Fig. 6.3).

Fig. 6.3 *The inside.*

The two meridians which represent this process are the Small Intestine and the Heart. The Small Intestine absorbs nutrients; it assimilates them in order to nourish the Heart, which in Oriental tradition is the core of our individual selves, our consciousness. By this means each being, whether amoeba, armadillo or human, is able to absorb what it needs from the environment in order to maintain presence, awareness and function in the world. According to the needs of each being, it assimilates what is appropriate, food, sense impressions, information, belief systems and emotional input.

The movement of energy in this process is inwards and the meridians involved are on the inner surfaces of the limbs, when we stand in the anatomical position. The catch phrase for this stage is, in Masunaga's words, "central control and conversion". The cycle of energy has now reached its central point, the Heart, the centre of identity, and the movement of energy, since the amoeba first differentiated itself from its environment, has been directed towards bringing nourishment to that centre.

Stage Four – flight from danger

The amoeba's cycle has now reached the stage where it is able to sustain itself and to respond to other stimuli in the environment. The next phase represents the most urgent of the circumstances in which it may find itself, that of danger. Let us imagine that, an evolutionary aeon further on in the primordial soup, an amoeba is under threat from a predator (Fig. 6.4).

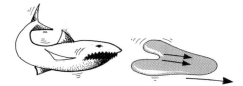

Fig. 6.4 *The back.*

The back (Fig. 6.4)

The urge for flight is perceived in the back; here we have a movement away from a given source of stimulus, whereas in Stage Two, that of desire or appetite for something in front of the amoeba, the movement was towards it. The Bladder and Kidney meridians embody this phase of the cycle and these are the meridians of the back. This strong source of movement originating from the back provided Masunaga with the key word in his catch phrase describing the activity of this stage: 'impetus'.

In TCM the Kidneys, through Kidney Yang and Source Ki, provide impetus for all our actions, functions and metabolic processes. If that impetus fails or slows, all bodily functions slow down and as a result stagnation can set in or residues build up. The Kidneys thus provide an impetus which purifies by maintaining flow and movement. In Western physiology, the purification of the blood is the main function of the kidney organ, while the fight or flight response is the domain of the adrenal glands, which sit on top of the kidneys. Masunaga's catchphrase for Stage 4, 'purify and give impetus', is thus appropriate according to both of these medical systems.

Stage Five – circulation and protection

Sudden attack is not the only danger threatening the amoeba; it has a day-to-day struggle to adapt to the environment, temperature changes, pollutants and other outside influences. We, too, need to shield ourselves from the same factors as well as from unwelcome intrusions into our emotional space. Stage Four is the surge of impetus that saves our backs; Stage Five is the provision of constant protection for the different layers of our being. Co-existing in a group is a form of protection, and yet this, too, requires adaptation. Each being in a group has its own individual identity and function, and yet it also needs to extend its consciousness outwards to make contact with others and contribute towards a group identity. We therefore need social and emotional mechanisms which can both extend the influence of the core self and withdraw it for greater protection when necessary. The Triple Heater and Heart Protector, currently not considered in TCM as having any major energetic identity, embody these mechanisms in Zen Shiatsu theory. The Triple Heater protects the surface from the hazards of the environment, including the influence of other personalities; the Heart Protector forms a "lining" to protect our emotional core (Fig. 6.5).

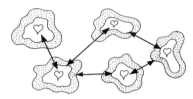

Fig. 6.5 *Surface and lining.*

These two zones of our energetic being, mentioned in the Chinese classic, Nan Jing,* are physically embodied in the arrangement of the meridians. If we adopt an enclosed, protective posture, sitting with our knees raised, our head lowered and our arms crossed over our knees, the extended meridian of the Triple Heater is visible in its entirety, protecting our whole body surface. The Heart Protector meridian, on the other hand, is invisible to an observer but visible to ourselves, since it forms the "lining" of the enclosed capsule formed by our protective body posture (Fig. 6.6).

In TCM the main function of the Triple Heater is to distribute the Source Ki and circulate fluids and that of the Heart Protector is to assist and protect the Heart. The main Western body system combining these functions is the circulatory system and

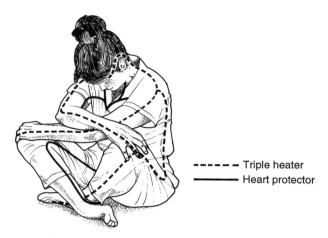

----- Triple heater
——— Heart protector

Fig. 6.6 *Protective body posture.*

Masunaga's catch phrase for this stage of the cycle is "circulation and protection".

Stage Six – choice of direction

The final stage of the cycle is also the preparation for a new cycle. The amoeba has so far learned to exchange Ki with the universe through its border; to go forward to find nourishment, and assimilate that nourishment; to save itself from danger; and to live in a community. The metabolic functions which have evolved in parallel with these developments have ensured a reserve stock of nutrients and energy but how to put them to best use?

It is the asking of the question, as much as the answer, which constitutes Stage 6. The Liver and Gall Bladder are the meridians involved and they are at the sides of the body, enabling us to turn from one side to the other in order to weigh up the possibilities of different courses of action. It is easier to visualize the human body in this situation than the hypothetical amoeba embodying the horns of its dilemma (Fig. 6.7).

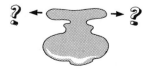

Fig. 6.7 *The sides.*

---

*"The master of the heart (Heart Protector) and the triple warmer become the surface and the lining...The master of the heart controls the lining. The triple warmer controls the surface." Nan Jing, 25; quoted in *Hara Diagnosis; Reflections on the Sea*, p. 121.

The metabolic activities of the amoeba in its cycle so far have built up a store of nutrients in reserve for this moment. According to Masunaga it is the Liver which stores them and the Gall Bladder which distributes them. At least in part, therefore, his theory accords with TCM, which has the Liver storing the Blood and ensuring the free flowing of Ki, and with physiological fact, which is that the liver stores glycogen for energy, iron and vitamins and that the gall bladder distributes bile. Thus in all three systems the combined activity of the Liver and Gall Bladder relates to storage and distribution of some kind. In Zen Shiatsu theory, however, the principal energetic function of these two meridians is to decide when to store and when to release the nutrients from storage for distribution around the body.

In Oriental medical tradition, the Liver is connected with planning, the Gall Bladder with decision-making. If we use the military wording traditionally associated with these "resolute organs" to make an analogy, the Liver can be compared to a general, marshalling reserves according to long term strategy, the Gall Bladder to an officer in the field, making moment-to-moment decisions on the deployment of those reserves, based on the current situation.

The area of life in which these plans and decisions take effect is that of action, any action. The nature of the Liver and Gall Bladder energy is to decide upon action, ideally in order to express the life plan of the being at a given moment in time. Anthropomorph-izing the amoeba, it could decide to invade a neighbouring amoeba community, write a novel, explore and colonize another area of the primordial soup or stay at home and engage in conflict with its nearest and dearest. The catch phrase for this stage in the cycle refers to the moment just before the decision to take action is made, while the options are still open; it is "irresolution".

This stage completes the life cycle of the amoeba, which was Masunaga's chosen method for explaining the phases of energy that succeed each other as each being pursues its individual path through life. To see it as a life cycle is to take the broad view; another perspective is to see each stage in the cycle as happening more or less continuously as a manifesta-tion of our physical, mental and emotional processes.

The first three phases of the cycle refer to the different ways in which we receive energy: from breathing or the natural flow of Ki exchange with the universe; from obtaining food or the satisfaction of our desires; and from absorption of that food or assimilation of physical, mental and emotional nourishment into the core of ourselves.

The last three phases describe the different ways in which we distribute energy throughout our being: the automatic reflex or adrenalin surge, which relates to survival; the constant, warm pulse of the circulation which nourishes and protects the different layers of our being; and the release and distribution of reserves of stored energy when we need it for a specific course of action.

The individual function of each meridian in the Zen Shiatsu system will be described in more detail in the chapters of Section Three.

The theory of Kyo and Jitsu

The interpretation of the functions of the meridians outlined in the life cycle is put to use through Zen Shiatsu diagnosis. Whereas TCM diagnosis encompasses the receiver's past health history with relevance to his or her present physical and emotional condition, Zen Shiatsu diagnosis and treatment deal with the immediate state and significance of the distribution of energy within the meridian network, as perceived by diagnostic palpation of the Hara or back. Diagnosis is explained in some detail in Chapter 12.

While this palpation generally reveals a complex picture of the different qualities and levels of Ki according to the condition of each meridian, only two factors are essential for diagnosis:

- the meridian with the greatest concentration of energy, called the most Jitsu, or full, meridian
- the meridian with the least concentration of energy, known as the most Kyo or empty, meridian.

Kyo and Jitsu not only exist on the Hara but are also constantly expressed in the whole body. Any body part can be predominantly Kyo or Jitsu, any meridian can be described as having a particular degree of Kyo or Jitsu and meridians can have different areas of relative Kyo or Jitsu along their length.

Although the words Kyo and Jitsu in translation mean roughly the same as "empty" and "full", Masunaga's principle of Kyo and Jitsu is more related to Yin and Yang than to the Excess and Deficiency category of the Eight Principles in TCM. Like Yin and Yang, Kyo and Jitsu are inseparable and interdependent states. Masunaga explained Kyo and Jitsu, once again, in terms of the simplest form of life, the one-celled animal (Fig. 6.8).

Stage One – the amoeba in a state of balance

The amoeba is in a state of inner balance, a temporary moment of stillness. Then, as is natural in the normal movement of life energy, a need develops.

Stage Two – the amoeba feels hungry

An emptiness or need manifests, which we will call Kyo. The need is essentially hidden; it is like a message written in invisible ink which can be read

only if another influence is brought to bear on it. Invisible ink can only be seen when heat is applied; the amoeba does not know that its emptiness is hunger until stimulated by the sight of food. Our own, human, "hidden" needs can be activated not only by the direct perception of a desired object but by a sensation or experience which triggers the unconscious memory of a past need and stimulates us to try and satisfy it, without knowing quite why.

Stage Three – the amoeba sees food

When a piece of food appears, the amoeba begins to move towards it by putting out a bulge (a pseudopodium or "false foot"). This is the visible manifestation of its emptiness and desire to satisfy it. This is what we can call Jitsu; a noticeable action, movement, symptom or distortion which is the messenger for the hidden Kyo.

Stage Four – the amoeba ingests the food

The natural purpose of the Jitsu action is to satisfy the Kyo need; then a temporary state of balance returns until the next need arises.

How Kyo and Jitsu affect our health

The meaning of this short sequence from an amoeba's day is related to the movement of Ki in the process of life, to the alternation of cause and effect, movement and stillness, need and action. Kyo and Jitsu manifest in human beings, as in amoebas, in health as well as in disease. In health, Jitsu actions are engaged in to satisfy our Kyo needs; it is part of the process of living. It is when the appropriate action cannot be taken to satisfy the need that we fail to recreate the state of balance. We may need something simple, like exercise or sleep; we may need something complex, like a sense of direction in life. If we cannot satisfy our need because of external or internal hindrance, our Jitsu will tend to take the form of behaviour which distracts us from our Kyo. Thus a pattern is set up of inappropriate energy expenditure, which manifests as behavioural characteristics and, eventually, as physical symptoms.

The different needs which we have at different times are expressed by the meridians according to

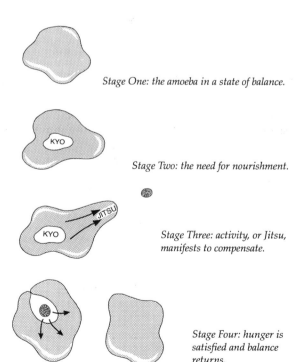

Stage One: the amoeba in a state of balance.

Stage Two: the need for nourishment.

Stage Three: activity, or Jitsu, manifests to compensate.

Stage Four: hunger is satisfied and balance returns.

Fig. 6.8

Masunaga's Chinese Clock, the life cycle of the amoeba. So Lung and Large Intestine embody the need for a strong sense of self, yet one which allows for exchange of Ki with the universe. Stomach and Spleen represent our need to be able to identify and satisfy our real hungers. Our Heart and Small Intestine need to assimilate messages from the external and internal environment and to integrate them into our emotional core. The Kidney and Bladder come into play when we need to produce impetus for survival and when we need to relax. The Heart Protector and Triple Heater help us with our need to extend ourselves towards others and to protect ourselves from environmental or emotional influences when necessary. The Liver and Gall Bladder embody our need to choose our own life path and express our creative individuality.

These are the basic needs of any one individual, at different points in time. Temporary circumstances in an individual's life will influence his Kyo and Jitsu patterns in the short term, but it is the circumstances in his early cultural or social environment which may tend to frustrate a particular need over a long period of time, leading to habitual patterns of Kyo and Jitsu. It is these habitual patterns which tend to lead to imbalances in the free flow of Ki and thus eventually to ill health of some description.

Kyo and Jitsu theory in diagnosis and treatment

Although symptoms result both from the Jitsu and the Kyo, the Jitsu symptoms often have a Yang quality of urgency, because of the greater investment of energy in the Jitsu. Many traditional Shiatsu styles are designed to deal with these urgent Jitsu symptoms,

often by fairly forceful means. In terms of the sequence described above, this would be analagous to finding the amoeba in Stage Three, with the obvious distortion of its pseudopodium, and trying to recreate the balanced state of Stage One by pressing the pseudopodium back into place (a). This treatment, however, would only take the amoeba back to Stage Two, with the Kyo still hidden inside (b), and after a very short time it would tend to recreate the same Jitsu in response to its unrecognized Kyo (c). The same thing happens in humans if the Shiatsu treatment concentrates on the Jitsu symptoms and ignores the Kyo (Fig. 6.9).

The Zen Shiatsu approach, however, asserts that the Kyo must be satisfied before the Jitsu will disperse. This does not mean that the Jitsu must not be treated but that the focus of the treatment is the Kyo. Ki must be brought to the Kyo and dispersed from the Jitsu to recreate a state of balance. Zen Shiatsu diagnostic procedure therefore aims to find the receiver's most Kyo and most Jitsu meridians at the moment of treatment, so that Ki can be tonified and dispersed, as appropriate. The reader is referred to Chapter 12 for diagnostic procedure, Chapter 13 for the interpretation of the diagnosis and Chapter 14 for tonifying and dispersing techniques.

Kyo and Jitsu compared with Excess and Deficiency

There are obvious temptations to make the assumption that Kyo and Jitsu meridians represent an organ in a Deficient or Excess condition according to TCM. In clinical practice, however, time and again, this is shown not to be so. In TCM, the term "Excess condition" applies when there is an excess of a pathogenic factor or one of the Vital Substances in one particular body part or organ, for example Blood stagnation in the chest or Damp-Heat in the Large Intestine. It always has physical symptoms. In Zen Shiatsu, Jitsu refers to a concentration of the receiver's Ki in one of the meridians and thus by implication in one of their energetic functions according to the life cycle of the amoeba. It does not necessarily produce physical symptoms. In TCM, a Deficiency condition refers to a Deficiency of one of the Vital Substances, or of Yin or Yang, or of a function of an organ. It can exist on its own, without an Excess,

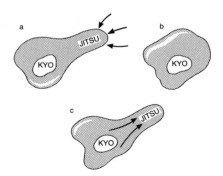

Fig. 6.9 *The cycle continues if only the Jitsu is treated.*

and produce physical symptoms and signs. In Zen Shiatsu, Kyo refers to a meridian (and thus to an energetic function of the individual) which is currently low in Ki, usually because it is neglected and underemphasized. It cannot, by definition, exist without relationship to a Jitsu and does not necessarily produce physical symptoms and signs.

Let us imagine that a receiver is beginning a cold. In Zen Shiatsu, this involves the Triple Heater meridian, which protects the body surface. Triple Heater may appear as either Kyo or Jitsu in the diagnosis. If you have diagnosed Triple Heater Jitsu, then the body is engaged in trying to fight off the cold; you have diagnosed during a phase of struggle. It does not necessarily mean that the receiver has a strong protective or immune system – it means that the immune system is currently in a reactive phase and working hard. If you diagnose Triple Heater Kyo, it means that the protective function is currently underactive and the body is not putting up resistance to the cold.

The above is an example of the body energy reacting on the physical level, without involving the receiver's consciousness. In connection with long term symptoms and chronic conditions, however, psychological tendencies often mirror the receiver's physical manifestations in the Kyo and Jitsu meridians. On the right is a typical, but hypothetical, case history in which a TCM Deficiency syndrome manifests as a Jitsu diagnosis.

CASE HISTORY

Ms X presents with typical symptoms of a Deficient Spleen in TCM terms. She has loose stools, feels tired, especially after eating, suffers from poor digestion and abdominal bloating, has a sweet tooth, is slightly overweight and has frequent, copious, clear urination. She is a motherly kind of person, a social worker, and suffers from stress since she worries a great deal about the well-being of the people under her care. Although she suffers from Spleen Yang Deficiency in TCM terms, the Zen Shiatsu Hara palpation diagnosis reveals the Spleen meridian very Jitsu, with the most Kyo meridian being the Bladder.

Obviously, in this case, the Spleen's physical activity is not in Excess. What the Kyo/Jitsu diagnostic picture represents is the receiver's own investment of energy in her life patterns. This receiver is identifying strongly with the Spleen energy, through enfolding others in her care, perhaps as a result of her own need for love and also through constantly churning over (as if digesting) other people's problems in her mind. The Spleen therefore comes up as Jitsu in the diagnosis. The area of her life which is being neglected (since it is hidden) is the Kyo Bladder, representing impetus. The receiver is investing energy in the meridians of her front, in her need to go forward towards others. She is neglecting her back, her survival instinct, care for her Source Ki, which gives impetus and energy. As a result, she feels anxious and stressed.

Interpretation of Zen Shiatsu diagnosis

Since Kyo and Jitsu are phenomena which accompany the movement of Ki and since the movement of Ki is necessary to the life process, a diagnosis of Kyo and Jitsu meridians does not imply disease. A Kyo/Jitsu diagnosis can relate to a mood lasting an hour, to a reaction to a situation lasting a month or so, to a personality characteristic ingrained since childhood but accompanied by few physical symptoms, or to any stage of physical illness.

Zen Shiatsu diagnosis is always based on the movements of energy outlined in the life cycle of the amoeba and physical symptoms can usually be traced back to these basic movements. Stomach Jitsu, for example, relating to indigestion caused by eating too fast, will have as its root cause the overactivity of the appetite factor represented by the Stomach in Stage Two of the life cycle. Perhaps the receiver was extremely hungry earlier in the day and thus bolted his last meal; perhaps, on the other hand, he has always eaten fast as a "displacement activity" to compensate for unfulfilled emotional or physical circumstances both in the long or short term.

It often happens that a diagnosis in Zen Shiatsu terms has no relevance whatever to the interpretation of the physical symptoms. At this point the giver can interpret the diagnosis as a recent overlay pattern on the emotional level, eclipsing the long term behavioural pattern which originally led to the physical symptoms. This situation is discussed in detail in Chapter 13.

Both the Kyo and the Jitsu meridians are important in Zen Shiatsu diagnosis, since both will manifest in the receiver's energy pattern as psychological or physical characteristics or symptoms. The diagnosis is always, therefore, of two meridians contributing to a composite energetic picture, one which is being overemphasized, one which is being neglected. In the case history discussed above, Ms X's physical symptoms according to TCM all stem from one cause, Spleen Yang Deficiency. These include the tiredness (Spleen not producing Ki from food), anxiety (thinking too much) and the copious urination (Spleen not transforming fluids). In Zen Shiatsu terms these symptoms are due to the Kyo Bladder which is the other "hidden" half of the diagnosis. TCM diagnosis and Zen Shiatsu diagnosis often vary for this reason, that the symptoms and signs which may be due to one root cause in TCM are always the result of the interactions of two meridians in Zen Shiatsu. The interpretation of the meridian functions may also vary between the two systems and these differences will be discussed in Section Three.

Harmonizing TCM and Zen Shiatsu theory

7

The Water Element – The Kidneys and Bladder

■ *"Under heaven, nothing is more soft and yielding than water. Yet for attacking the solid and strong, nothing is better. It has no equal."*

TAO TE CHING

Element associations: life, depth, flow, power, purification

Water seems the most contradictory of the Elements. For every adjective that we can call to mind describing it, the opposite is also true: deep, shallow; gentle, powerful; clear, murky; still, moving. But perhaps its qualities are not contradictory but all-encompassing; perhaps water holds these opposites within itself without contradiction. For this reason, perhaps, the Water Element is the basis of both Yin and Yang in the human bodymind.

We know that water is the essential basis of our physical substance and that we can survive only for a very short time without it; that without water not only we but all life forms around us cease to exist. Life depends on water and water is the source of life; modern Western understanding of the beginnings of life on this planet in the ocean of primordial soup bears this out, as does the Oriental concept that it is the "moving Ki between the Kidneys" which creates life.

Although not all water is deep, water will always sink to the deepest level. In the human body, the Water Element governs the deepest structures and tissues, the bones and their marrow and the spinal cord. In terms of time, it also reaches back to the individual being's deepest past, the emergence of life from the void at the moment of conception.

Although that moment seems to us like a beginning, to Chinese thought it is part of a continuum. As the water in a river flows continuously, each drop clinging to the next in an appearance of unity, always different yet always the same, so we can view the Kidney Essence of each individual as part of the larger flow of ancestry, handed down from generation to generation, merging, diversifying, taking on different forms, yet still the same inheritance of life.

It is movement and flow also which give water its ability to cleanse; it washes through sludge and flushes away dirt. In the same way, the Water Element purifies by supplying energy to prevent stagnation in the mind and body. Ki which flows and does not stagnate is pure Ki and to experience that flow and movement is to experience purification.

The continuous flow of water also means power. Even the smallest drip, over time, can wear away stone and the power of that continuous movement is incalculably greater when allowed to gather momentum in a larger space like the ocean. It is the Water Element which gives the human body its power and energy and the human mind its will to continue.

Spiritual capacity of the Element: will

The Water Element, being the source of life, also confers the will to survive. It is said in the texts that "The kidneys are like the officials who do energetic work, and they excel through their ability and cleverness" (*The Yellow Emperor's Classic*, p. 133). This cleverness is activated in life-threatening situations and gives the cool strategic ability to take appropriate steps for survival. The Kidneys also provide a storehouse of vital reserves of Ki and Essence, on which we draw in situations where endurance is required; they give us the strength to go on and on and on, like water.

If the Water Element is out of balance, we may feel that our survival is threatened at every turn and endow quite ordinary projects with a compelling significance. The will takes over and does not know when to stop; this is the condition of the person who continues to work even when exhausted and whose response to stress is to drive himself even harder, often drawing further upon his vital reserves with the use of stimulants such as coffee. Another manifestation of a water imbalance can be lack of will, with low motivation and inaction accompanying the feeling of exhaustion which makes the simplest tasks appear too much to tackle. Guilt, timidity and self-abasement, which result from giving another person's will priority above our own, may also accompany lack of will.

The will to survive, to act and to accomplish is the Yang manifestation of the will of the Water Element. According to Ted Kaptchuk (Lecture in Oxford, UK, November 1991), the Yin aspect of Water also has a will. Since Yang is active and Yin receptive, the "Yin will" is the ability to flow with the natural course of events, to follow our destiny. Here, too, the "ability and cleverness" of the Kidneys is required but in a different way, as we must take a detached view and consider where our life path is taking us. With the Yin will and courage of the Water Element, we can then go forward in harmony with events, without swimming against the tide. The balance between the Yang will which acts and the Yin will which allows is the gift of a healthy Water Element and ensures the highest use of our ancestral inheritance of Ki and Essence.

Movement of Element energy: downwards

Water continually seeks the lowest level and the natural flow of all water is downwards, first into the earth, to enable it to give life, and finally into the sea, the great reservoir, whence it can be recycled to fall again as rain and continue its downward flow. This process is mirrored in the human body, as the fluids we take in find their way downward, moistening and cooling in the process, until we expel the waste fluids. In patterns of disharmony, body fluids collect in the lowest part of the body, causing oedema.

The downward movement of the Water Element is intimately connected with its capacity to store. In winter, the season of Water, the Ki of nature withdraws deep within the earth, to rest and regenerate before the outward thrust of Spring. The place of the Water Element and its meridians is in the lower body, the Hara, and this is where our Essence and Source Ki are stored. This is also where we receive and anchor the Ki of Heaven, which the Lungs take in as breath, and which is received and held in the Hara by the Kidneys. The downward pull of Water roots and steadies us, enabling us to breathe deeply and replenish ourselves from our Source.

Element emotion: fear

Fear is part of our survival instinct. Intense fear causes a release of Source Ki from the Kidneys, which we would call an adrenalin rush, the "fight or flight" response. Body wastes are jettisoned, digestive processes are suspended and we are ready for action. It is a normal reaction in a life-threatening situation. With an imbalance in the Water Element, however, this kind of fear may be felt at the sight of a spider, a dentist's chair or a letter from the taxman. Phobias or other neurotic or obsessive fears and anxieties often accompany an imbalance in Water.

Many of the Elements can manifest fear. Earth has the fear of insecurity, Fire the fear of loss of control, and Wood the timidity of indecision. All of these are more likely to manifest openly than the fear belonging to the Water Element, which comes from the roots of our being and is often too powerful to be acknowledged, manifesting instead as a desire to control events before they control us. This may masquerade as the aggression of the Wood Element or as the caring of the Earth Element and it may indeed be mingled with these, since Water creates Wood and is controlled by Earth, according to the Five Element cycles (see p. 81). Fear combined with the will to survive, however, impart an intense quality to situations which is recognizable as a steely undertone of determination. It is not a refusal to let go, as in a Metal imbalance; it is a refusal to give up.

Element colour: blue/black

The classics variously describe the colour associated with Water as blue or black or a combination of the two. When the Water Element is out of balance, a blackish or bluish tone overlays the natural complexion. Like all the hues, this can be hard to see on a face in isolation, especially a black face, and it is easier to compare several different faces at the same time in order to see the subtle hues. Easier to see on a white skin are the blue-black circles under the eyes which are a classic sign of fatigue (a Water symptom).

Element sound: groaning

The sound of a pronounced Water imbalance can be the most striking of all the voices. The groaning voice often has a characteristic rasping catch to it which demands our attention. Occasionally, however, it manifests as a monotone which drones on like water itself. If a receiver is particularly tired, his voice may develop a temporary hoarseness characteristic of Water which disappears after rest.

Element odour: putrid

The putrid odour of a Water imbalance is the faint but unmistakable ammoniac smell of stale urine. When perceived around a receiver's lower parts, it may simply be that, but it can sometimes be smelt around the chest, head or shoulders.

Element sense organ: the ear

The sense of hearing is closely linked with fear. Loud and sudden noises make us start with fright and can cause babies to cry with terror; when we are alone at night, what we can hear is much more frightening than what we can see; if we turn the sound off when a horror film is showing on television, it loses its effect. The sense of hearing affects us in a particularly powerful way, as if it reaches in to our Essence. It also declines as we get older, in the same way as our kidney Essence, and the deafness of old age is linked to the Kidneys.

Whereas disorders deriving from infection or inflammation of the ear may be related to the local meridians, the Triple Heater, Gall Bladder or Small Intestine, problems such as deafness and tinnitus which are not traceable to these Exterior causes are treated as a dysfunction of the Kidneys.

Element taste: salty

We now know that salt causes the body to hold on to its water content and augments the volume of fluid in the blood and tissues, so that in Western terms the salty taste gives the kidneys more work to do. In the Chinese model, the salty taste has a downward-moving action, so that it can supplement the downward movement of a weak Water Element. When there is an imbalance in the Water energy, therefore, the receiver often craves the salty taste. The Shiatsu giver may need to suggest a lowered salt intake, but should add that as the Water Element rebalances, the craving for the salty taste will naturally subside.

Element season: winter

Winter is the season when energy in nature moves inwards and lies dormant in preparation for rebirth. Plants and trees take a rest period; all their Ki has gone into producing the seeds which lie deep within the earth, waiting to be activated by spring. Many animals hibernate; the rest engage in mimimal activity in order to stay alive. In rural societies, the year's work is mostly finished and only maintenance needs to be done until the new season. According to Chinese thought, human beings should mirror the Ki of nature in their conduct, consciously avoiding activity.

■ *"The three months of Winter are called the period of closing and storing... People should retire early at night and rise late in the morning, and they should wait for the rising of the sun. They should suppress and conceal their wishes, as though they had no internal purpose, as though they had been fulfilled."*

(YELLOW EMPEROR'S CLASSIC, p. 102)

Element climate: cold

Cold has an observable effect upon the kidneys and bladder, since as we sweat less we urinate more. The connection is significant according to the Chinese medical model, since Water is the coldest, most Yin of the Elements. The vital Fire within the Kidneys, the pilot light for the warming system of the whole body, must be encouraged by warmth and it is considered essential to keep the kidney area and lower body covered and warm. It would be anathema to an Oriental to expose bare flesh between T-shirt and jeans, especially when lifting, as Western workers do; it would be to invite back strain and deplete Kidney Yang, at the very least.

It is the warming nature of Yang, powered by Kidney Yang and the fire within the Kidneys which derives from the Source Ki, which keeps our bodies warm. If Kidney Yang is Deficient, then we will feel cold and be unable to get warm. As our Source Ki and Kidney Yang decrease as we get older, so we feel the cold more and more. Many old people in the Far East have special kidney-warmer belts.

Element time of day: 3–7 pm

The time of the Water Element is in the afternoon, when workers have used up the morning energy which the Spleen and Stomach provide. The time of the Bladder is from 3 to 5 pm and that of the Kidney from 5 to 7 pm. Now is the time when adequate Kidney Yang and the Bladder's function of transforming Ki are essential, if energy levels are not to reach rock bottom during the last working hours of the day. The endurance and will epitomized by the Water Element must also come into play.

In clinical practice, many receivers with a Water imbalance will report a sudden drop of energy levels at round 5 pm and it may be worthwhile to consider treating these people with Shiatsu earlier in the day, when there is more Ki available to work with.

The Kidneys in TCM

The kidney organ is one small part of the TCM Kidney system, which encompasses all life functions, procreative capacity and indeed the individual's own basic constitution as part of the genetic chain of evolution. The Kidneys are considered to be the foundation of both the Yin and the Yang of the body and they contain our ancestral inheritance of both, the Yang in the form of Source Ki, the Yin in the form

of Essence. Essence and Source Ki are essentially the same, the Yin and Yang sides of a single coin. Essence is the substantial aspect, Source Ki the energetic aspect of the root of life in the body. Essence has the qualities of Water, as the source of form, Source Ki has the qualities of Fire, as the source of activity. In ancient times, it was thought that the Fire was stored in the right Kidney, the Water in the left, but later both Essence and Source Ki were thought to be stored "between the Kidneys". The Yang qualities are accessible at the point on the spine between the Kidney Yu points (see p. 239), known as Ming-Men or Gate of Vitality. The Yin qualities of our ancestral package lie deep within the belly, in the Hara, where the reproductive organs release Essence to be passed on to our children.

The philosophical underpinnings of Chinese medicine are evident if we consider the Kidneys as symbolic of the destiny of the individual within the race; our Essence embodies within us the urge of the human species to reproduce itself, our source Ki gives the potential for individual action and contribution within that wider process.

Storing Essence: the foundations of health

Oriental medical philosophy has it that we are all born with an inherited "survival kit" stored between our Kidneys, which gives us sufficient Essence and Source Ki to last our lifetime – the sand in our hourglass, so to speak. How long that lifetime can be and what the quality of our physical existence may be during it depend both on the quality of the package and how carefully we conserve its contents.

The first variable depends on factors which we would call genetic; the Chinese call them "ancestral". Our parents' age and state of health at our conception, our mother's health during pregnancy, the circumstances of our birth and the 6 months or so after it, while we are still effectively fused with our mother's Ki, determine the quality of our Essence and Source Ki thenceforth. If the predetermining circumstances are good, we will have strong, healthy constitutions with plenty of robust energy. If they are not so good, we will have more delicate constitutions and less stamina. If Essence and Source Ki are seriously damaged or depleted, due to any of the above factors, there may be birth defects or hereditary disease.

The second variable depends entirely on ourselves. Essence and Source Ki can never be augmented, only conserved and supplemented by Ki from correct breathing and eating. Those most likely to waste their Essence are those with strong constitutions, since the more delicate individuals know from childhood that they must take care of themselves. There are certain times in life when it is easier both to strengthen and weaken the constitution (see p. 71). Moderation is the key to conserving Essence; avoiding overwork, stress and stimulants, eating and exercising regularly but in moderation, paying attention to breathing and maintaining a quiet mind.

Storing Essence: growth

A child born with a good supply of Essence and Source Ki will grow normally into a healthy adult; if they are insufficient, growth may be retarded both physically and mentally. Since it is the gradual using up of our Essence which constitutes the ageing process, signs of ageing may begin earlier; if there is less sand in the hourglass, it will run through sooner. Prematurely greying hair may be one manifestation; premature senility is another, fortunately rarer, possibility.

Storing Essence: reproduction

Our inheritance of Essence from our parents determines our ability to reproduce, since it is that Essence which we pass on to our descendants. Insufficient Essence can affect reproduction in several ways: sexual development and maturation may be incomplete, as in congenital hormonal imbalance; infertility can also be an effect; or there may be a sexual dysfunction, such as impotence or low sexual energy. (There can be other causes for these apart from insufficient Essence, however, and the giver should check for confirmatory signs of Kidney weakness.) Since Essence is used up in procreation, excessive sexual activity can deplete it and for women, childbearing diminishes the supply.

The bones

Since the Kidneys are the foundations of our energy system and since, as pertaining to the Yin Water Element, they rule that which is deepest and densest, or most Yin, within the body, they govern the bones; this also includes the teeth, the "bones of the mouth". Bones which develop poorly in childhood are a sign of weak Essence; brittle bones which fracture easily and are slow to heal indicate weak Kidney function and osteoporosis in later life may be caused by the decline of Kidney Essence with age, which also causes the teeth to deteriorate.

The marrow

"Marrow" is a broadly descriptive term, not only for the bone marrow found within the long bones, but for the substance of the spinal cord and the brain, found within the vertebral column and the skull respectively. Since the Kidneys govern the deepest, most Yin structure within the body, the bones, they also rule the substances found even deeper, within the bones; thus not only the bone marrow but the central nervous system, including the brain, which the Chinese called the Sea of Marrow. Marrow, therefore, nourishes not only the physical body in terms of the bones and the blood but also, through the brain and nervous system, our thought processes, awareness and alertness. Slow reactions or poor coordination, dizziness or being "prone to slip and fall prostrate" can result from insufficient marrow. It is debatable whether the marrow aids the brain's capacity for intellectual thought, since the intellect is the province of the Spleen, but it assists memory and clarity.

Control Water

The Kidneys and Bladder are assisted in controlling Water by the Spleen, which extracts it from food, the Lungs, which disperse it to the skin, and the Small Intestine, which helps to purify it. It is the Yang energy of the Kidneys which enables these metabolic transactions to take place, since Kidney Yang is the foundation of all bodily activity. Kidney Yang ensures that the Fire of each organ is not drowned out and supervises the discharge of excess water by the Bladder. If this function is impaired, there may be chilliness, oedema in the lower part of the body and frequent pale urination. Kidney Yin enables the organs and tissues to retain and hold all the Water they need to keep them moist and lubricated; if it is Deficient, urination will be scanty and dark and there will be other symptoms of Empty Heat (see p. 79). Deficiency of either Kidney Yin or Kidney Yang will lead to urination at night.

Anchoring Ki

It is the Kidneys which allow us to retain the Ki taken in from Heaven by the Lungs. Breathing into the Lungs (upper chest) alone is relatively less beneficial than abdominal or Hara breathing, which utilizes the strength of the Source Ki, resident in the Hara, to "root" the Ki of the indrawn air in the lower body. Less Source Ki flowing from the Kidneys to the Hara results in shallow breathing, which means that the Triple Heater's function of activating and distributing the Source Ki is inhibited. Asthma can therefore result from a Kidney Deficiency, as the Ki from the inbreath cannot be held down and rises to produce a sensation of suffocation.

The two Yin

The "two Yin" is the Chinese euphemism for the two lower orifices (three in women). We have already seen how the Kidneys are in charge both of sexual activity and urination; they are therefore responsible for the condition of the urethral and vaginal outlets and, by extension, for the whole surrounding area, including the anus. In general, therefore, problems such as incontinence, soreness or itching in this area are usually due to Kidney Deficiency. There is always the possibility of Liver involvement, however, since the Liver meridian runs through the genitals (see p. 129), so the practitioner should check for other signs of Kidney weakness. Urgent diarrhoea before the normal time of rising can be sign of low Kidney Ki failing to rule the two Yin.

The hair

The luxuriance and health of the head hair is taken to be an outward sign of the health of the Kidneys. Hair thins, greys and falls with the decline of Essence and Source Ki in later life. Premature greying or thinning of the hair is often a sign of deficient Kidney Essence and hair in poor condition may reflect a weak Kidney energy.

The ears

The sense organ associated with the Kidneys is the ear, which resembles a Kidney in shape. Although external causes of diseases, such as ear infections, may attack the ear through one of the meridians around it, the Gall Bladder, Small Intestine or Triple Heater, the Kidneys are chiefly responsible for the quality of our hearing, which often deteriorates with the decline of Essence. Tinnitus results from Kidney Yin not nourishing the ears and is usually treated through the Kidney meridian.

Primary Yang, primary Yin: a reminder

The Kidneys embody the qualities of both Fire and Water and these opposite tendencies can be seen throughout not only the body but also the mind. The balance between Yin and Yang is crucial to health and the Kidneys help to maintain it by supplying the Yang energy for fight or flight or the Yin nectar of relaxation when stress is removed. If Kidney Yang is depleted, then the Yang of other organs such as the Spleen or Heart will suffer, leading to coldness and sluggishness in their function. Conversely, if Kidney Yin is affected, then the Yin of the Liver, Heart or Lungs is not supported, leading to symptoms of Heat and restlessness.

The Kidneys in Zen Shiatsu theory

Masunaga's concept of Kidney function is rooted in classical theory, yet he was also influenced by Western physiology and the idea of the Kidneys as the foundation of the constitution and the root of Yin and Yang does not figure in his theoretical model.

The Kidney and Bladder phase in the Cycle of the Meridians relates to impetus, the ability to respond to stimulus and to summon up energy when we need it. The Kidneys in Zen Shiatsu theory have an equal partnership with the Bladder in providing impetus by sending orders throughout the body, the Kidneys through hormones, which are liquid messages, the Bladder through the nervous system, with which its meridian connects (see p. 111). They are still in a sense, therefore, the root of all bodily, mental and emotional processes but the significance of this is less emphasized in Zen Shiatsu and the TCM roles of Source Ki and Essence become aspects of hormonal activity.

Hormones

Hormones are one of our principal sources of impetus. Not only can hormones, such as adrenalin, provide us with sudden bursts of energy when we need it, but they supply the stimulus for growth, sexual maturity and reproduction, which take us through our lifespan and, in average circumstances, ensure our posterity. This is very much the role of the Source Ki in TCM. Hormones also act as messengers which facilitate bodily processes such as digestion and regulate the fluid content of the blood and tissues, so that their sphere of activity closely approximates to that of Kidney Yang and Yin in the Oriental medical model. "The kidneys ... control the whole body through hormonal regulation" (*Zen Imagery Exercises*, p. 68). There are three areas where the hormones are most significant in Zen Shiatsu theory and their correspondence to the TCM understanding of the Kidneys: namely water metabolism, sexual activity and response to stress.

Water

The kidneys in health, under the direction of hormones from the pituitary gland, control the balance between water excreted from the body as urine and the water remaining in the tissues. Masunaga maintains the ancient Chinese view that the left Kidney controls water metabolism, while the right is connected with the endocrine system*. However, this aspect of the theory is not stressed and in practice both Kidneys are treated alike. Problems which occur when the Kidneys are not controlling water are oedema, overhydrated or swollen skin,

frequent or sparse urination and densely coloured urine. Prostate problems may also occur.

Sex

The sexual hormones are under the control of the Kidneys, particularly the right Kidney which, according to Masunaga, governs the endocrine system. The Kidneys thus influence the condition of the reproductive organs to some extent, although the female reproductive system is also influenced by the Stomach, Spleen and Bladder. In health, a feedback system ensures that a state of hormonal balance is maintained. This balance extends into the psychological state and sexual desire is commensurate with sexual capacity. When the hormones are disrupted, which may be the case with a Kidney diagnosis, the result may be loss of sexual balance. Desiring sex but being unable to obtain fulfilment, as in impotence, is a sign of disruption of hormonal messages; excessive sexual activity, abstention from sex or "thinking but not doing" can be ways of disrupting the hormonal messages. Any imbalance between desire and fulfilment is what Masunaga means by the phrase "abnormal sex life" (*Zen Shiatsu*, p. 45).

Stress

In Zen Shiatsu, as in TCM and indeed in Western physiology if we include the adrenal glands, the Kidneys help us adapt to stress. It is the Yang aspect of the Kidneys which reacts to stress via the "fight or flight" response of the sympathetic nervous system. Masunaga calls this "controlling spirit and energy to the body". The ability to recover from stress and relax is the Yin capacity of the Kidneys. A deficiency of the adrenal functions means that our reaction to stress is characterized by lack of determination and extreme fatigue. There is continual anxiety and the receiver is jumpy and easily startled. This manifestation is similar to Kidney Yang Deficiency in TCM. When there is an inability to recover from stress and relax, then the symptoms are "workaholism", impatience, restlessness and nervous sensitivity, all of which are similar to Kidney Yin Deficiency. In either case, the family or occupational stress which causes such symptoms is usually relentless and severe and the receiver is likely to suffer from lack of sleep.

---

*In the Nan Jing, the right Kidney is identified with Ming-Men, the Gate of Vitality, and thus with the Source Ki while the left Kidney is linked with the Bladder and the function of transforming Water.

Fear

A Kidney imbalance tends to produce the deep fear associated with the Water Element. Phobias or irrational fears may manifest and there is often a continual fear of what the future may bring, which leads to further stress and over-reaction. Since the Kidneys also confer will, however, a Kidney diagnosis may ensure that the receiver also demonstrates extreme courage, overcoming fear to accomplish goals against the odds.

Bones and back

Since the Kidneys rule the bones, and especially the lower back, lower back pain is a symptom of Kidney (or Bladder) imbalance in Zen Shiatsu as well as TCM. When the Kidneys are Kyo, the backache is accompanied by feelings of cold and by poor circulation in the hips and Hara. As in TCM, weak or brittle bones may accompany a Kidney imbalance.

Miscellaneous Kidney symptoms

Many of the symptoms which Masunaga listed in his books as indicative of Kidney imbalance are related to TCM. Blackish colour in the face is a Five Element association. Inflamed throat, poor hearing when drugs are taken, ringing in the ears and proneness to inflammation are all classically caused by Kidney Yin Deficiency. Thirst, bitterness in the mouth, bad breath, vomiting and blood in the saliva are signs of Heat in the Stomach when the Kidneys do not provide enough fluid for digestion.

The Kidney meridian and how to treat it

The traditional Kidney meridian begins on the sole of the foot, in the hollow where the instep meets the ball of the foot. It ascends the inner aspect of the foot to a point between the ankle bone and the Achilles tendon, circles back on itself around the inner surface of the heel, then ascends again by way of Sp 6, up the inner curve of the calf muscle to the point at the back of the knee on the medial side where two tendons of the hamstring join. It goes straight up the medial surface of the thigh, posterior to the adductor muscles, to the area where the groin joins the perineum. It goes internal at this point, re-emerging on the abdomen immediately above the pubic bone and about half an inch from the midline and then ascends the torso, widening to outline the edges of the sternum and ending in the hollow below the medial end of the collar bone.

Masunaga not only extended the Kidney meridian throughout the body, but also slightly altered its pathway. The path of the traditional meridian between the back of the knee and the groin is academic as far as acupuncturists are concerned, as there are no points between the back of the knee and the pubic bone. Masunaga felt that the Kidney Ki and sensations of the meridian did not follow this pathway, but traced them instead diagonally across the back of the knee and up the lateral part of the hamstring, over the biceps femoris muscle. In the classical meridian system, this is part of the Bladder meridian. In the lower leg, while the Zen Shiatsu meridian still goes to Sp 6, the circle around the heel and ankle is omitted. The Zen Shiatsu Kidney also runs down the lateral border of the erector spinae muscles on either side of the spine. There is a branch of the Kidney meridian in the hips, which closely follows the outline of the sacrum. On the front of the torso, the lower part of the meridian is replaced by the Hara diagnostic areas. The upper pathway of the Kidney meridian remains the same, on the outer borders of the sternum. It is drawn lateral to the Heart in the charts, though in practice the Kidney and Heart on the chest are both on the outer borders of the sternum; it is the different angles of pressure which differentiate them and not the surface location. A new branch running along the lower border of the clavicle leaves the meridian at its classical exit point and another ascends the throat between the Heart Protector and Stomach, medial to the sternocleidomastoid (SCM) muscle. From the outer end of the clavicle, the meridian goes internal to emerge at the top of the axillary crease, on the posterior surface of the arm. It travels down the arm, posterior to the Small Intestine meridian, and along the edge of the ulna on the forearm to the centre of the mound on the ulnar side of the palm.

The Hara diagnostic area for the Kidney is a horseshoe shape surrounding the circular Spleen area

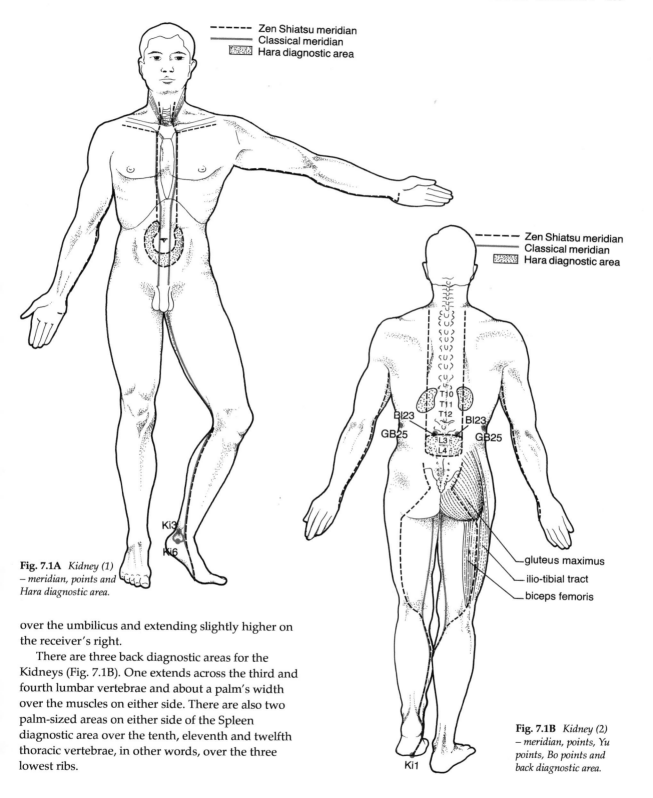

Fig. 7.1A *Kidney (1) – meridian, points and Hara diagnostic area.*

Fig. 7.1B *Kidney (2) – meridian, points, Yu points, Bo points and back diagnostic area.*

over the umbilicus and extending slightly higher on the receiver's right.

There are three back diagnostic areas for the Kidneys (Fig. 7.1B). One extends across the third and fourth lumbar vertebrae and about a palm's width over the muscles on either side. There are also two palm-sized areas on either side of the Spleen diagnostic area over the tenth, eleventh and twelfth thoracic vertebrae, in other words, over the three lowest ribs.

Treatment procedure

The meridian is most accessible in the prone and supine positions. Note: when working in prone, the meridian is treated downwards, according to the Zen Shiatsu approach, finishing at the starting point of the Kidney on the sole of the foot. In my experience, this does not adversely affect the treatment (see p. 253).

1. The meridian on the back lies along the outer border of the erector spinae muscle, lateral to the Yu points. The upper portion can be worked in the sitting position with thumb or elbow, but the whole meridian can be worked in prone, either one or both sides at a time, with palms, thumbs or elbows (Fig. 7.2). When working one side at a time, it is advisable to treat the side nearest you and change to the receiver's other side to treat the other. When working both sides together, if there is a pronounced slope to the receiver's shoulders, it can be difficult to attain the correct angle of penetration for the upper back from the position shown. It is best to start at the first horizontal point and work down the back, then to treat the upper back later in the routine from behind the receiver's head.

2. The meridian in the hips follows the outline of the sacrum, diagonally downwards and inwards. The angle of pressure is directed down and medially, under the edge of the bony ridge of the ilium and the sacrum. The thumb and elbow are the most suitable tools and the meridian is treated one side at a time, with the giver's mother hand resting on the lumbar area. The meridian then moves outward and downward across the lower buttock to the lateral edge of the thigh. This portion is treated with palm, thumb or elbow, with perpendicular pressure (Fig. 7.3).

3. The Kidney in the back of the thigh is on the lateral edge of the horizontal surface of the leg – "the side of the top" – in the prone position. (Compare the Large Intestine, which is on "the top of the side" in the prone position; the posterior edge of the vertical surface of the leg, just anterior to the Kidney.) With the giver's mother hand on the sacrum, it can be worked with the palm, thumb, elbow or knee. When using the knee with the receiver in prone, hold the receiver's foot and flex the leg slightly towards the opposite buttock, as on p. 34.

4. At the point where the tendon of the biceps femoris begins to be felt, the meridian begins to cross the knee diagonally. (This part of the meridian should be worked only with the thumb and with the minimum of physical pressure.) Having crossed to the medial side of the calf it descends the belly of the medial head of the gastrocnemius (in other words, the fullest bulge of the calf muscle on the medial side) and follows straight down from there to the hollow between the medial malleolus and the Achilles tendon. The thumb is most suitable for treating this part of the meridian and it is easiest to do if the giver turns her hand and grasps the calf so that her thumb falls upon the meridian. When using modified body weight, she is applying gentle pressure to the back of the calf, while focusing her Ki through her thumb on the Kidney meridian.

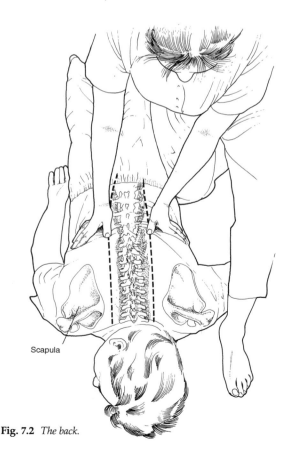

Scapula

Fig. 7.2 *The back.*

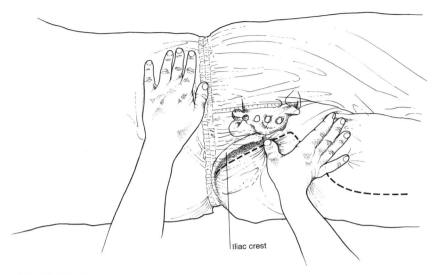

Iliac crest

Fig. 7.3 *The hips.*

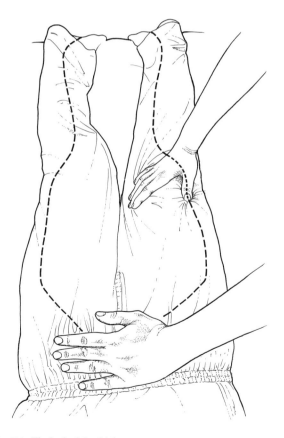

Fig. 7.4 *The back of the thigh.*

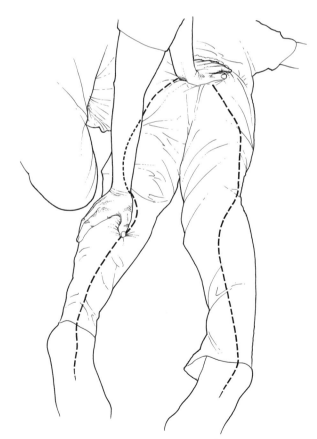

Fig. 7.5 *The calf.*

5. From the hollow between the Achilles tendon and the medial malleolus, the meridian crosses to the sole of the foot and Ki 1, the point in the depression between the ball of the foot and the instep. This part of the meridian is best worked with the thumb, either following on from technique 4 above or as part of a separate foot treatment, as shown.

6. The meridian in the chest is reached in the supine position, with the giver kneeling or in the lunge position beside the receiver's chest. The lower part of its pathway occupies the same surface area as the Heart meridian on the borders of the sternum, but instead of angling the pressure inwards under the sternum, as when working the Heart (see p. 153), the angle is perpendicularly downwards. This means that at the level where the giver's pressure contacts the receiver's meridian, below the surface, the Kidney is in fact lateral to the

Heart (although not as lateral as is indicated on the Masunaga charts). It is treated in the same way as the Heart, with the ulnar edge of the hand (one or both sides at a time) or with perpendicular fingertip pressure (usually both sides at once).

Unlike the Heart, the Kidney meridian carries on up to the sternoclavicular joint and then moves out in the hollow under the clavicle. This part of the meridian can be treated with the heel of the hand or the thumb, usually both sides at once, as shown.

7. The Kidney meridian in the arm lies on the division between the Yin and the Yang sides of the arm, between the Small Intestine and the Heart. It can be treated together with the Bladder (see p. 117) or singly, as shown. The arm is laid in its meridian stretch, higher than that of the Small Intestine, but preferably not across the receiver's throat. The sternoclavicular joint is a good area to

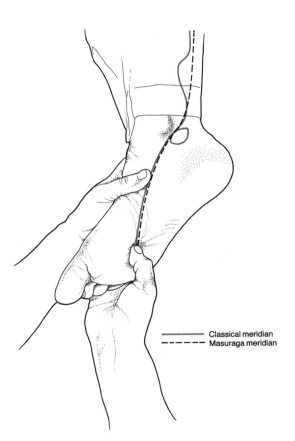

Classical meridian
- - - - - Masuraga meridian

Fig. 7.6 *The sole of the foot.*

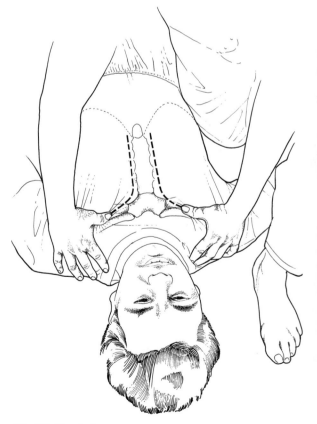

Fig. 7.7 *The chest.*

aim for. The meridian is then treated in the same way as the Small Intestine (see p. 161).

8. The path of the Kidney meridian in the throat is the deepest hollow between the carotid artery and the SCM muscle, between the Heart Protector and the Stomach meridians. Great care must be exercised to penetrate deeply without pain or constriction of this area or without causing fear in the receiver. The giver sits behind the receiver's head, supporting the head or neck with her mother hand, and works gently but deeply down the meridian with her thumb, one side at a time.

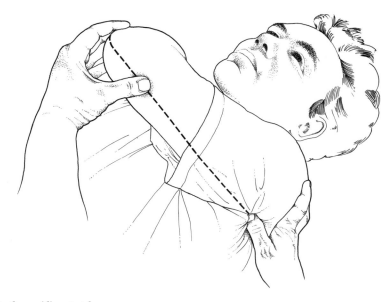

Fig. 7.8 *Working the arm in the meridian stretch.*

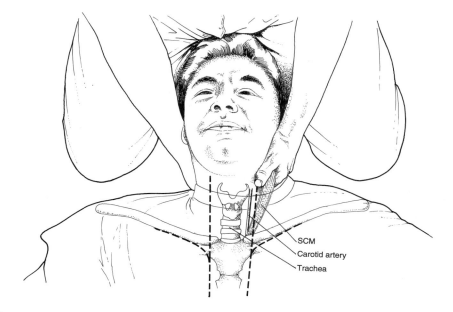

SCM

Carotid artery

Trachea

Fig. 7.9 *The throat.*

She may, if in doubt as to the quality of her pressure, ask for feedback from the receiver. She should feel the pulsing of the carotid artery on of her thumb and the resistance of the SCM muscle on the other.

Major points on the Kidney meridian

Kidney 1

In the depression between the middle third and distal third of the sole, when the foot is plantarflexed.

Actions

- Tonifies Yin
- Clears Heat
- Subdues Wind and restores consciousness (revival point)
- Calms the Shen

Kidney 3

In the depression between the medial malleolus and the Achilles tendon, level with the tip of the medial malleolus.

Actions

- Source point
- Tonifies the Source Ki and Essence
- Tonifies the Yin and Yang of the whole body
- Tonifies the Kidneys
- Regulates the uterus
- Strengthens the lower back and knees

Kidney 6

One thumb's width below the medial malleolus.

Actions

- Nourishes Yin and fluids
- Cools the Blood
- Calms the mind and promotes sleep
- Tonifies the uterus

Kidney Yu point

Bl 23 – two fingers' width lateral to the midline of the spine, level with the lower border of the second lumbar vertebra.

Kidney Bo point

GB 25 – on the side of the abdomen, at the lower border of the free end of the twelfth thoracic (floating) rib.

The Bladder in TCM

The Bladder, whose organ function is the storage and excretion of urine, has a meridian function of far greater importance. The Transporting points of the Bladder meridian, known in Japanese as the Yu points, directly influence the workings of all the bodily organs and functions. They lie on either side of the spine down the two pathways, inner and outer, of the Bladder meridian, in most cases at a location near the organ which they govern. The inner row of points is thought to govern the physical functions of the organs, the outer row of mental and emotional aspects of the same organs. Acupuncturists needle these points for a strong and rapid effect on the organ function and they are among the most frequently used points in the repertoire. Even the Zen Shiatsu practitioner, who does not rely on prescribed points for treatment, may find it useful to know the locations of the Yu points, since they are often significant aids to diagnosis, whether the giver perceives them as areas of distortion or the receiver finds them tender (see p. 239).

Yang aspect of Kidneys

All the Yang organs can be regarded as embodying the energetic function of their paired Yin organs. It is the Yu points which indicate that the Bladder meridian represents more than the physical bladder organ, acting as a vehicle for the Yang functions of the Kidneys. Kidney Yang supplies energy to all the organ functions; the Bladder meridian tonifies all the organ functions. An imbalance in Bladder function is thus likely to resemble Kidney Yang Deficiency in its symptomatology: coldness or sluggishness in any body part or function, usually accompanied by copious, clear urine.

Transforms and excretes urine

The Bladder receives impure fluids from the Kidneys, which it transforms into urine, then stores and excretes. This function can be hampered by Kidney Yang Deficiency, if there is not enough available Ki to transform the fluids into urine. The Bladder function is also affected by Spleen Deficiency. If the Spleen does not process fluids correctly, they either pass straight through the body, supplying the Bladder with more fluids than it can deal with, which gives rise to excessive urination, or they form Dampness, which can obstruct the Bladder, causing difficult urination and scanty, cloudy urine. The Bladder can also be influenced by the Small Intestine, with which it is associated in the Six Divisions (see p. 82). The Small Intestine can receive Heat (often from emotional causes) from its paired organ, the Heart, and impart the Heat to the Bladder, causing scanty, dark urine, and sometimes painful urination.

The uterus

Because the Bladder is the executive of the Kidneys, which govern reproduction, and because the organ is situated very close to the uterus, Bladder Ki influences uterine function and a deficiency can result in infertility or painful menstruation.

The back

The Bladder, with the Kidneys, influences the bones and the meridian runs the length of the spine. Any long term imbalance in Bladder Ki will thus affect the back. When this begins early in life, the structure of the back may be distorted, resulting in such symptoms as scoliosis or curvature of the spine. In other cases, back pain is the result, usually lower back pain or sciatica with pain radiating down the Bladder meridian in the leg. Sometimes there is tightness or pain along the whole spine or pain in other areas of the back. When Kidney Yang is Deficient, the pain is often associated with a chilly sensation. The energy in the Bladder meridian also influences posture, since it gives strength and support to the back.

The Bladder in Zen Shiatsu theory

In Zen Shiatsu theory, the Bladder, together with the

Kidneys, embodies impetus, the survival instinct and response to stimulus. Its characteristics and functions are subtly differentiated from those of the Kidneys, however, and are largely related to the meridian pathway. The Bladder meridian begins in the deepest part of the eye socket, on a level with the pituitary gland which governs the autonomic nervous system, and then descends on either side of the spine, close to the spinal nerves. This suggests that it is involved with the nervous system response which governs all body processes and voluntary activity. Masunaga, when describing Bladder symptoms, frequently uses the word "nervous" in its descriptive sense as well as its anatomical one, implying that Bladder Ki in disharmony tends to manifest as tension and overreaction.

Nervous system

The Bladder, via the autonomic nervous system, provides the body's response to stimulus or information. If the Bladder function is underactive, there is no impetus to respond to information received by the nervous system; in Masunaga's words, "although one feels the need to do something, one has no stamina to act" (*Zen Imagery Exercises*, p. 200). If the Bladder function is hyperactive, the nervous system is extremely sensitive to information and overreacts to it, draining the body's reserves. Both of these conditions cause intense stress and exhaustion. With a Bladder imbalance, the receiver's nerves are on edge and quite ordinary irritations become sources of stress. Because of nervous sensitivity, the receiver may be easily startled, anxious or restless and in severe cases these symptoms may reach the level of neurosis or paranoia.

Will, determination and intensity

The level of nervous tension which a Bladder imbalance generates is extreme and intensifies with stress. The nervous system is sensitive both to outside stimuli and to the internal impetus of will, the spiritual capacity of the Water Element, so that it is under double pressure.

A Bladder imbalance may arise temporarily, as the result of a period of overwork or stress, but a long term Bladder imbalance will ensure that the overwork and stress are permanent conditions, as the receiver is continually aware of imperatives both from without and within. There are always tasks to perform and self-imposed deadlines to meet for someone with a Bladder imbalance, whether he accomplishes them or merely frets because he cannot. These imperatives create an intense atmosphere around him, so that other people are influenced by his tension and urgency. This is most commonly seen in work situations, but it can as easily arise in a family environment. Wherever it happens, it creates further stress, not only for the individual with the Bladder imbalance but also for those around him.

Fatigue

The Bladder meridian is frequently diagnosed on a short term basis when the receiver is tired and temporarily lacking in impetus. As it is the Yang meridian of the Water Element and therefore more superficial, the temporary depletion of Ki involved tends not to be as deep as that linked to a Kidney imbalance and does not necessarily affect the internal body processes. When Bladder energy is persistently out of balance, the fatigue becomes chronic and is likely to alternate with a Kidney diagnosis as it penetrates deeper into the system.

Fear

Fear, the emotion of the Water Element, often accompanies a Bladder diagnosis. It is not usually a conscious fear, however, tending to manifest more as tension, anxiety and restlessness. The receiver may experience fear in particular situations, such as fear of flying, fear of heights or fear of being alone at night; fears which are considered "normal" and have not yet reached the irrational level of phobias. When under particular stress, however, the receiver may be aware of a different level of free-floating panic, with no particular cause.

The back

The Bladder meridian governs the spine and the physical structure of the back. The two other long Yang meridians, the Stomach and the Gall Bladder,

together with the Bladder, form as it were energetic guy ropes which work together to support us in an upright posture. A weakness in any of them is likely to affect the others, altering postural balance and creating further patterns of tension or discomfort. The Bladder connects at the sacrum with the Gall Bladder to secure an even alignment of the hips and lower back and in this area it is particularly vulnerable to distortion, which then affects the rest of the spine. Tightness in the back muscles, lower back pain and sciatica are problems which can result from a Bladder imbalance. These problems are often accompanied by a chilly sensation and may be made worse by cold.

On the psychological level, as well as epitomizing our "backbone" or determination, the Bladder embodies many aspects of ourselves that we put behind us. Fear, jealousy or repressed sexual longings, the emotions which we are reluctant to acknowledge, are pushed into the back of our minds while we show the world a very different front. These emotions cause further fear and tension and until recognized and accepted, they may affect the balance of the Bladder.

The urinary and reproductive systems

A Bladder disharmony often, though not always, results in urinary problems. Excessively frequent urination is common, and also difficult or obstructed urination. Bladder is often diagnosed in cases of cystitis. Because of its proximity to the uterus, a Bladder diagnosis may be linked to gynaecological problems such as excessive, scanty or irregular bleeding, discharge or painful menstruation. In men, the Bladder meridian can be related to impotence.

The meridian pathway

On such a long meridian there are many potential sites for discomfort. Eye problems, sinusitis and hayfever may affect the pathway in the face; occipital headaches and neck tension may relate to the Bladder meridian. Pain, discomfort or stiffness along the spine and in the sacrum are discussed above.

The Bladder meridian and how to treat it

The classical Bladder meridian arises at the hollow above the inner canthus of the eye and travels up the forehead, widening slightly just within the hairline, and over the crown of the head to the occipital ridge. It then descends on either side of the vertebral column, about two fingers' width from the midline of the spine, a line which on most people falls on the ridge of the erector spinae muscles. Descending in a vertical line to the level of the lowest sacral foramen, it ascends once more to the top of the sacrum to descend again on a more medial and diagonal line, directly over the sacral foramina to the tip of the coccyx. It then crosses the buttock to the middle of the transverse gluteal fold and descends the midline of the back of the thigh, veering outwards for the last third of the length of the thigh to the lateral side of the popliteal fossa, then to the centre of the popliteal fossa. The meridian then goes internal and its next appearance is once again at the occipital ridge. It ascends to the upper back and descends the medial border of the scapula, then the back, on a vertical line about four fingers' width from the midline of the spine, to the level of the fourth sacral foramen. It then curves laterally across the buttock and down the back of the thigh on a more lateral pathway than before, curving inward to reconnect with the first branch of the meridian at the centre of the popliteal fossa*. It descends centrally to the middle of the calf, then laterally to pass between the Achilles tendon and the lateral malleolus, around which it curves to travel along the lateral edge of the foot to the lateral side of the little toenail.

Masunaga's Bladder meridian is simpler and straighter but in essential points not very different from the classical Bladder. It takes the same pathway to the occipital ridge, but descends the back directly lateral to the spinous processes of the vertebrae, on the medial border of the erector spinae muscle; in other words, next to the spine, rather than two fingers' width lateral*. There is no outer pathway down the back; it has been replaced by the Kidney meridian and the zigzag over the sacrum is omitted, since the whole of the sacrum and the fifth lumbar vertebra constitute the Bladder diagnostic area.

From the lower borders of the sacrum, the meridian descends in the shortest line between two points to the middle of the transverse gluteal fold, then down the midline of the thigh, knee and calf, to end at the little toe. An extra branch goes from C7 out over the top of the scapula, following the line of the scapular spine (and mirroring the branch of the Kidney at the front which follows the lower border of the clavicle) to the front of the shoulder and down the radial edge of the arm, between the Lung and Large Intestine and opposite the Kidney, to end in the centre of the thenar eminence.

The Hara diagnostic area is a horseshoe shape encircling the Kidney and extending from the pubic bone up beside the umbilicus to the upper abdomen. The end of the horseshoe on the receiver's left is lower than on the right because of the descending shape of the Stomach diagnostic area.

---

*This is a recent rearrangement of the Bladder meridian pathway, which in previous versions went internal at the tip of the coccyx, re-emerged at the top of the shoulders and descended in a vertical line down the medial border of the scapula, the back, the buttock and the centre of the back of the thigh, deviating laterally for the last third of its pathway to the lateral side of the popliteal fossa, then to the centre as before. The newer version incorporates a branch down the outer part of the thigh which approximates to the Zen Shiatsu Kidney meridian, while keeping, through the intersection of the two thigh pathways, a central meridian down the back of the leg which is the same as the Zen Shiatsu Bladder. It has altered the numbering of the points between Bl 35 and Bl 54.

*This difference in pathway, which causes much anxiety to Shiatsu students, is not as radical as it appears. In ancient times, this was the pathway of the Bladder meridian, established by the physician Hua Tuo. When the Bladder was moved out to its present position, the points next to the spine were retained in the acupuncturists' repertory, and renamed the Hua Tuo points. Because of the position of the spinal nerves, all points level with a particular intervertebral space, regardless of latitude, influence the same meridian. It is traditionally considered that the closer to the spine the point is, the more directly physical its influence. Thus the Hua Tuo points influence the organs and tissues in a more physical way than the Yu points, while the outer Bladder points influence more the spiritual qualities of the organs.

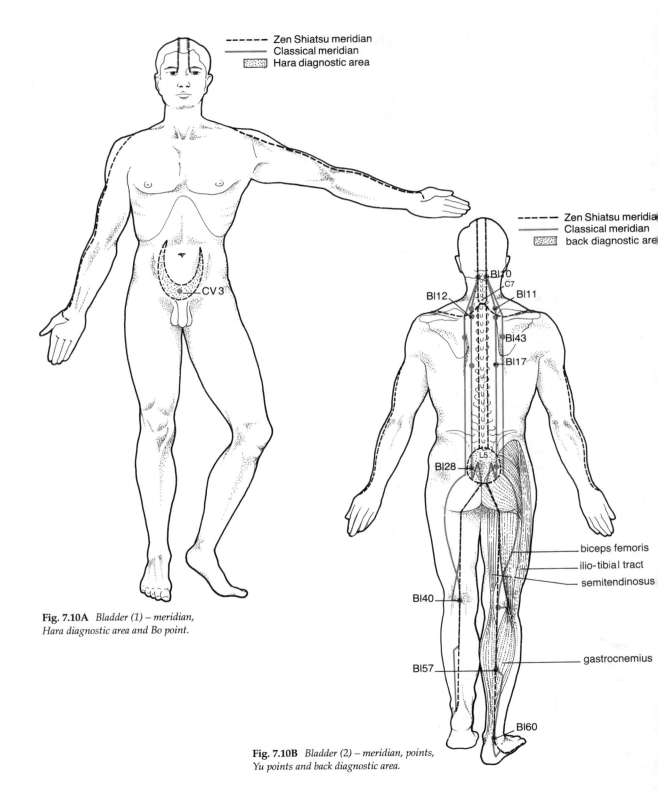

Zen Shiatsu meridian
Classical meridian
Hara diagnostic area

CV 3

Zen Shiatsu meridian
Classical meridian
back diagnostic area

Bl70
C7
Bl12
Bl11
Bl43
Bl17
L5
Bl28

biceps femoris
ilio-tibial tract
semitendinosus

Bl40

gastrocnemius

Bl57

Bl60

Fig. 7.10A *Bladder (1) – meridian, Hara diagnostic area and Bo point.*

Fig. 7.10B *Bladder (2) – meridian, points, Yu points and back diagnostic area.*

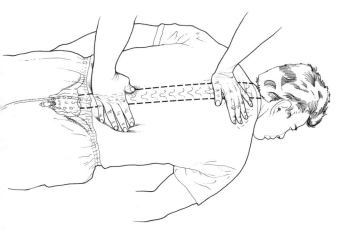

Fig. 7.11 *The back.*

The back diagnostic area for the Bladder is a circle including the whole of the sacrum and the fifth lumbar vertebra.

Treatment procedure

The meridian is most effectively treated in the prone and supine positions, although it can also be worked in the side and sitting positions.

1. The Bladder in the back is treated in the same way as the Kidney. It can be worked with palm, thumb or elbow, either one or both sides at a time. If working one side at a time, as shown (Fig. 7.11), it is best for the angle of penetration (vertical) to work the side of the spine nearest to you and change sides to do the other. If working both sides at a time, and if there is a pronounced slope in the receiver's shoulders, it is best to work from the mid-shoulder plateau downwards and move behind the receiver's head to treat the shoulders separately from a more convenient angle.

2. The Yu points lie about a thumb's width lateral to the Zen Shiatsu Bladder meridian. They are treated with the thumbs, both sides at once, from a lunge position at the receiver's side (Fig. 7.12A). If there is a pronounced slope to the shoulders, the three upper Yu points are best treated from behind the receiver's head (Fig. 7.12B).

3. To treat the sacrum, the giver kneels in the lunge position beside the receiver's hips and faces his head. The sacrum is best worked with palms and

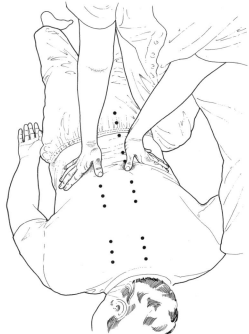

Fig. 7.12A *The Yu points, treated from the side.*

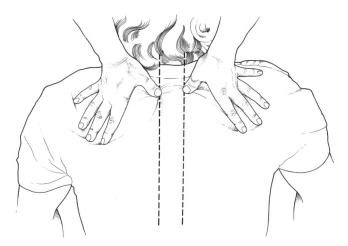

Fig. 7.12B *The Yu points, treated from behind the receiver's head.*

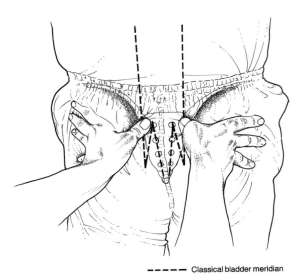

- - - - - Classical bladder meridian

Fig. 7.13 *The sacrum.*

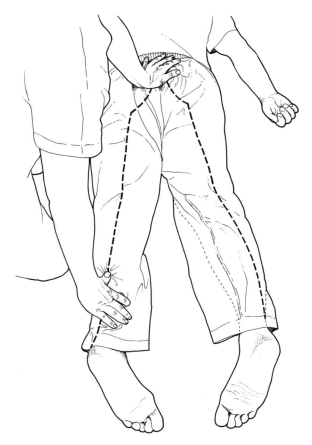

Fig. 7.14 *The back of the leg.*

thumbs, both sides at once in order to ascertain the alignment of the sacrum. With practice, it is possible to feel two vertical lines of tsubos, just medial to the posterior superior iliac spine, which include the Small Intestine and Bladder Yu points.

4. To treat the back of the leg, the giver kneels facing the receiver's thigh, with her mother hand on the sacrum. The meridian, which lies on the midline of the leg, will vary considerably in apparent location according to the position of the receiver's leg and the giver should check the location of the ischial tuberosity and the midpoint between the dimples at the back of the knee to ascertain its true pathway. If the receiver's foot turns outwards, it should be supported with cushions to make the midline of the leg more available. The meridian can be treated with palm, thumb, elbow, knee or Dragon's Mouth on the thigh, remembering to lighten the pressure drastically when approaching the back of the knee. The back of the knee requires minimal pressure, the calf only light pressure and this part of the meridian is best treated with palm and/or thumb.

5. The Bladder meridian in the feet and ankles is best treated from a sitting or kneeling position at the receiver's feet. It is useful to press Bl 60 and Ki 3, on either side of the Achilles tendon, together with both thumbs, then to work down the Bladder on the side of the foot with the

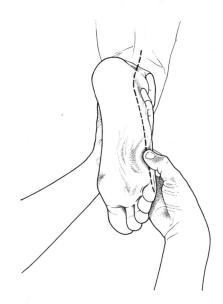

Fig. 7.15 *The feet and ankles.*

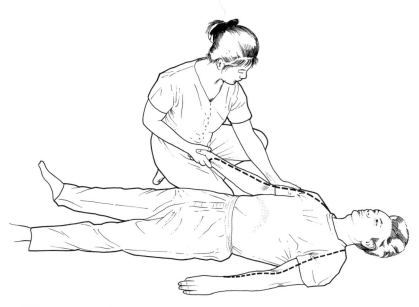

Fig. 7.16 *Bladder and Kidney together in the arms.*

thumb, as shown, finishing by stretching and pressing the little toe.

6. The meridian in the arms is most easily treated in the supine position, as follows. The giver takes the receiver's nearest hand with her own nearest hand, as if shaking hands. In this position, the Bladder and Kidney meridians in her own arm are in alignment with those in the receiver's arm, which makes it easier to know where to place her grip on the receiver's upper arm meridians. Exerting a gentle stretch to straighten and lift the receiver's arm, she grasps the upper arm with her thumb on the Bladder, her fingertips on the Kidney, and works them both together down the arm to the wrist. The meridians on the forearm are on the two bony edges and are easy to find (Fig. 7.16). She finishes by laying the back of the receiver's hand on her knee and working with both thumbs from the sides of the wrist towards the inner palm.

7. The Bladder in the neck can be effectively treated in the sitting position with the thumb, one side at a time, as shown. The giver should be at arm's length from the receiver, grasping the back of the receiver's neck so that her thumb falls on the Bladder meridian, and with her mother hand on the shoulder on the side being treated. The pressure can be carried down the meridian to the

level of the mid-back, with the mother hand holding the receiver steady. The Bladder in the neck can also be treated in the supine position by placing both sets of fingertips on either side of the cervical vertebrae and penetrating upwards against the weight of the receiver's head.

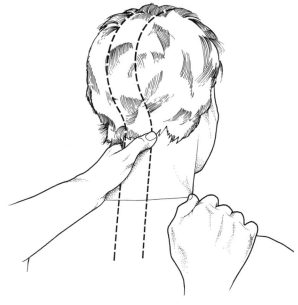

Fig. 7.17 *The neck.*

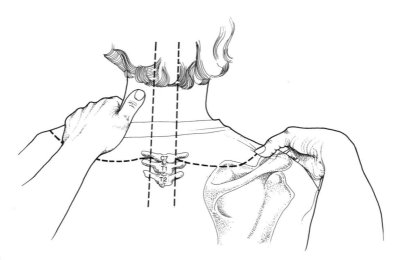

Fig. 7.18 *The shoulders.*

8. The meridian in the shoulders can be treated with the thumb in the sitting position, one side at a time, with the giver's mother hand supporting the opposite shoulder. Work from the lower borders of C7 out to the tip of the shoulder and over it to the clavicle, using the line of the scapular spine as a guide. This part of the meridian can also be treated in the prone position but less of it is accessible.

9. The top and back of the head can be worked in the prone position with the receiver's forehead resting on a small pillow, but the meridian in the

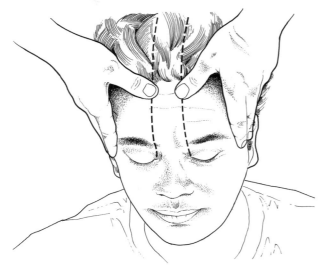

Fig. 7.19 *The face and the top of the head.*

face and head is usually worked in the supine position. A cloth can be used. Bl 1, in the deepest part of the eye socket, is usually treated with the little fingers, then the meridian from the medial end of the eyebrow up the forehead and over the top of the head is worked with both thumbs at once, as shown (Fig. 7.19).

Major points on the Bladder meridian

The Yu points

For the location of the Yu point of each meridian, see the section on how to treat that meridian.

Actions of the Yu points. The Yu points can be used in diagnosis, as explained on p. 239. In treatment, they can be used to:

- strongly tonify the organ system concerned, especially in chronic disorders
- treat the sense organ corresponding to the organ system concerned (e.g. nose: Lungs)
- subdue Rebellious Ki in the case of the Stomach and Lungs.

Bladder 10

In the suboccipital groove, within the posterior hairline, just under two fingers' width lateral to the midline of the spine.

Actions

- Expels Wind
- Treats headache, stiff neck and lower back
- Benefits the eyes and brain

Bladder 11

Two fingers' width lateral to the midline of the spine, level with the lower border of the spinous process of the first thoracic vertebra.

Actions

- Expels Wind and releases the Exterior
- Nourishes the Blood
- Strengthens the bones and soothes the muscles

Bladder 12

Two fingers' width lateral to the midline of the spine, level with the lower border of the spinous process of the second thoracic vertebra.

Actions

- Expels and prevents Exterior Wind
- Releases the Exterior
- Stimulates the Lung dispersing function
- Stimulates the Defensive Ki

Bladder 17

Two fingers' width lateral to the midline of the spine, level with the lower border of the spinous process of the seventh thoracic vertebra.

Actions

- Tonifies Ki and Blood
- Nourishes Blood (especially with moxa)
- Moves Blood
- Subdues Rebellious Stomach Ki

Bladder 40

In the centre of the popliteal fossa.

Actions

- Clears Heat and Summer Heat
- Cools the Blood
- Resolves Dampness from the Bladder
- Benefits the lower back

Bladder 43

Four fingers' width lateral to the midline of the spine, level with the lower border of the spinous process of the fourth thoracic vertebra. It is quite likely that this point, the outer Bladder point level with the Heart Protector Yu point, relates to the information-carrying function of the deep fascia (see p. 174). Its Chinese name means "the Yu point of Gaohuang" – Gaohuang being translatable both as "the vitals" and "fatty membranes".

Actions

- Nourishes Essence
- Tonifies and strengthens Deficiency (especially with moxa)
- Invigorates the Shen
- Benefits Lung Yin and stops cough (no moxa)

Bladder 57

Halfway down the calf, in the depression immediately below the belly of the gastrocnemius.

Actions

- Clears Heat
- Moves Blood
- Sphere of influence is lower back, buttocks and anus

Bladder 60

In the hollow between the lateral malleolus and the Achilles tendon, level with the tip of the lateral malleolus.

Actions

- Expels Wind
- Benefits the back, neck and shoulders
- Clears Heat from the Bladder
- Moves Blood

Bladder Yu point

Bl 28 – Two fingers' width from the midline of the back, at the level of the second sacral foramen.

Bladder Bo point

CV 3 – On the midline of the abdomen, one thumb's width above the upper border of the pubic bone.

8

The Wood Element – The Liver and Gall Bladder

■ *"the force that through the green fuse drives the flower."*

FERN HILL, DYLAN THOMAS

Element associations: energy, cooperation, adaptability, organization, self-expression

The Wood Element is the only one in the Oriental model which expresses individual identity as well as being a force of nature. The plant world as a whole has a group energy – Aristotle spoke of the "vegetable soul" to describe a certain level of consciousness – but each plant species and each individual plant within that species has its own unique form and design.

Plant life has an irrepressible urge to reproduce and establish itself and the energy of the blade of grass which pushes up through the asphalt or the tree which grows sideways out of a wall is the same energy which produces the prodigious luxuriance of a tropical rainforest. Plant energy is almost impossible to destroy; it can lie dormant for years or aeons and burst into life again like the flowers which spring up in the desert after rain or the seeds which germinate after 8000 years in an Egyptian tomb. The primal strength of the urge to live and grow is the characteristic of the Wood element and its representatives in the human being, the Liver and Gall Bladder. (The name "liver" suggests that Western traditions, too, associate this organ with life.) Because of the force of Wood Ki, the Liver and Gall Bladder are often given a military character in ancient writings and are called, respectively, "General" and "Lieutenant". The Wood energy in nature is not specifically aggressive, however, in spite of its competitive strength. A few

plants may be poisonous, though many more are healing, and others may defend themselves with spines or thorns, but on the whole the plant world is benevolent rather than otherwise. Above all, when many plants are found together there is a strong sense of community and cooperation, as well as competition. A walk through mixed woodland reveals lichens colonizing the branches of trees, fungi and ferns enjoying the damp, shady spots beneath them and dead trees playing host to mosses and more mushrooms during the slow process of their disintegration. This capacity for harmonious coexistence is one of the most important aspects of Wood in the human body and mind, together with its complement, the urge for individual self-expression.

Plants can live harmoniously together because of their adaptability and this quality also serves the solitary plant. Trees can send roots hundreds of feet into the earth to seek for water or grow an equal distance upwards to compete for light. Creepers show almost human cunning in seeking for support and any plant will change the direction of its growth if it meets with an obstacle. Wood is flexible because it is alive; and it is alive because it is flexible. The ability to plan and make decisions is a facet of the Wood Element in the human character, similar to the strategy of the tree and the creeper; it represents the choice of the optimum direction for growth. But it is essential that the plans and decisions adapt to changing circumstances. We, too, have to be flexible or our plans lose their living purpose.

Plant life is also organized, each plant a miracle of design which is also a part of its function; the parachutes of thistledown, the fronds of a fern, the gills of a mushroom, all have a function in the individual life of the plant and all are examples of perfect design. It is the organization, the design of the plant world, which allows most efficient expression of the boundless energy of Wood. In the same way, the capacity to organize our efforts effectively is our human way of harnessing our creative energy and represents an aspect of the Wood Element within us.

Organization is as evident in the coexistence of plants together as it is in the plant in isolation; the design is part of a larger design, as ecologists emphasize. Wood energy allows us to attain our maximum potential for self-expression, if we use it well; but individual self-expression is only significant when others in the group or culture can relate to it. We may not know what our individual purpose on this earth is, but the gift of the Wood Element is to urge us to strive equally for our own well-being and for that of the other life forms which share or create our environment; only with this balance of emphasis is our survival ensured.

Spiritual capacity of the Element: Ethereal soul

The Liver houses the ethereal soul or Hun (for much of the information on this, I am indebted to Ted Kaptchuk for his inspiring lecture in Oxford, November 1991). The Hun, housed in the Liver, is a kind of "soul-personality", which survives after death. This concept is common to Confucianism, Buddhism and Taoism. To the Chinese, it has the sense of a "thread"; it binds the Shen to the physical body and personality which enacts the individual's life purpose. It is also considered to be the part of our consciousness connected with our "ren" or benevolence during our lifetime. After leaving our body at death, it does not dissolve for three generations, as it is nourished by the remembrance of our descendants. It then joins the clan ancestral spirit, or a cosmic deity, according to different beliefs.

This concept of Hun clearly illustrates the essential role of the individual in harmonious relationship with the group, which is central to our understanding of Wood. Our spiritual existence, according to this idea, is not only our own; it is nourished both by our own "benevolence" during our lifetime and that of our descendants after our death. As individuals, we are part of a larger community also on the spiritual level.

Movement of element energy : upwards

The growth of plants is essentially in all directions; the roots grow downwards and outwards, the shoots upwards and outwards. Similarly, when in a state of balance, the Liver ensures the free moving of Ki in all directions in the body. Wood Ki, however, has all the strength of spring, birth and new beginnings and can easily become too Yang in nature. The movement of Yang is upwards and this is the direction which Wood energy often takes in disharmony. The other imbalanced expression of Wood is stagnation, which usually manifests in a horizontal plane, and this is discussed further in the following section.

Element emotion: anger

Given the basically benevolent nature of Wood, why is anger its characteristic emotion? It is partly because of the strength of the energy involved, as with the blade of grass pushing up through the asphalt in the city. The urge for life and self-expression is so strong that it cannot bear obstruction. In an ideal human culture, this urge would be balanced by an emphasis on the complementary Wood quality of peaceful coexistence. However, it is more usually repressed in our earliest childhood, by the authority figures who surround us. In these circumstances, anger is a way of demanding to be heard.

It is the balance between the strength of the Wood energy and the force of the repression which determines the way in which anger will manifest and the direction of Ki flow which accompanies it. If the urge to live and express is strong the Ki will push upward, like the blade of grass through the asphalt, with the additional impetus of anger behind it. The Nei Jing states that "excess anger causes the Qi to ascend" (Nei Jing Su Wen, Ch. 39, p. 221). If this is our habitual mode of expression, we will manifest anger openly, describing ourselves as having a "short fuse" or a quick temper. The upward movement of Ki which accompanies this tendency may result in violent headaches, eye problems, a red face, high blood pressure and the ensuing complications.

If the force of repression is stronger than the urge to grow, then the anger cannot manifest openly; if the asphalt is too thick, the blade of grass must direct its energy horizontally or in upon itself, seeking expression yet weakened because it cannot get the light and air it needs. Similarly, the movement of Ki in the human body often slows down and creates horizontal blockages, particularly in areas where the body structure is already primarily horizontal, namely the throat, the diaphragm and the pelvic floor. This is where symptoms associated with repressed anger, linked in Oriental medicine with the Liver and Gall Bladder, may manifest. Repressed anger is very common in our society, particularly in women who have been traditionally encouraged to suppress their natural assertiveness; the anger bottled up inside often turns against the self, becoming depression.

When the individual is truly recognized and encouraged to be his or her self, neither anger nor depression is an issue; then the positive qualities of Wood – creativity and harmonious coexistence – can function to their best advantage.

Element colour: green

Green is the colour of the plant kingdom. It is also the diagnostic colour perceived in cases of Liver or Gall Bladder disharmony, around the eyes or mouth. The Chinese word for this colour means "blue-green" and the subtle hue can be this shade, but it is also common to see yellowish green.

These subtle colours come and go – they are not the same as the skin tone, but there is also a particular skin tone common in chronic Liver imbalance which is often described as "sallow" or "olive". It is dark, with a greenish or yellowish tinge.

In some cases, where the Liver or Gall Bladder Ki is rising too strongly, the skin tone can be florid – an unvarying, uniform red.

Element sound: shouting

Shouting is the tone which we adopt when we want to draw attention to what we have to say. We can "shout" in different ways, by amplifying our voice, by projecting it with force or by clipping and shortening our words to convey emphasis.

Most of us do any or all of these things when the occasion calls for it, but when any of them becomes a permanent feature of our speaking voice, it usually indicates a Liver or Gall Bladder imbalance. A voice can be loud or emphatic without sounding angry; it can be clipped without sounding angry; but it is still a shouting voice. When we repress our anger, on the other hand, we usually also repress any tendency to raise our voice or sound assertive, so that a gentle, soft, placatory tone of voice is our invariable mode and this in itself is an indication of a disharmony in Wood. A gentle voice is not in itself a bad sign; it is the inability to depart from it which suggests a problem.

Element odour: rancid

Although the smells which indicate disharmony are usually difficult both to classify and to detect, the smell of Liver and Gall Bladder is the easiest. It is strong, like Wood energy, and has a slight undertone of rotting meat. If you notice an unpleasant smell when you are giving Shiatsu, it is most likely rancid.

Element sense organ: the eyes

Our sense of sight allows us to seize the broad scope of the situation before us, in order to choose a course of action, to "see a clear way forward". This is true on many levels, the practical, physical level, the intellectual level of "far-sighted" planning and decision-making, and the intuitive level on which, through images, we may receive "second sight". Because we must see how the land lies before we can act, the eyes are the domain of Wood.

Problems affecting the eyes, therefore, often indicate a disharmony in Wood. Blurred or fuzzy vision, whether short- or long-sighted, is often a sign of Deficiency of Liver Blood and so are "floaters" in the eyes. Dry, gritty-feeling eyes accompany Liver Yin Deficiency. Red or painful eyes may be a result of Liver Fire and yellowing of the whites of the eyes is associated with Damp Heat in the Gall Bladder.

Element taste: sour

The taste classically associated with Wood is the sour taste, which is astringent or contracting. We can thus relate it to the experience of constriction which arises through unexpressed emotion; often the sensation of a lump in the throat or a knot in the stomach is accompanied by a sour taste, which is the physical manifestation of unpleasant emotions. Imagine sucking a lemon and see what kind of grimace begins to form. Think also of the language we use to describe people who carry repressed anger: "a vinegary old woman", a "sourpuss". Sometimes the sour taste manifests from within, as a permanent taste in the mouth; sometimes the sour taste in foods is particularly craved or, alternatively, disliked.

Element season: spring

It is in spring that the force of Wood can best be seen. There is a particular moment in spring when shoots push up through the soil at a visible rate, a time when the rapidity of change all around can induce a feeling of disorientation. Spring is a time of rebirth after the quiescence of winter; new growth cycles begin and our adaptability and motivation are challenged. For those whose individuality has been suppressed and who feel themselves to be "dead wood", the sap springing all around can be too much to bear. Spring is a revitalizing time for many people, but for those whose Liver or Gall Bladder Ki is out of balance it can bring an intensification of physical and mental discomfort and often symptoms such as headaches get worse at this time.

Wood is associated with all times of beginning, not only with the spring season. Each morning is the beginning of a new cycle and people who feel out of sorts at this time may be experiencing a Liver or Gall Bladder disharmony. The power "to give birth" is traditionally ascribed to Wood and any major life change, whether outer, such as a change of career, or inner, such as a new relationship, can test our adaptability. Men tend to experience this more in the field of achievement of goals; women are also made aware of it in the hormonal cycles within their bodies; each menstrual cycle potentially involves the power to give birth. Wood is linked with the menstrual cycle and also with the menopause, which is a beginning as well as an end, the time when a woman "gives birth" to her mature self.

Element climate: wind

Wind is the aspect of the weather which most resembles Wood, in its force and its ability to change direction. Trees respond to wind; it shakes, strips, prunes and strengthens the strong ones while the weak trees fall. People with an imbalance in Wood often suffer in windy weather. Wind is the most dynamic and penetrating of the climatic influences and can combine with Heat or Cold to "blow" them into the body (see p. 72), giving rise to sudden aches and pains, head colds or other acute infections. Those whose Liver or Gall Bladder Ki is out of balance may be particularly susceptible.

Wind can also affect our moods; the general incidence of depressive illness rises sharply after a prolonged bout of strong wind and certain European countries have their own malefic regional winds such as the French mistral, the Italian tramontana and the Swiss fön, which bring illness and malaise.

A Liver or Gall Bladder imbalance can also allow a condition known as Internal Wind to arise, causing symptoms to move around confusingly, appear and disappear and change without warning. Internal Wind can also cause tremors, spasms or tics to manifest like leaves and branches shaken by the wind. Severe Internal Wind can cause "Wind-Stroke", which the West also calls a stroke, with loss of consciousness and subsequent paralysis or other complications.

Element time of day: 11 pm to 3 am

Although our Wood Ki determines how we face the beginning of our day, the specific times of the Gall Bladder and Liver meridians according to the Chinese Clock (see p. 86) are 11 pm to 1 am and 1 am to 3 am respectively. The diagnostic significance of this is often an increase in energy, so that the individual with a Wood disharmony is wakeful at these times. This tendency to stay awake late, combined with malaise in the morning, often leads to a sense of being a "night person" and a lifestyle which accommodates this preference.

The Liver in TCM

The Liver has vital roles to perform both in connection with Blood, which it stores, and Ki, whose smooth flow it regulates. It therefore has both a storing, or Yin, function and a moving, or Yang, one. However, the tremendous force of energy which the Wood phase embodies means that the Liver and Gall Bladder, the Wood organs, tend to a preponderance of Yang. Even when the Liver fails in its Yang function of moving the Ki, the result is stagnation which is in itself an excessive, or Yang, symptom.

Stores the blood

The Liver is considered to act as a reservoir for the Blood of the whole body. When the body is at rest, all Blood flows back to the Liver where it is stored until needed. When the body requires Blood to nourish the tissues for action, it flows out from the Liver. The Liver can fail in this function in three ways: it can be slow in making the Blood available when it is needed; it can fail to make it available, causing Blood Deficiency; and if the Liver is hot, it can impart Heat to the Blood.

Blood not readily available

If the Liver is slow to release Blood to the muscles when it is required for action then symptoms, particularly stiffness and pain, are worse after rest (the Blood returns to the Liver at rest). Typically, this means that they are worse in the morning on rising, but it can mean that they are worse after sitting down for some time. (This symptom may also arise from a failure of the Liver to move Ki, causing stagnation.)

Blood Deficiency

This can arise as much from the Liver's failure to make the Blood available as from the Spleen's failure to make enough of it. Typical symptoms of general Blood Deficiency are dull, dry skin and hair, a sallow complexion, dizziness, inability to get to sleep, depression and poor memory. In women, menstruation is scanty, with pale blood, or there may be no periods at all. When the Liver is involved, there may be blurred vision, spots in front of the eyes ("floaters"), weak and brittle nails and a tendency to strained or weak tendons.

Heat in the Blood

When the Liver imparts Heat to the Blood, the Blood tends to "move wildly", causing profuse or violent bleeding. Often this manifests as heavy, flooding menstruation but it can also be seen as sudden, heavy nosebleeds, profusely bleeding piles or sudden bleeding from anywhere in the body. In general, bleeding caused by Liver Heat is more violent than bleeding caused by the Spleen's failure to contain the Blood, which is usually characterized by slow leakage. A further symptom of Heat in the Blood can be red and itchy skin disease, such as urticaria.

Governs free flowing of Ki

The Liver is responsible for maintaining a free flow of Ki throughout the meridian network and the whole body. Its action in this respect is described in the texts as "sprinkling" rather than pumping. When the Liver is distributing Ki well, the flow is relaxed, spontaneous and even. When it is not, the result is stagnation, which can occur in any part of the body. Stagnation of Liver Ki is responsible for a host of symptoms, commonest among which are pain accompanied by a feeling of distension, mood swings, depression, premenstrual irritability with painful breasts, menstrual pain, the feeling of a lump in the throat or difficulty in swallowing. There can also be many digestive symptoms such as nausea, hiccups, abdominal distention or pain, constipation or diarrhoea, caused by the stagnant Liver Ki invading the Stomach, Spleen or Intestines. Discomfort in the chest, breathlessness and cough can result from Liver Ki stagnation affecting the Lungs. Characteristically, the symptoms come and go depending on the person's emotional state. If Ki stagnates over a long period of time, it can lead to stagnation of Blood, which is often a more serious condition.

Affected by emotions

If we remember that the nature of the Wood phase of energy is the expression of the individual self, we can see that repression of feelings must affect the Wood organs. In TCM, emotional problems are usually thought to affect the Liver. Disharmonies of Liver Blood and Liver Ki are commonly caused by emotional problems , which impair the Liver's ability to store Blood and "sprinkle" Ki. It is usually the suppression of the emotions which causes the problem, rather than their free expression, and suppressed anger and resentment are the commonest causes of all. Depression is a symptom of both Blood Deficiency and Ki stagnation and this compounds the emotional factor which caused the condition in the first place. It may be difficult for a receiver to "see" the emotional origin of his symptoms, so that "stagnation of Liver Ki" can be a useful concept for explaining the mind–body connection in TCM, thus allowing the receiver to make that connection within himself.

The eyes

The eyes are the sense organs associated with the Wood Element and eye problems are most often part of a Liver or Gall Bladder disharmony (although the Water meridians can also be responsible). The problem can be with vision itself, as in the blurred vision and "floaters" of Blood Deficiency, or with the physical aspect of the eyes: red or bloodshot eyes, dry eyes, painful eyes (see p. 123).

Liver Yin is vulnerable

On the physical level, the energy of the Liver tends to be strong and forceful, or Yang in nature. On the emotional level, the Liver asserts our individual right to growth and self-expression, a Yang function. Therefore, the Yin physical attributes of the Liver which are mainly concerned with the nourishing qualities of Liver Blood, and its Yin emotional attributes, softness, vulnerability and sensitivity to others, are often compromised. If the Yin of the Liver is Deficient, the Yang becomes relatively preponderant and rises upwards, giving symptoms such as headaches on the top of the head, tinnitus or vertigo, accompanied by irritability. Liver Yang rising can also result from deficient Kidney Yin, which fails to nourish the Yin of the Liver (Wood is the "child" of Water in the Creative Cycle of the Elements).

The tendons

The tendons are the body tissues dominated by the Wood Element; the word can also be translated as "sinews" or "muscles". What is meant is the connective tissue which confers strength and elasticity to the muscles and roots them to the bone. When Liver Blood is deficient, the tendons are not nourished and can be easily damaged or strained. Repetitive strain injury is an example of deficient Blood (often depleted by overuse of the eyes at a computer screen) which fails to nourish the tendons. Tendons surround the joints and help to hold them together, so that joint problems may involve the Liver or Gall Bladder.

The nails

The nails are a "residue" of the Wood Element. In clinical practice, cracked, brittle or flaky nails are a sign that Liver Blood is deficient and not nourishing the nails.

The ethereal soul

When reading in the texts that the Liver houses the ethereal soul (Hun in Chinese), one should remember that Chinese philosophy does not, like Western thought, admit the existence of only one soul. The ethereal soul is one of many aspects of the human spirit and is the counterpart of the Po, or corporeal soul, which is housed by the Lungs. The Lungs come at the beginning of the cycle of the meridians and the Po comes into being with the first breath and leaves with the last. The Liver ends the cycle of the meridians and the Hun, which it houses, survives the body after death, though not for ever; the survival time of one's Hun is influenced by the virtue of one's ancestors and the dutiful remembrance of one's descendants. The Hun can leave the body during sleep; this concept of the soul's astral travels is also found in some Western mystical traditions. It is also said to follow the Shen in its comings and goings.

The Liver in Zen Shiatsu theory

The Liver ends the Chinese Clock and thus ends Masunaga's life cycle of the meridians. The physical body has been created and fed, its core of consciousness established; the individual knows how to reproduce, survive threats and how to live in a community. What is there left? The answer could be any or none of the exploratory and creative activities available. The traditional function of the Liver as general, together with the Gall Bladder as assistant officer, is to plan a course of action and put it into practice. To this end, their main physical functions are described by Masunaga as "storing and distribution of nutrients". The Liver is more in charge of storing, the Gall Bladder of distribution, although their roles often overlap. We can see that these two functions reflect the traditional Chinese ones of storing (the Blood) and distributing (the Ki). In Western physiological terms, the liver is in charge of detoxifying, which is the process of storage and distribution in reverse; the liver intercepts toxins and inactivates them before sending them away for disposal. Zen Shiatsu sees all these activities as serving the choice and execution of a life plan – Wood's purpose.

Which way to turn?

The Liver and Gall Bladder meridians run down the sides of the body and the two sides reflect our ability to choose – this way ...or that way? The Liver energy gives us our ability to plan our life path and choose the direction in which we must go. Once the choice has been made, Liver energy gives us the capacity to work hard at realizing it. When the Liver is in harmony, plans are made and executed efficiently and thoroughly but without drama or fuss, since the plans are simply a way of setting in motion our creative self-expression. When the Liver is in disharmony, there may be much discussion of plans without any action being taken or a hyperefficient mapping out of time without any room for spontaneity or an inability to think or plan ahead at all.

Excessive behaviour and detoxification

When, in very early life, the growth of our creative self-expression is repressed and we are not encouraged to make our own choices, our life path does not unfold before us in a natural way. We find ourselves in unfamiliar territory, literally unable to see a way forward to express our creative self. In this situation, working to someone else's plan or expectations and often unaware that there is any alternative, we experience frustration, tension and depression. If we are in the double bind of repressing our feelings, then all the emotional force of the Liver energy will be diverted into some form of distraction. Since we are not in a situation where our spontaneous self-expression can manifest, we develop a conditioned response, a habit pattern. It is very common for people with a Liver imbalance to exhibit patterns of "excessive behaviour". Excessive drinking comes immediately to mind in this connection, but excessive eating may also be a compensatory factor in Liver imbalance. Recreational

drug-taking may be another option. All these patterns temporarily numb emotional pain and anger, but all of them strain the Liver's detoxifying capacity and weaken its physical function. The toxic condition induced by excessive abuse of the body results in headaches and heaviness of the head. If the Liver is extremely weak, even one glass of wine will induce a feeling of being poisoned.

Uneven energy

The Liver plans when to store energy and nutrients and when to release them for distribution. If distribution is poor, the individual will experience bursts of motivation and hard work, followed by periods of extreme fatigue. If there is a stagnation problem, there may be a general loss of vitality, not because there is no energy present but because it is not being distributed. In both cases, there is no healthy alternation between activity and rest.

Uneven emotions

The Liver and Gall Bladder store and distribute emotional as well as physical energy. Emotional inconsistency, mood swings and bursts of emotional display which are swiftly controlled characterize these meridians in imbalance. A classic example of the uneven flow of emotions is premenstrual syndrome. Anger or bad temper is traditionally associated with the Liver meridian, but this is not always the case. Heightened emotional reactivity of any kind may be shown, causing feelings which appear unusually intense in the circumstances (e.g. excessive jealousy) or inappropriate (bursting into tears at the thought of a loved one). When the Liver is not appropriately distributing emotional energy, feelings may surface too suddenly to be expressed diplomatically and the Liver imbalanced person may acquire a reputation for tactlessness and inappropriate remarks. Often the unmanageable feelings are covered up or repressed, however, and it is the repression of emotion which is the most harmful, since it may manifest instead as physical symptoms.

Aggression or timidity

The Liver makes us sensitive to others, in keeping with the group connectedness of the Wood Element.

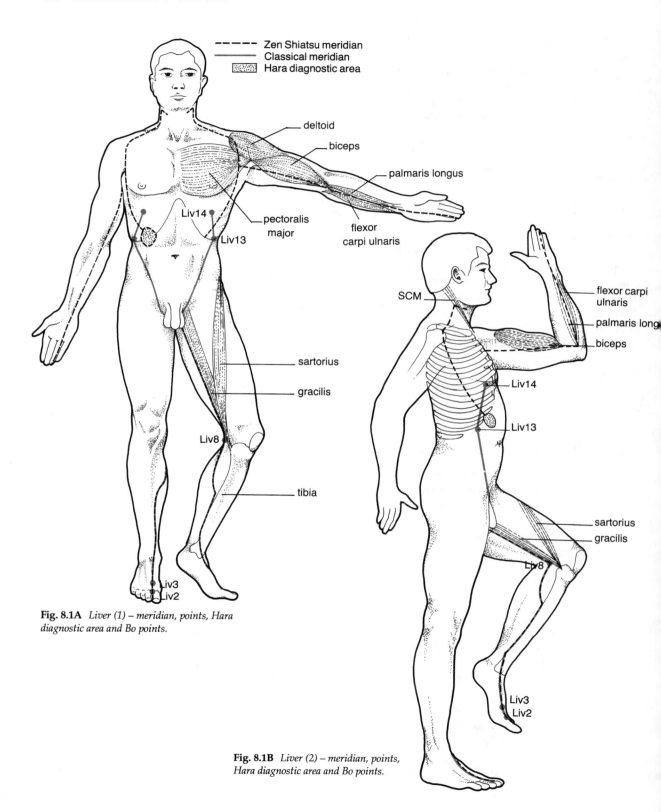

Zen Shiatsu meridian
Classical meridian
Hara diagnostic area

deltoid
biceps
palmaris longus
flexor
carpi ulnaris

Liv14
Liv13

pectoralis
major

sartorius
gracilis

Liv8

tibia

Liv3
Liv2

SCM

flexor carpi
ulnaris
palmaris long
biceps

Liv14

Liv13

sartorius
gracilis

Liv8

Liv3
Liv2

Fig. 8.1A *Liver (1) – meridian, points, Hara diagnostic area and Bo points.*

Fig. 8.1B *Liver (2) – meridian, points, Hara diagnostic area and Bo points.*

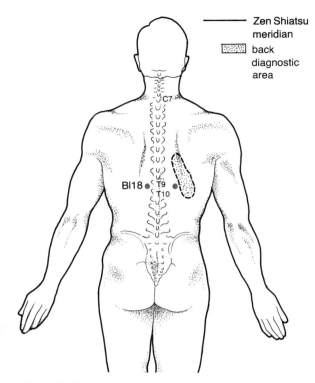

Zen Shiatsu meridian

back diagnostic area

Fig. 8.1C *Liver (3) – back diagnostic area and Yu points.*

In harmony, the Wood energy allows peaceful coexistence with others, each individual expressing his or her self in the context of the group. If it is in disharmony, the way in which we perceive others is directly influenced by our own capacity for self-expression. We may see others as mere obstructions in our path, to be brushed aside; or we may see them as powerful and potentially threatening figures to be placated; it depends on how powerful we feel ourselves to be. In the former case, our own life path is seen to be more important than anything else and we act agressively; in the latter, our own life path and choices have very low priority and we are unable to assert ourselves.

Genital and reproductive problems

The Liver meridian runs through the genitals and problems in this area, and in the pelvic floor generally, may result from a Liver imbalance. Pain in the testicles, prostate problems, inflammation of the female reproductive organs and impotence are all

mentioned by Masunaga as being Liver-related. Pain in the sacrum and coccyx and haemorrhoids are also local conditions, resulting from muscular pulling on the pelvic floor.

Stiffness of muscles

A Liver disharmony means a lack of flexibility in body and mind. In TCM, the Liver rules the tendons and Liver Blood nourishes them. In Zen Shiatsu, too, general stiffness and inflexibility and weak joints come from a Liver imbalance.

The Liver meridian and how to treat it

The traditional Liver meridian begins on the lateral side of the big toenail and ascends the dorsum of the foot between the first and second metatarsals, to the medial side of the ankle. From there it runs on the posterior border of the tibia to a point two-thirds of the way up the leg, where it begins to curve away from the bone towards the medial end of the knee crease. It runs up the inside of the thigh, under the gracilis muscle, through the genitals, up the groin and the lateral abdomen to the sixth intercostal space.

Masunaga's extended version travels from the Liver diagnostic area on the right of the Hara (and from the equivalent position on the left side), up the side of the body, posterior to the Spleen meridian; it follows the line of the axillary fold up in front of the shoulder, from where a branch travels down the arm, in the seam between the triceps and the biceps, in a line between the Heart Protector and Heart meridians to the fourth finger. From the front of the shoulder the meridian goes up the side of the neck, in the groove between the sternocleidomastoid and the trapezius. A branch travels horizontally towards the pharynx and the meridian ascends above it to meet the Gall Bladder meridian where the earlobe joins the jaw.

The diagnostic area for the Liver on the Hara is below the ribcage on the right side, over the Liver organ itself.

The diagnostic area on the back lies to the right of the spine, roughly from the seventh to the tenth

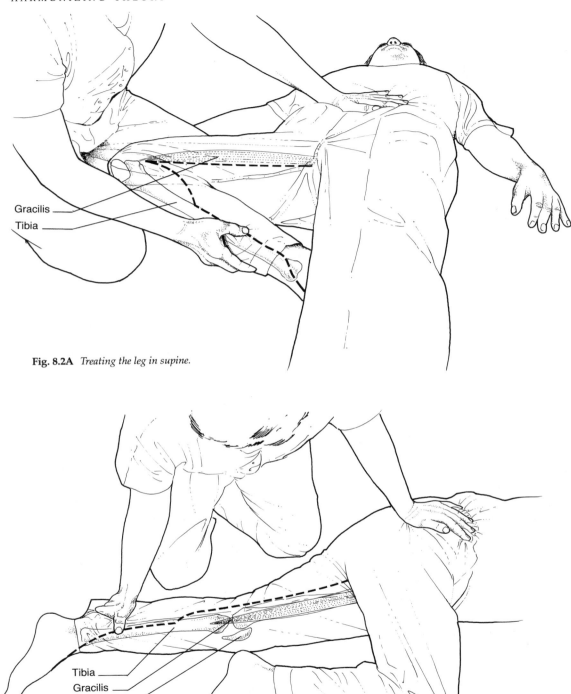

Gracilis
Tibia

Fig. 8.2A *Treating the leg in supine.*

Tibia
Gracilis
Patella

Fig. 8.2B *Treating the leg in side position.*

thoracic vertebrae, sloping laterally out under the inferior angle of the right scapula towards the Small Intestine meridian.

Treatment procedure

1. On the leg, the meridian can be treated in supine when placed in the meridian stretch with the toe laid to the opposite knee. The giver may need to support the leg by anchoring it between her own. With her mother hand on the receiver's Hara, the giver works the meridian with her plam or thumb, angling her pressure to reach under the gracilis muscle on the midline of the inner thigh. Her hand turns to grasp the shinbone when working the meridian down the edge of the tibia on the lower leg (Fig. 8.2A).
2. Alternatively, the meridian is exposed on the lower leg in the side position and can be worked with palm and thumb, with the giver's mother hand resting on the uppermost hip or the sacrum. (Fig. 8.2B)
3. On the torso, the Liver meridian curves up the ribcage between the Spleen and the Large Intestine. It is best treated bilaterally in supine with the fingertips, to accommodate the spaces between the ribs (Fig. 8.3A).

4. It can be treated in the side position, with perpendicular pressure of fingertips or thumb, the mother hand supporting the top of the shoulder. This technique can lead into treating the meridian in the shoulder, as described in point 5 (Fig. 8.3B).
5. The giver's mother hand supports the scapula, while the thumb of her working hand penetrates

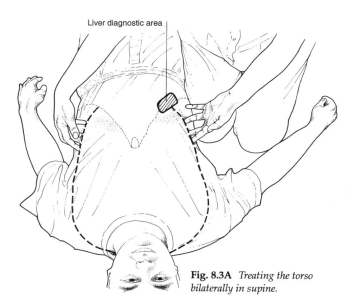

Fig. 8.3A *Treating the torso bilaterally in supine.*

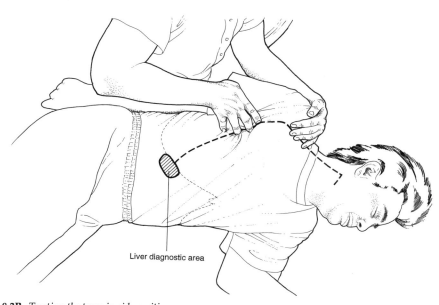

Fig. 8.3B *Treating the torso in side position.*

deeply into the groove between the humerus and the upper ribs, at a horizontal angle (Fig. 8.4).

6. The meridian in the neck is most easily felt in supine, with the head turned to open the valley between the sternocleidomastoid and the trapezius. When working down the side of the neck with a straight thumb, the horizontal branch of the meridian is perceived as a flatter area pointing towards the Adam's apple. When the giver's thumb is lying on this horizontal flat area, the vertical part of the meridian travels down the neck in a line level with the base of her thumb. The meridian is worked with gentle thumb pressure, either in this position (Fig. 8.5) or in the side position, with the giver facing the receiver's head and supporting the top of his shoulder with her mother hand.

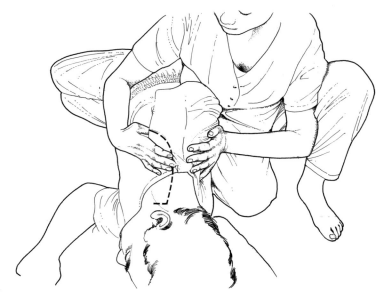

Fig. 8.4 *The shoulder.*

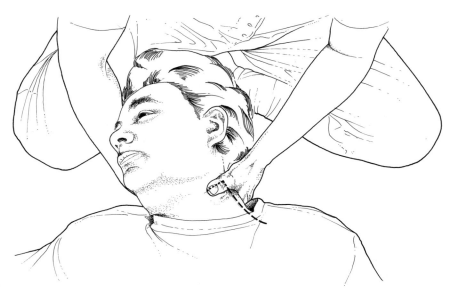

Fig 8.5 *The neck.*

Major points on the Liver meridian

Liver 2

At the base of the lateral side of the big toe, just distal to the joint between the metatarsal and the phalanges.

Actions

- Cools Blood
- Clears Liver Fire and subdues Liver Yang

Liver 3

On the dorsum of the foot, just distal to the junction of the first and second metatarsals.

Actions

- Source point
- Promotes the smooth flow of Liver Ki
- Expels Interior Wind (spasms, cramps and tics)
- Subdues Liver Yang
- Calms the mind

Liver 8

At the medial end of the knee crease when the knee is flexed, posterior to the medial condyle of the tibia.

Actions

- Eliminates Dampness from the Bladder and Lower Burner
- Nourishes the Blood

Liver 13

On the side of the abdomen, below the free end of the eleventh floating rib.

Actions

- Bo point of the Spleen
- Eliminates stagnation
- Harmonizes Liver and Spleen

Liver 14

On the nipple line, between the sixth and seventh ribs.

Actions

- Bo point of the Liver
- Cools the Blood
- Harmonizes Liver and Stomach

Liver Yu Point

Bl 18 – two fingers' width from the midline of the spine, level with the lower border of the spinous process of T9.

Liver Bo Point

Liv 14 – see above.

The Gall Bladder in TCM

The Gall Bladder, being the only Yang organ which does not open to the exterior or process food or waste products, occupies a special place in the TCM system. It is also the only Yang organ to be formally allocated any mental or spiritual capacity. It aids the Liver in many of its functions, but its sphere of influence is mainly the Yang one of Ki and it does not have the Liver's profound involvement with the Blood.

The Gall Bladder meridian is one of the three long Yang postural meridians and supports the sides of the body, as the Stomach supports the front and the Bladder the back. For this reason, and because the Wood Element governs the tendons, it can be very important in postural problems.

Stores and excretes bile

This function, which is the only role of the gall bladder in Western terms, is part of the Gall Bladder's responsibility as assistant to the Liver. Through this function, it helps with the smooth distribution of Liver Ki in the abdominal area and if it fails to do so, symptoms of Ki stagnation obstructing the Stomach, Spleen, Intestines or Lungs may result (see p. 125). Because bile is a "pure" fluid, in other words it does not enter the body as food nor leave it as waste, it is considered to impart clarity and impartiality to the Gall Bladder for its mental and spiritual roles.

Decision-making

Whereas the Liver, the general, makes long term plans, the Gall Bladder, the officer in the field, makes moment-to-moment decisions. Occupations which place undue strain on the decision-making faculty over a long period, such as high-level executive positions, can result in Gall Bladder disharmony with resulting physical symptoms, the commonest of which are neck and shoulder tension and headaches.

Clarity and organization

The clarity associated with the pure bile, together with the swift decision-making capacity of a healthy Gall Bladder, combine to give the ability to set physical and mental environments in order. "The Gall is the palace of tidiness" (Nan Jing 16, Yu Shu's Commentary, p. 226). Careful organization and tidiness occur naturally as a result of healthy Gall Bladder function, but can become an obsessive concern when the Gall Bladder is in disharmony. If spontaneity and creative decision-making are impaired, the Wood energy can be channelled into creating a rigidly organized environment instead.

Gall

We use the word "gall" in English to denote daring (as in "How you have the gall to tell me..."). In both the Chinese and Japanese languages, the same usage occurs. The decision-making of the Gall Bladder must necessarily involve the ability to take risks, as well as the determination to stand by the decisions once made. When the Gall Bladder is deficient, there is timidity, hesitation and a reluctance to take risks.

Eyes, tendons and joints

The meridian begins at the eyes and since the Gall Bladder, with the Liver, rules the tendons and the elasticity of the muscles, it enables us to make the connection between our perception and our physical response, in order to make decisions and carry them out. Poor vision and poor muscular coordination may make us clumsy and accident-prone. Weak tendons and poorly circulated joints may make us inactive physically and susceptible to injury, and arthritis is also a possibility later in life.

The meridian

The Gall Bladder meridian is geared towards action. It gives to the physical body what the Gall Bladder energy confers on the mental level: flexibility, coordination and balance. It runs down the sides of the body, so that whenever we lift one foot off the ground, in walking and running, it supports the other side to stop us overbalancing. It keeps the hips level, gives side-to-side flexibility to the torso, strengthens the shoulders and supports the sideways bending of the neck. The flexibility of all these areas is compromised if the Gall Bladder is in disharmony. The meridian also covers the sides of the head several times, indicating its importance in mental decision-making. If the Gall Bladder is out of balance, temporal headaches are a common symptom and migraine headaches affecting one or both sides, with the associated visual disturbances, may also result.

The Gall Bladder in Zen Shiatsu theory

The Gall Bladder has a fairly fleshed-out portrait in TCM, for a Yang organ, and the Masunaga model does not have to elaborate much upon it, only to refine it. The psychological characteristics are already there in TCM; by an unusual reversal, it is Zen Shiatsu which adds a category of physical symptoms, those of digestion.

The sides

More significantly than the Liver, the Gall Bladder's domains of influence are the sides of the body. Whereas the Liver makes choices on a long term, internalized, Yin basis and its meridian is on the insides of the legs near the midline of the body, the Gall Bladder in its Yang, decision-making capacity requires the scope of a 180° angle in order to turn from one direction to another and its meridian runs down the lateral sides of the body. Among the physical problems related to the meridian pathway (such as eye disorders, headaches and hip, neck and shoulder pain), pain or problems in the flanks (the sides of the abdomen and ribcage) are very common with a Gall Bladder imbalance, whether or not they are related to an actual gall bladder disorder.

Occasionally, when looking at the receiver's energy (see p. 231), a split can be seen between the left and right sides of the body, so that each side expresses a different quality of energy and different physical characteristics. In practice, this often reflects a conflict between two facets of the receiver's personality which the receiver is unable to resolve. Instead of harmonizing (for example) his feeling nature with his analytical approach to life and expressing both, the receiver feels impelled to choose one or the other. Since we cannot suppress a part of our nature in this way, the rejected "side" will often seek expression in the bodily energy and posture, leading to a left–right split. This is often seen accompanying a Gall Bladder disharmony. The major point of conflict is often in the hips and sacrum, where the two sides meet, via a deep Gall Bladder pathway to the sacrum, and sciatica or hip pain is often a result.

Control of digestive juices

The Gall Bladder is considered in Zen Shiatsu theory to control and regulate the release not only of bile, but of the other secretions necessary for digestion (the production and quality of these is the province of the Spleen). Consequently it is involved in many aspects of digestive dysfunction, which would be explained in TCM terms as the Liver invading the Spleen. In clinical practice, a Gall Bladder diagnosis usually accompanies a variety of digestive symptoms, such as heartburn, nausea, constipation or diarrhoea, pain or hyperacidity, belching and flatulence.

Inflexibility

The Gall Bladder promotes our physical suppleness as well as our psychological flexibility. The general tone and looseness of our framework is influenced by the Gall Bladder so that muscular stiffness or, less frequently, hypermobility, can result from an imbalance in its energy. The Achilles tendon is often treated in Zen Shiatsu to release and strengthen the joints and tendons. Although it is on neither the Gall Bladder nor the Liver meridian, it exerts a strong influence on all the tendons, by virtue of being the largest tendon in the body.

Discrimination and impartiality

In order to make decisions, the Gall Bladder must have a keen ability to discriminate – clear and accurate vision. In order that this faculty is not coloured by bias or clouded by emotion, a high degree of impartiality is also needed. In a Gall Bladder disharmony, it is possible that either or both of these qualities are deficient or overemphasized.

Without discrimination between potential courses of action it is impossible to decide correctly, so that we are either tormented by indecision or we make the wrong decision. Either way, there is a tremendous feeling of threat and pressure and a desire to escape the necessity to decide. Without impartiality, on the other hand, we make decisions on the basis of our emotions at the time, without reference to the wider view of events or the needs of others. Such decisions, although they may solve our short term dilemmas, do not serve our ultimate life purpose and may harm other people.

If we invest too much of ourselves in the qualities of discrimination and impartiality, without regard to their purpose, which is to help us make decisions to further our life plan, the result is overconcern for details and an attitude which is colloquially described as "being unable to see the wood for trees".

The Gall Bladder meridian and how to treat it

The classical Gall Bladder meridian begins at the lateral corner of the eye and descends to the jaw before zigzagging twice over the side of the head, including the mastoid process and the forehead in its path. After reaching the occipital ridge, it then descends the upper border of trapezius down the neck to the midpoint of the shoulder, where it goes internal, re-emerging below the armpit to take a zigzag path diagonally covering the ribcage, waistline and hips. From the lateral side of the buttock it descends the midline of the lateral aspect of the leg, following the iliotibial tract in the upper leg and the fibula in the lower leg, crossing in front of the lateral malleolus to travel between the fourth and fifth metatarsals to the lateral side of the fourth toe (Fig. 8.6A).

The Masunaga Gall Bladder meridian diverges from the classical one in three respects. Firstly, where the classical meridian travels upward from the jaw to the temporal region and from there posteriorly around the ear down to the mastoid, Masunaga's meridian does the opposite. It moves from the jaw below the ear (where it connects with the Liver) to the mastoid process, then down to the back of the neck, whence it ascends to cover the side of the head, in roughly the same pathway as the classical meridian but in the opposite direction. This change of direction makes little difference to the treatment of the meridian.

Secondly, where the classical meridian travels internally between the top of the shoulder and the ribcage, Masunaga traces its pathway from the top of the shoulder around the vertebral border of the scapula and across to the midaxillary line on the ribcage, before it crosses around the back of the arm to follow a straight pathway down the midline of the Yang surface of the arm to the middle finger. (In keeping with the Gall Bladder's military character, if we stand to attention with the middle finger pointing down the outside trouser seam, the meridian describes a straight pathway down both arm and leg, from shoulder to ankle.) The addition of the pathway around the scapula is very useful in practice for treating Gall Bladder-related shoulder problems, since it incorporates the sensitive scapular edge into the meridian.

Thirdly, Masunaga's Gall Bladder pathway over the torso and hip is substantially different from the classical meridian. Whereas the classical meridian comes forward on to the nipple line on the front of the ribs, then goes back to the free end of the twelfth rib, behind and slightly above the waistline, Masunaga's meridian does not go to the front of the body at all and on the back it goes to the end of the eleventh, not the twelfth rib, according to the charts. This may be due to inaccurate annotation or simply to the flexible Japanese attitude towards meridian and point location, mentioned on p. 86.

The classical meridian goes forward on the hips to within the anterior superior iliac spine and then back to GB 30 on the side of the buttock before taking its straight course down the lateral leg. Masunaga's meridian takes a straight path down the side of the body from the end of the eleventh rib, down the gluteus medius and straight over the greater

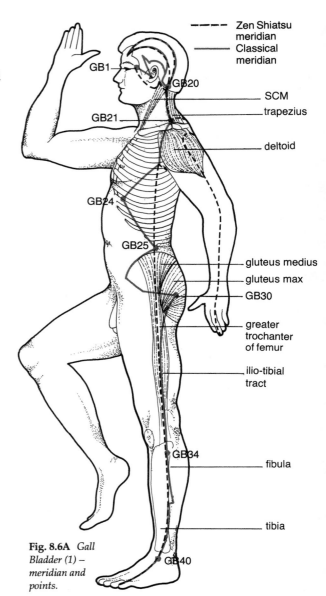

Fig. 8.6A *Gall Bladder (1) – meridian and points.*

trochanter of the femur down the side of the leg. The major difference between the two versions of the meridian on the torso is that the classical Gall Bladder makes pronounced zigzags towards the front and back of the body, almost as if sewing them together, and the Masunaga meridian does not. A possible explanation is that the classical Gall Bladder meridian is alone in supporting the sides of the body, while the Stomach holds up the front and the Bladder supports the back. In the Zen Shiatsu meridian network,

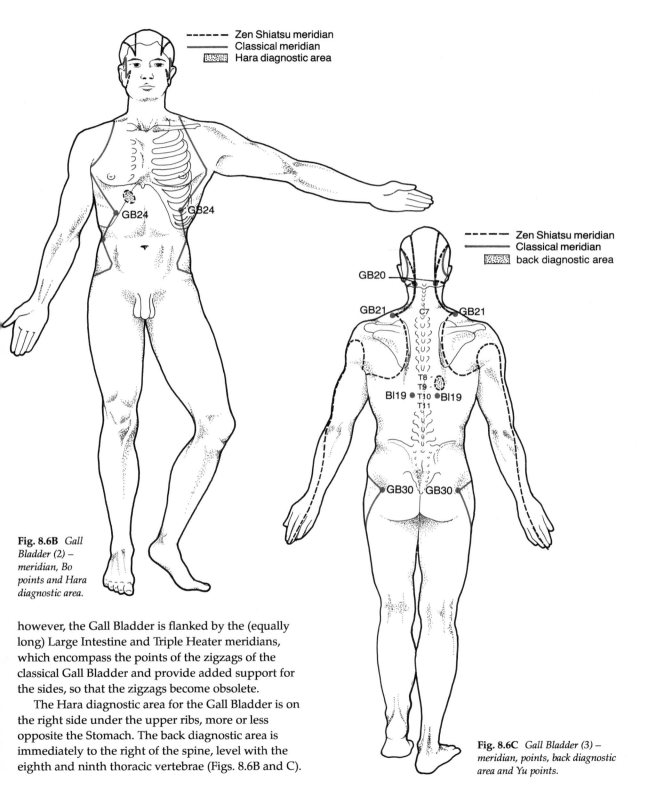

Zen Shiatsu meridian
Classical meridian
Hara diagnostic area

GB24

GB24

Zen Shiatsu meridian
Classical meridian
back diagnostic area

GB20

GB21   C7   GB21

T8
T9
Bl19 T10 Bl19
T11

GB30 GB30

Fig. 8.6B *Gall Bladder (2) – meridian, Bo points and Hara diagnostic area.*

Fig. 8.6C *Gall Bladder (3) – meridian, points, back diagnostic area and Yu points.*

however, the Gall Bladder is flanked by the (equally long) Large Intestine and Triple Heater meridians, which encompass the points of the zigzags of the classical Gall Bladder and provide added support for the sides, so that the zigzags become obsolete.

The Hara diagnostic area for the Gall Bladder is on the right side under the upper ribs, more or less opposite the Stomach. The back diagnostic area is immediately to the right of the spine, level with the eighth and ninth thoracic vertebrae (Figs. 8.6B and C).

Treatment procedure

The Gall Bladder meridian is most accessible in the side position, but most of it can also be treated in prone and some parts in supine and sitting.

1. The meridian on the side of the head is only really accessible in the side position. The lower of the two pathways of the meridian is discernible as a groove in the temporal area, approximately 1½ inches away from the border of the ear, and can be palmed and thumbed with the giver in the lunge position with her mother hand supporting the receiver's forehead (Fig. 8.7).

2. The uppermost of the two head pathways is easier to reach in the supine position. It travels in a straight line up from GB 14, one-third of the distance between the midpoint of the eyebrow and the natural hairline, lateral to the Bladder meridian. It is thumbed only, not palmed (Fig. 8.8).

3. In the neck, the meridian can be reached in side position, as shown (Fig. 8.9), pulling the receiver's shoulder slightly downwards with the mother hand to stretch the meridian. From GB 20 it descends the groove between the sternocleidomastoid and the trapezius, slightly anterior to the border of the trapezius. It can also be worked in supine, by turning the head to expose the meridian and supporting it in that stretch (see p. 48) while the meridian is thumbed. It can also be worked with the receiver in the sitting position.

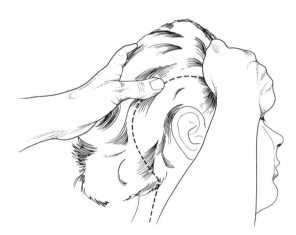

Fig. 8.7 *The side of the head.*

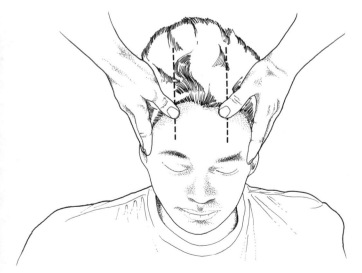

Fig. 8.8 *The forehead and top of the head.*

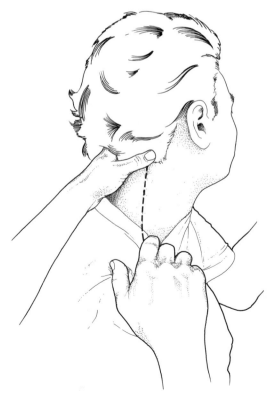

Fig. 8.9 *The neck.*

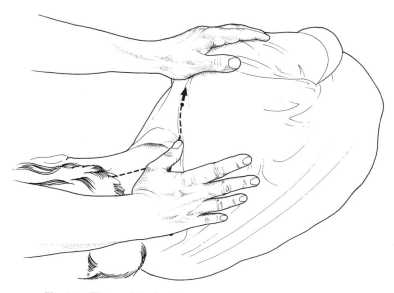

Fig. 8.10 *The top of the shoulder.*

4. On top of the shoulder, the meridian can be palmed and thumbed from behind the receiver's head in the side position, as shown (Fig. 8.10), pushing the receiver's shoulder slightly downwards to stretch the meridian, or in the prone position, and it can be worked with the elbows in sitting position (see p. 56). It runs along the upper border of the trapezius.

5. The Gall Bladder around the scapula can be reached in prone, side or sitting position by means of the "shoulder slash". This is illustrated in Chapter 4 for both side and sitting positions. Here is the prone version. The receiver's arm is in a half nelson. The giver's working thumb is angled towards the palm of the supporting hand. The movement from the supporting hand as it lifts the joint should be less than the pressure downwards from the working hand. The meridian lies just underneath the edge of the scapula and the slight lifting movement is necessary to expose it (Fig. 8.11).

6. In the arm, the Gall Bladder is most accessible in the side position when, if the receiver's arm is laid along his side, it is on top of the arm, on the midline. It can also be elbowed in the sitting position, with the receiver's arm laid over the

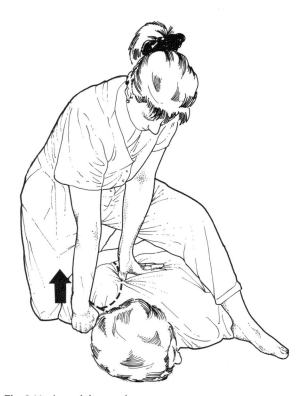

Fig. 8.11 *Around the scapula.*

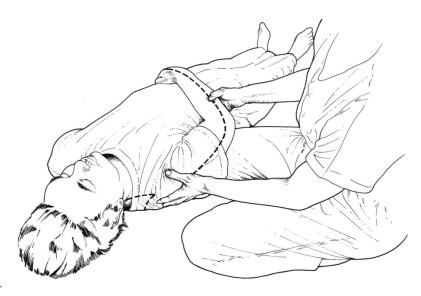

Fig. 8.12 *The arm meridian stretch.*

giver's raised thigh (see p. 58). In Fig. 8.12, the
supine position is illustrated, with the receiver's
arm stretched over his body towards the opposite
hip. The meridian follows the midline of the arm,
taking the insertion of the deltoid muscle and the
middle finger as landmarks. It can be palmed and
thumbed. Care should be taken to support the
receiver's arm with a mother hand on the
shoulder and the giver's knee underneath
(Fig. 8.12).

7. The Gall Bladder on the side of the torso can only
   be reached comfortably in the side position. It can
   be worked as shown in Chapter 4 (p. 54) or with
   both hands together, using the Dragon's Mouth
   (double) as shown, instead of palming (Fig.8.13),
   and both thumbs together for thumbing.

8. In the hip, the meridian goes straight down from
   the side of the waist over the gluteus medius and
   just behind the greater trochanter of the femur. It
   is most easily reached in the side position, where
   it can be palmed, thumbed and elbowed, though
   it can also be worked in the prone position, as
   shown, with the giver lowering her centre of
   gravity in order to achieve perpendicular
   penetration, which in this instance means
   horizontal penetration (Fig. 8.14).

9. The meridian in the leg is easily palmed and
   thumbed in the side position, as shown, where it

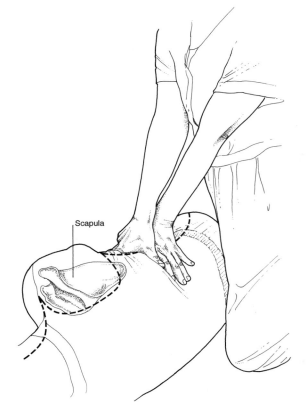

Scapula

Fig. 8.13 *The side of the torso.*

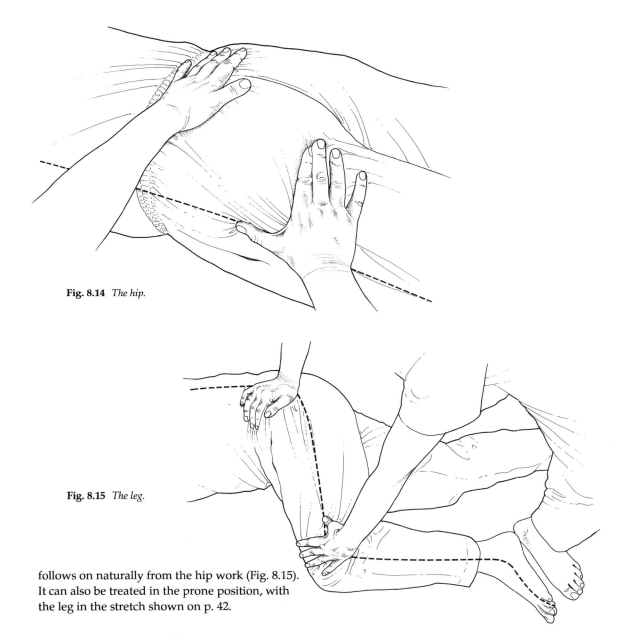

Fig. 8.14 *The hip.*

Fig. 8.15 *The leg.*

follows on naturally from the hip work (Fig. 8.15). It can also be treated in the prone position, with the leg in the stretch shown on p. 42.

Major points on the Gall Bladder meridian

Gall Bladder 1

In the depression just lateral to the orbit, level with the outer canthus.

Actions
An effective local point for all eye problems and for migraine headaches.

Gall Bladder 14

On the forehead, one thumb's width above the midpoint of the eyebrow.

Actions

- Eliminates Exterior wind
- Local point for one-sided headaches

Gall Bladder 20

Below the occiput, within the hairline, between the trapezius and the sternocleidomastoid.

Actions

- Expels Interior and Exterior Wind
- Subdues Liver Yang
- Benefits the eyes and ears
- Clears the brain

Gall Bladder 21

On top of the shoulder, halfway between GV 14 and the acromion.

Actions

This point has a strong downward movement and is thus helpful in:

- reducing neck and shoulder stiffness
- helping in labour and delivery (at the pushing stage)
- increasing the let-down of milk in nursing mothers.

   DO NOT USE DURING PREGNANCY

Gall Bladder 24

On the nipple line, between the seventh and eighth ribs (one rib below Liv 14).

Actions

- Bo point of the Gall Bladder
- Clears Damp Heat from Gall Bladder and Liver
- Encourages the free flow of Liver Ki

Gall Bladder 25

On the side of the torso, on the lower border of the free end of the twelfth floating rib.

Actions

- Bo point of the Kidney

Gall Bladder 30

One third of the distance between the greater trochanter of the femur and the sacral hiatus.

Actions

- Tonifies Ki and Blood
- Removes Damp-Heat from the groin and anal area
- Meeting point of Bladder and Gall Bladder (thus an important point for aligning the hip area)

Gall Bladder 34

 In the depression anterior and inferior to the head of the fibula.

Actions

- Relaxes the tendons
- Encourages the free flow of Liver Ki

Gall Bladder 40

In the depression anterior and inferior to the lateral malleolus.

Actions

- Source point of the Gall Bladder
- Encourages the free flow of Liver Ki

Gall Bladder Yu Point

B1 19 – Two fingers width lateral to the midline of the spine, level with the lower border of the spinous process of T10.

Gall Bladder Bo point

GB 24 – see above.

9

The Fire Element – The Heart, Small Intestine, Heart Protector and Triple Heater

■ *"Having purified the great delusion, the heart's darkness, the radiant light of the unobscured sun continuously rises".*

H. H. DUDJOM RINPOCHE

Element associations: transforming power, light, warmth, excitement, movement, responsiveness

Fire is one of the contradictory Elements (the other being Water). It has been one of mankind's great benefactors, warming our hearths, cooking our food, forging our metal; and at the same time it is the swiftest and most ferocious destroyer, whether raging out of control in a dry forest or powering bullets and bombs. Even the sun itself, source of all our light, warmth and well-being, can parch and burn if we do not guard against its power. The ultimate form of Fire as annihilator is the nuclear weapon, "brighter than a thousand suns".

The nature of the power of fire is its capacity to transform. It is the agent of swift and irreversible change: wood burns to leave charcoal, then ash; dough expands and solidifies to become bread; clay hardens into porcelain; chemicals combine to create new substances. Fire destroys one form in order to create another. This power of transformation, which we now take for granted, was so astonishing to early peoples that they worshipped fire as a divine manifestation. As philosophies and theologies became more sophisticated, many, including Taoism, adopted the metaphor of fire as a symbol of transformation and rebirth, through the destruction of physical form in order to obtain the pure essence of spirit.

Although we no longer think of fire as divine power, it remains a dominant symbol in religious imagery but its destructive aspect is now usually ignored. Light, fire's accompaniment, is continually used as a metaphor for divinity and some form of fire is present at most religious ceremonies, from the candles of the Christian church to the butter lamps of Tibetan Buddhism. It is as if the radiance, the glow and warmth of these man-made lights are symbolic of the same qualities in the human spirit, of what is sometimes called "the divine spark within".

Gazing into a fire is one of the best ways of attuning the conscious mind to the unconscious. The movement and flicker of fire provides a natural strobe effect which encourages the mind to produce alpha waves, those associated with calmness and insight, and to flow in creative ways. For this reason the hearth has traditionally been the focus for social groups to express both their sense of community and their creativity by telling stories and singing songs. The warmth and comfort of the fire encourages relaxation and togetherness; the flickering, moving light induces a peaceful and creative frame of mind.

When fire is burning in a contained situation, as in a hearth, its Yang power is tamed and it exhibits the Yin quality of responsiveness. The slightest breath of air causes the shape of the flame to change and move. It also has an affinity for that which it consumes, its source; watching a sheet of flame wrap itself around the underside of a burning log, we can understand the name of the Fire hexagram in the *I Ching*, "Li, the Clinging".

When a fire burns fiercely and high, however, it has a more excitatory effect. It is the most Yang of the elements and its heat, movement and energy can encourage excitement at a time when passions are running high. Fire always accompanies riot and rebellion; it is a quick and easy means of destruction and it also mirrors, reaffirms and excites the feelings of the mob.

Both aspects of Fire are expressed in Oriental medicine. On the one hand, the meridians of the Fire Element embody the light, radiance and responsiveness of Spirit as contained in human consciousness; on the other, Fire can exist within the body as uncontrolled destructive energy, often fuelled by emotion. The latter kind of Fire is not exclusive to the Fire meridians, since it can originate in the Stomach or Liver, as well as the Heart. To distinguish it from the body's intrinsic Fire Ki, I have called it "pathogenic Fire" throughout.

The inter-relationship of the Fire meridians

Since Fire is the only Element to be represented by two pairs of meridians, an examination is necessary here of the dynamics of their relationship.

The central Fire function is that of the Heart, which houses the Shen, or consciousness. It is at this point that medical theory merges with Oriental cosmology and philosophy. Inasmuch as consciousness belongs to the Fire element, it is equated metaphorically with light, with the divine spark within each sentient being which is unique to each individual, yet is a part of the greater radiance of universal consciousness. Although sometimes translated as Spirit, the Shen, the light of consciousness, does not have to be spiritual; it is the awareness and presence which guides our every action, however ordinary.

The various organs are often referred to in the medical texts as government officials. In this context, the Heart holds the place of Emperor. The Emperor was considered to be the Son of Heaven in ancient China, the embodiment on earth of divine authority. Similarly, the Heart, in housing the Shen, provides a physical home for the divine part of ourselves.

As the emperor, the central figure in the government of the bodymind territory, the Heart requires protection. All the other meridians of the Fire Element are in different ways protectors of the

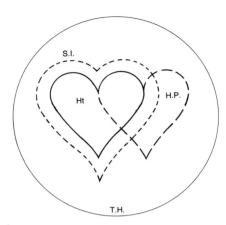

Fig. 9.1 *The inter-relationships within the Fire Element.*

Heart or messengers which help to extend its influence. Their boundaries therefore overlap and all the Fire meridians are to some degree extensions of the Heart energy.

The Small Intestine protects the Heart by fending off immediate danger, like the official taster who intercepts poisoned food. The Heart Protector protects in a different way, by mediating between the Heart and the surface via the circulation; in the texts, the Heart Protector is likened to an ambassador, but since it also takes on some of the Heart's workload, we could think of it as a deputy for the Emperor on a more significant level, as a Prime Minister or Grand Vizier. The Triple Heater also has an ambassadorial function, conveying the Source Ki to all the organs of the Three Burning Spaces, thus mediating between the three districts of the realm.

We could depict these relationships in a diagram (Fig. 9.1). The Heart, or emperor, occupies the central position, closely protected by his bodyguard, the Small Intestine. The place of the Prime Minister, the Heart Protector, overlaps with that of the Heart and its sphere of influence is carried further by that of the Triple Heater, which represents the Fire Element throughout the bodymind territory.

These functions and inter-relationships will be discussed further when dealing with the individual meridians of the Fire Element.

Ming-Men

The metaphor of the Heart as Emperor in the classical texts is carried further by the differentiation of the

Fire Element into "sovereign Fire" (the Heart) and "ministerial or helping Fire". The ministerial Fire is variously interpreted by different commentaries as the Heart Protector, which extends the "will of the Heart" throughout the body, or as Ming-Men, the Fire within the Kidneys. This tiny but fiercely burning flame is appropriately named the Gate of Vitality (the literal translation of Ming-men). Ming-Men, which is discussed further in the section on the Triple Heater, signifies the union of Fire and Water, Yang meeting with Yin. Since consciousness is Yang and form is Yin, the Fire within the Kidneys, which unifies the two, is at the root of our existence; it is also represented by the "moving Ki between the Kidneys" which is the generative force in the Hara. Form (Yin) needs energy (Yang) to activate it and help it grow. The Source Ki and Essence, which are the basis of Yang and Yin in the body, emerge via Ming-Men, the Gate of Vitality.

Spiritual capacity of the Element: Shen

According to some authorities, the Shen is best translated as 'spirit', according to others as 'mind'; in which case, how does one interpret 'mind'? It is not the thinking intellect, which is the Spleen's domain. It represents consciousness but so, in one form or another, do all of the spiritual capacities of the Elements, for example the ethereal soul belonging to the Liver, which is said to follow the Shen in its comings and goings. It has a connection with virtue, whose Chinese character contains the Heart radical, and its nature is to radiate or shine out.

Although Chinese medicine derives from the pre-Buddhist era, it seems that the concept of Shen is similar to the Buddhist idea of mind as pure awareness in its unattached state, sometimes called Buddha-nature. Buddha-nature exists in all beings and, according to Buddhist teaching, enlightenment comes with recognition and identification with that awareness in its pure state within oneself. It is therefore both divine and rooted in the physical body; a treasure unique to each living being, yet present in all beings.

Awareness is Buddha-nature only when it is completely pure and unattached – "empty" is the unappealing translation often used. So, too, the mind is Shen only when free of attachment. It provides a clear, aware space in which all our spiritual and

mental capacities can operate to produce action and fulfil our individual destiny. This may be why the collective name for the spiritual capacities is the "five Shen"; they are grouped together under the Shen of the Heart, which contains them all yet is itself spacious, clear and luminous, like the sky.

Yet the Shen of the Heart must remain anchored in reality, responding to the demands of all physical circumstances. This is the nature of "propriety", the virtue which results from correct use of the Heart's spiritual capacity. When pure awareness, free from attachment, engages with the demands of physical existence, correct and appropriate behaviour results. In this way, the Shen is the link between Heaven and Earth, as the emperor, the Son of Heaven, was considered to embody heaven on Earth in his rulership.

Movement of element energy: outwards

The movement of Fire has similarities to the movement of Wood in that both, being Yang, have a tendency to go upwards when the Element is out of balance. Fire, when it rages out of control, roars upwards and pathogenic Fire creates symptoms in the upper part of the body, such as headaches, red or painful eyes in the case of Liver Fire, mouth ulcers in the case of Heart Fire or bleeding gums in the case of Stomach Fire. In all these cases, it also creates mental restlessness and agitation, often with insomnia, as the Fire rises up to disturb the Shen.

In balance, however, the Fire Element's energy radiates outwards, like light, as it extends its influence through the circulation to all parts of the body. Its characteristic manifestations, however, are in the complexion and the eyes, both in the upper part.

Element emotion: joy

The Chinese character for the emotion of the Heart is perhaps mistranslated as "joy", since "Etymological study yields the meaning of "joy and pleasure derived from eating" "(*Fujido's Etymological Dictionary*, from *Hara Diagnosis; Reflections on the Sea*, p. 33). The emotion of the Heart in tranquillity, therefore, is a kind of contentment, without overt or noisy expression.

Excessive joy is one of the causes of disease (Chapter 5) and has to be avoided. Too much elation or excitement, as from good news or celebrations, can cause imbalance or illness.

There are times, also, when excessive elation without apparent cause can be a symptom of illness. An extreme example of this is seen in mania, when there is great excitement but the sufferer is not grounded in reality or responding appropriately to circumstances, indicating that the Shen is disturbed. It is more common, however, for the Shiatsu giver to meet receivers with a Fire imbalance who remain almost inappropriately cheerful in spite of pain or distress. Contentment is a quality of the Shen, but so also is an ability to respond appropriately.

The Nei Jing Su Wen says that "Excessive Shen is laughter that does not stop; empty Shen is grief", and sometimes lack of joy can indicate a problem with the Fire element. This can be distinguished from the grief of the Metal Element by the receiver's responsiveness to warmth from others, in this case the giver. If there is a problem in Metal, the receiver remains cut off, unresponsive. A receiver with a problem in Fire will become more animated in response to cheerfulness from the giver, but will soon relapse into "lack of joy" if the stimulation stops.

Element colour: red

Red is the colour which we naturally associate with Fire. Being the colour of oxygenated blood, it is also the colour which, diluted to pink, accompanies a healthy heart and circulatory system.

A florid skin tone of unvarying red is likely to indicate the pathogenic Fire which accompanies extreme Heat in the Stomach, Liver or Heart, rather than an imbalance in the Ki of the Fire meridians themselves. A Fire imbalance may cause easy blushing, as the Heart responds too readily to emotional stimulus, or there may be a permanent, though slight, rosy tinge to the face around the eyes or mouth.

Element sound: laughing

We saw in the quote from the Su Wen above that "Excessive Shen is laughter that does not stop". Excessive or inappropriate laughter may well be a sign that the Fire Element is out of balance. Because we accept that laughter is a natural way to ease awkwardness in social situations, we may forget that

it is also a diagnostic sign; after all, people with a Metal imbalance or a Wood imbalance are unlikely to resort to laughter when nervous or embarrassed, since they have their own characteristic ways of reacting. Laughter is also winning and appealing, so that it is easy to overlook the inappropriateness of a receiver's laughter when speaking about the death of her father (this is a factual example), since the constant laughter or giggling appears to be, indeed is, part of an attractively bubbly personality. In this type of Fire manifestation, the laughter may actually become part of the tone of voice, so that it seems to have a constant gurgle of laughter behind it and the speech is often extremely fast.

The other side of the Fire imbalance is the second half of the quote – "empty Shen is grief". If Fire appears to be lacking, the receiver will often seem quiet and almost mournful and laughs little unless encouraged by a display of warmth from another person.

Element odour: scorched

This is not often encountered in clinical practice, but some receivers with a Fire imbalance may smell like scorched ironing.

Element sense organ: the tongue

The Fire Element is connected to the tongue because of its ability to communicate, as the organ of speech, and not as the organ of taste, which is related to the mouth and the Earth Element. Of course, speech is not the only means of communication between humans; a more intimate and open way of speaking one to another is with the eyes and in fact the Shen is said to be visible in the eyes*.

---

*Another means of communication which was not available to the Chinese in ancient times is the sign language used by the deaf and dumb and there is evidence that this is governed by the same area of the brain which normally affects speech. Film taken of a young deaf-mute woman who had suffered a stroke which had damaged the speech area of her brain (Broca's area) showed that she was unable to sign afterwards, although her movements were perfectly fluid and coherent when not attempting to sign. This shows that our speech function in fact covers other forms of communication and we can assume that the Fire Element does the same.

The tongue is the means by which we "speak our hearts" to each other and express our emotional responses to the outside world. Since the Fire Element governs our responsiveness, its connection with the tongue is appropriate. Speech problems, such as stuttering or dumbness, are usually treated via the Fire meridians. Excessive laughter or very fast speech are signs of a Fire imbalance, as are confused or incoherent speech or the delirium of a high fever or mental disorder.

The tongue is considered to be a "sprig of the Heart" and although it is mainly the tip of the tongue which reflects the Heart's condition in tongue diagnosis, tongue ulcers anywhere on the tongue body are a sign of pathogenic Fire in the Heart.

Element taste: bitter

The bitter taste of medicinal herbs is "drying and hardening", like Fire. In the West, common foods preferred by those whose Fire Element is out of balance are black coffee, Campari and bitter chocolate; some may also like bitter vegetables, such as Brussels sprouts.

If there is pathogenic Fire present, there is often a bitter taste in the mouth.

Element season: summer

The hottest season of the year is obviously that which belongs to Fire. It is the season of light and heat, of Yang at its peak of expansion and richness of manifestation. Energy has extended itself as far as it can go, out to the flowers and fruits of each plant; animals and birds have reared their broods of young. It is at this point, or rather after the 10 days of Earth stillness at the end of this season (see p. 185), that the transition to Yin, the return to the cool, the dark, the still, must begin; there is nowhere else to go.

It is unusual for the Fire-starved peoples of the Northern world to dislike summer but the Northern summer is a mild and temperate affair. In more tropical latitudes, the extended period of heat can be a great strain on health, especially if there is already pathogenic Heat or Fire within. Those who dislike hot weather or whose symptoms worsen after a holiday in a hot climate are more likely to be suffering from internal Heat; these signs would not on their own be reliable pointers to an imbalance in any of the Fire meridians.

Element climate: hot

As mentioned above, excessive external Heat can place the body under strain. The fire meridians suffer particularly, since the blood must move faster around the circulatory system to cool itself at the exterior, which puts pressure on the Heart and Heart Protector, and the Triple Heater must attempt to maintain a constant body temperature. A prolonged stay in a hot climate may produce an imbalance in these meridians.

The adverse effects of a hot climate will be felt first by those who already have internal Heat symptoms or a constitution which tends to be Hot. To those with a Cold constitution or with internal Cold, a hot climate will be beneficial. If there is Dampness present, however, it is likely to combine with the Heat and symptoms of discomfort will result.

Element time of day: 11 am to 3 pm and 7–11 pm

The Heart and Small intestine meridians have their peak of energy at midday, the hottest, lightest and most Yang time of day. Chinese tradition considers it unhealthy to work during this time, and a rest after lunch is thought to be necessary to refresh the mental and digestive powers.

The time of the Heart Protector, "from whom joy and pleasure derive", and its companion, the Triple Heater, is in the evening, after the day's work is done and there is time for family and social relationships. If one of these meridians is out of balance, there may be a drop in energy during this time which is different from everyday tiredness, since the energy may revive again after 11 pm. It is important, if the receiver has a consistent Heart Protector or Triple Heater diagnosis, that he endeavours to go to bed while this tiredness lasts, since a Fire meridian imbalance affects the quality of sleep in general.

The Heart in TCM

In TCM, the Heart is *the* Fire meridian; all the other Fire meridians are protectors or agents of the Heart. By a curious paradox, the Heart actually does very little compared with, say, the Spleen or the Liver. Its main function is to provide a home for our Shen. According to Ted Kaptchuk (lecture in London, November 1989) the "job specification" of the Emperor, the Son of Heaven, was similarly undemanding. He had to participate in certain rites at certain specific times, as mediator between Heaven and the Empire; a high-profile function, but with little actual work. The performance of these rites, however, was thought to prevent the catastrophes which, according to Chinese philosophy, result from disharmony between Heaven and Earth – floods, epidemics, famine and so on. In providing a physical home for the Shen, the "divine spark" of consciousness, the Heart has a similar function, that of unifying Heaven and Earth in Man.

The home of the Shen

As has already been extensively discussed, the Shen is that quality in us which is variously translated as spirit, mind, consciousness or awareness. In order for the Heart to house the Shen, it must itself be tranquil and empty of disturbing emotions*. Much of Taoist spiritual practice and meditation was designed to nourish and root the Shen, since the Shen's presence was necessary for health and long life; if the Shen became scattered or left, it was impossible to recover from a disease.

In ancient China, many conditions where the Shen or consciousness became scattered or left would now be classified as shock, coma or critical states of illness with delirium and many of these are still fatal, although technological methods of intensive care do often result in recovery. Other disorders where the Shen is scattered are nowadays classed as mental illnesses, such as schizophrenia, where the sufferer lives in another reality, his Shen is elsewhere, and recovery is as difficult today as it was then.

Epilepsy is another condition in which the Shen is affected and this was thought to be due to Phlegm

misting the holes in the Heart. Less serious states in which the Shen is affected are blackouts or periods of amnesia, although these can also be due to Deficiency of Blood, which then fails to nourish the brain or anchor the Shen.

Shen/Blood relationship

In fact, the tranquil resting place for the Shen in the Heart is provided by the Blood. Deficiency of Blood in general, either from failure of the Spleen to provide enough Food Ki and Essence for its manufacture or from inefficient storing by the Liver, can result in the Heart's not holding enough Blood to nourish and anchor the Shen. We must remember here that Blood is not just a red fluid, however life-giving and full of nutrients and oxygen. It has a spiritual, psychological component in that it provides us with our sense of satisfaction and completion. If there is enough Blood in the Heart, the Shen is happy to be there, to be securely linked to a physical body in which it can function. If there is not enough Blood, the link becomes more tenuous and the Shen is anxious; symptoms can manifest such as depression or insomnia (although usually once the person falls asleep he can stay asleep, which is not the case in Yin Deficiency insomnia), anxiety and poor memory.

Conversely, the Shen can influence the Blood. If the Shen is strained by emotional problems over a long time, the Heart function can itself suffer. Since the Heart is the place where Food Ki is transformed into Blood, the production of Blood can be disrupted by the insecurity of the Shen.

Emotions and the Heart

The Heart does not have the same emotional connotations in TCM as it does in Western tradition, since all the organ pairs in the Five Element system are connected with an emotion and the burden of repression of these emotions is mainly carried by the Liver. The Heart, in ideal circumstances, is an embodiment of the spaciousness of pure, unattached consciousness; in such conditions, emotions may come and go but they do not affect the Shen, which radiates out accompanied by contentment ("joy") and compassion. In the normal course of events, however, our consciousness is attached to our emotions, so that

---

*"In your Heart there is love, don't love too deeply. In your Heart there is hate, don't hate too deeply, because too much of any of these will attack the Shen." Sun Simiao, *The One Thousand Ducat Prescription Book*, quoted in *Five Elements and Ten Stems*, Kiiko Matsumoto and Stephen Birch, Paradigm, 1983.

they stay and register with us for a while and tend to produce physiological effects in our Ki and Blood. The Heart can therefore be affected by all the emotions.

Heart Blood

Blood is made in the Heart, so that problems with the Heart function affect the Blood and problems with the Blood affect the Heart. It is common for too much thinking and worry to deplete the Blood, because it exhausts the Spleen which provides Food Ki and Essence for the making of Blood. Repressed or unacknowledged emotion of any kind can also affect the Liver, causing Blood Deficiency, which depletes the Blood in the Heart. When Heart Blood is deficient, the general symptoms of dizziness, insomnia, depression and poor memory are accompanied by anxiety and palpitations.

Heart Blood can also stagnate as a result of repressed emotion which causes stagnation of Ki and then Blood in the chest. This causes stuffiness, constriction or discomfort (stagnation of Ki) or severe fixed pain (stagnation of Blood) in the chest, with palpitations, as well as the other general symptoms of Ki or Blood stagnation.

Heart Fire

Heart Fire often results from the rising of Liver Yang or Liver Fire which accompanies anger, although any of the emotions will cause a build-up of Heat over time which can overheat the Heart and cause Heart Fire. Its characteristic symptoms are agitation, insomnia, thirst, palpitations and ulcers on the tongue.

Empty Heat

This is caused by Deficiency of Heart Yin, an increasingly common condition which results from emotional stress accompanied by the depleting effects of our modern lifestyle on Kidney Yin. Heart Yin Deficiency or Empty Heat in the Heart may manifest with any of the general symptoms of Yin Deficiency, together with insomnia, restlessness, anxiety and palpitations.

Heart Ki and Yang

Sadness or emotional frustration over time can affect the Ki of the Heart, via the Lungs, which partner the Heart in the Big Ki of the Chest. This results in fatigue, shortness of breath and slight palpitations. When Heart Ki is deficient, it may progress to Heart Yang Deficiency which manifests as poor circulation, chilliness and discomfort in the chest as well as the above symptoms. Kidney Yang Deficiency from overwork can also affect Heart Yang.

Sweating

Any condition involving the Heart may be accompanied by sweating, since the secretion corresponding to the Fire Element is sweat; not overall sweating, however, such as the spontaneous sweating which accompanies Ki Deficiency or the night sweats of Empty Heat. Characteristically, Heart-related sweating occurs as a result of emotional disturbance or nervousness; sweaty palms are the classic Heart indication, but the armpits and feet may also sweat.

Circulation

The Heart is said to "govern" the Blood in TCM. Apart from the transformation of Food Ki into Blood, which takes place in the Heart, the Heart is ultimately responsible for the circulation of the Blood and the condition of the blood vessels, "ultimately responsible" because this function is shared by the Heart Protector. The pericardium or Heart Protector was thought to assist the Heart's pumping action by constricting it, as is indicated by one of its alternative names, Heart Constrictor.

The complexion and the eyes

The condition of the Heart is said to manifest in the complexion and this depends to a great extent on the circulation. If the condition of the Blood and the circulation is good, the complexion will be healthily tinged with pink and the skin soft and supple, whereas a face of unvarying red may indicate Fire in the Stomach or Liver, as well as the Heart. The Heart also has a connection with the eyes, since the Shen is manifested in them, and presence, vitality and expression are the characteristics of Shen in the eyes.

Speech

Our hearts speak to each other through our tongues. Since the Heart is said to "open into the tongue", speech problems such as stammering or aphasia (dumbness) are treated as Heart related in TCM.

The Heart in Zen Shiatsu theory

Masunaga's concept of the Heart's function differs very little from the classical version. In the Zen Shiatsu cycle of the meridians, the Heart and Small Intestine complete the work begun by the Stomach and Spleen; in other words, they assimilate and integrate the material which the Stomach and Spleen have taken in and processed. The Heart integrates what the Small Intestine has assimilated and transforms it into an aspect of the physical and emotional manifestation of each unique individual.

Core of emotional being

An ancient Chinese fable about a legendary physician tells how he performed surgery to cure two men of their conditions by transplanting their hearts one into the other. But when the men returned home their whole physical identity had altered, so that their families did not recognize them. This shows the integrative power of the Heart in the Oriental medical tradition. Our consciousness, the Shen stored in our Heart, shapes and forms our bodies as well as our minds.

Anything which we assimilate into the mental and physical complex of our being alchemically becomes us as our Shen animates it – the transformative power of Fire at work. Masunaga's concept of the Heart as integrating what the Small Intestine assimilates reflects the same view of the Heart as the centre and creator of our individual being.

Emotional response

According to Masunaga, who followed the ancient texts closely in his interpretation of the Heart's function, the Heart works to integrate the input from the five senses and generate appropriate internal responses. If our Heart, our centre, is unstable, our responses are inappropriate. Psychological symptoms then develop, such as tension and neurosis, jumpiness, oversensitivity, poor concentration and memory and paranoia. These will express themselves in physical symptoms such as sweaty palms, palpitations and a nervous stomach.

Emotional and physical tension

Where the Heart is weak and vulnerable, the body will develop physical tension and armouring in an attempt to protect it. Masunaga ascribes many of the classical Heart symptoms to physical tightness, such as stammering caused by tightness in the tongue and a feeling of oppression in the solar plexus caused by tension of the abdominal muscles. He also includes the sensation of something stuck in the throat, which in TCM is a typical Liver stagnation symptom of emotional origin, and rigid palms; both of these are associated with the meridian pathway.

Meditation and reflection

The movement of energy in the Heart and Small Intestine stage of Masunaga's interpretation of the meridian cycle is inwards, assimilating sense impressions into the emotional core. He explains this as the "resting" phase of the Heart, the Yin period of stillness which alternates with Yang in the rhythm of the heartbeat. The posture which he chose to symbolize this stillness is the position of prayer, which emphasizes the Heart and Small Intestine meridians. Withdrawal into the core of our self must alternate with outward responsiveness in order to maintain balance in our emotional life.

The Heart meridian and how to treat it

The traditional Heart meridian emerges from the deepest part of the armpit and travels down the arm between the biceps and the triceps (on the medial part of the anterior surface of the arm in the anatomical position), towards the little finger, where it ends at the lateral side of the little fingernail.

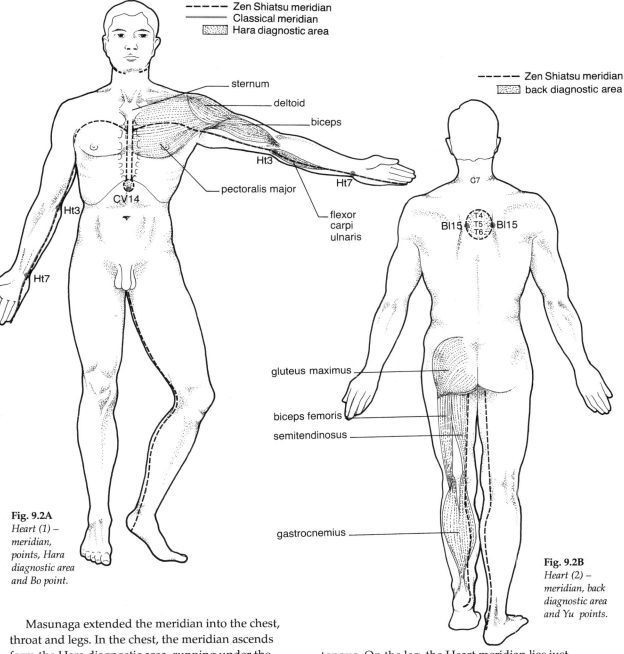

Fig. 9.2A
Heart (1) –
meridian,
points, Hara
diagnostic area
and Bo point.

Fig. 9.2B
Heart (2) –
meridian, back
diagnostic area
and Yu points.

Masunaga extended the meridian into the chest, throat and legs. In the chest, the meridian ascends form the Hara diagnostic area, running under the edges of the sternum to the approximate level of the third intercostal space where it branches, curving laterally over the chest towards the armpit before taking its traditional path down the arm. In the throat, the meridian runs along the edge of the floor of the lower jaw, connecting with the root of the tongue. On the leg, the Heart meridian lies just posterior to the traditional Kidney meridian, on the posterior surface of the thigh adductors, medial to the semitendinosus muscle, in a straight line down the medial portion of the gastrocnemius on the lower leg and on the medial side of the calcaneum, to curve under the foot into the pad of the heel (Fig. 9.2B).

The Hara diagnostic area is a small circle just below the sternocostal angle. The diagnostic area on the back is the area surrounding the fourth, fifth and sixth vertebrae (Fig. 9.2B).

Treatment procedure

Note: If there are current emotional problems connected with the Heart diagnosis, the receiver may feel too vulnerable if the meridian is worked in the supine position throughout. It would be better to work as much as possible in the side position to stabilize the Heart Ki before finishing with the chest and throat areas, which can only be worked in supine.

1. The Heart meridian in the arm can be palmed and thumbed in the supine or side positions, as long as the receiver's arm is taken as far as possible above his head, which brings the meridian to the surface. It can also be worked in a similar stretch in the sitting position, with the fingertips of the giver's hand reaching into the meridian as she grasps the receiver's arm, which is bent behind his head. For ease of illustration, the supine position is shown here (Fig. 9.3).
2. The legs are an excellent place to approach the Heart meridian without unnerving or upsetting the receiver. The easiest way to locate the meridian is to imagine the leg as a long box, with the meridian on the top surface of the medial corner. To locate it by muscle anatomy, it follows the medial border of the semitendinosus and takes a straight line down till it curves under the foot into the centre of the heel. The angle of pressure is straight down to the floor in prone position, horizontal in the side position (Fig. 9.4).
3. The first part of the meridian in the chest lies just under the edges of the sternum, up from the Hara diagnostic area to roughly the level of the third rib. The giver must angle her pressure from the edges of the sternum underneath the bone to reach the meridian. Here she uses the ulnar edges of her hands, but fingertips between the intercostal spaces also work well (Fig. 9.5A).
4. The fingertips are the most suitable tool for working the rest of the meridian in the chest. It curves in a heart shape outwards from the sternum, somewhat like the shape of a Fifties' strapless dress. On large-breasted women, the meridian may lie on the outer breast tissue, so that excessive pressure should be avoided and focus, intention and Hara should be used to aid penetration (Fig. 9.5B).

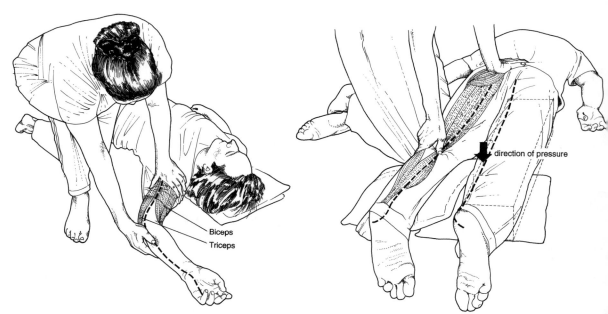

Fig. 9.3 *The arm meridian stretch.*

Fig. 9.4 *The leg.*

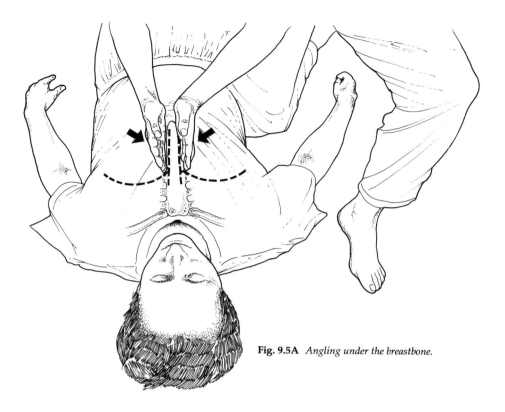

Fig. 9.5A *Angling under the breastbone.*

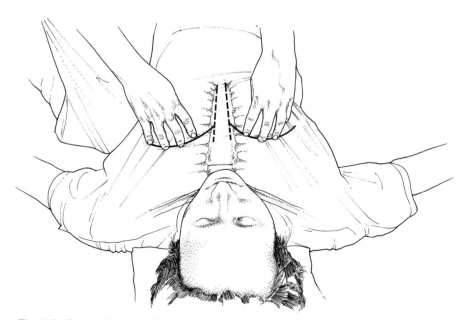

Fig. 9.5B *Treating the chest with the fingertips.*

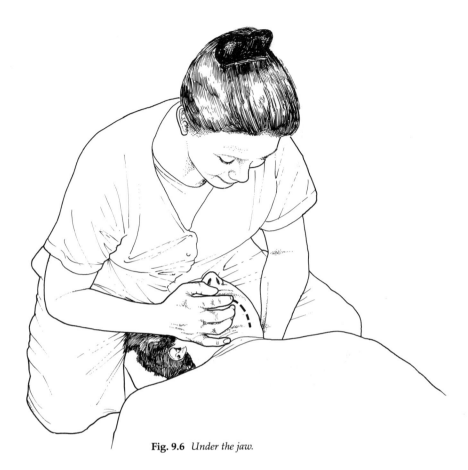

Fig. 9.6 *Under the jaw.*

5. Depending on the size of the area under the chin, the meridian here can be worked with the fingertips of one or both hands. If one hand is used, the mother hand should support the back of the neck. If two hands are used, they can work alternately, with consecutive running pressures from all the fingertips (Fig. 9.6).

Major points on the Heart meridian

Heart 3

At the medial end of the elbow crease, in the depression anterior to the medial epicondyle of the humerus.

Actions

- Clears Heat from the Heart (Full or Empty)
- Calms the Shen

Heart 7

At the medial side of the wrist crease, between the pisiform bone and the ulna, on the radial side of the tendon of flexor carpi ulnaris.

Actions

- Source point
- Tonifies Heart Blood
- Calms the Shen and clears the mind

Heart Yu point

BL 15 – two fingers' width from the midline of the spine, level with the lower border of the spinous process of T 5.

Heart Bo point

CV 14 – on the midline of the abdomen, about three fingers' width below the junction of the sternum with the xiphoid process.

The Small Intestine in TCM

The pairing of the Heart and Small Intestine is an odd one in physiological terms, even stranger than that of the Lungs and Large Intestine, and TCM does little to explain it. Perhaps there was some understanding of it in ancient times of which no written record remains. Modern research makes it easier to establish a connection between the two, however; on the one hand is the connection between the Small Intestine and the blood (see p. 157) and on the other the development in the embryo of the heart and the intestines from the same layer of tissue (*Hara Diagnosis: Reflections on the Sea*, p. 171).

The potential for projecting psychological functions of the organs, parallel to their physiological action, is not obvious in TCM. The ancient texts work more with metaphor and subtle techniques of allusion to describe the organs and their functions than with the method of direct analogy which is more accessible to the modern mind and which is a cornerstone of Masunaga's theory. Since the Small Intestine is traditionally associated with mental clarity, however, it is likely that it has a psychological function in TCM which reflects its physical one.

Receiving, being filled and transforming

This function refers to the Small Intestine's capacity to assimilate nourishment. In TCM terms, since the Spleen is the chief organ in charge of the transformation and transportation of Food Essence and Food Ki, the Small Intestine works to the orders of the Spleen in this, its principal function.

On the physical level, it receives food from the Stomach and, under the direction of the Spleen, separates it into "pure", which is transported to the organs and limbs by the Spleen, and "impure", which is sent down to the Large Intestine for excretion.

Fluids are similarly separated into "pure", which are sent up to the Lungs by the Spleen, and "impure", which are sent down to the Bladder, with which the Small Intestine is connected in the Six Divisions.

Abdominal problems

Small Intestine problems usually manifest with abdominal pain, often accompanied by changes in bowel habit such as constipation or diarrhoea and symptoms such as flatulence. Occasionally urinary problems, which are usually of a Hot nature, arise from Heart Fire, communicated to the Bladder by the Small Intestine. A typical example would be burning urination accompanied by insomnia, following on from emotional problems.

Clarity

Since the Small Intestine "receives, is filled and transforms", we can imagine, although TCM does not spell this out, that it does with sense impressions and other input what it does with food, separating the pure from the impure and assimilating the pure. As a result, the information received by our centre of consciousness is pure or appropriate to our needs.

This clarity is even more important than that of the Gall Bladder, since the Gall Bladder makes decisions on the basis of the information which the Small Intestine has assimilated. The Small Intestine is like a filter, allowing only useful material through into the bodymind and screening out the rest. If it fails in this function, the Heart, representing our central consciousness, may integrate information which is impure into our psychological make-up. This information might include wrong beliefs concerning ourselves and others, or concerning our environment and our relationship with it, thus leading to emotional and mental confusion.

Meridian problems

The Small Intestine meridian zigzags across the shoulderblade and is particularly important in the treatment of shoulder pain and a stiff neck. Other problems associated with the meridian are tinnitus and deafness or ear infections, since the meridian ends in front of the ear.

The Small Intestine in Zen Shiatsu theory

The Small Intestine's TCM role is highly amplified in Zen Shiatsu theory. On the one hand it ceases to be an assistant of the Spleen and acquires its own role in the digestive system, as in Western physiology, and on the other it is recognized for its relationship with the Heart, both in assimilating information for the Heart to integrate and also in providing a link between Heart and Hara. Its connection with the blood is also stressed and as a result, many symptoms which in TCM would be associated with the Liver or the Spleen are in Zen Shiatsu related to the Small Intestine.

Assimilation

This is the function which is not quite spelled out in the TCM phrase "receiving, being filled and transforming". The Small Intestine takes food and environmental stimuli, both emotional and sensory, in to the territory of the individual bodymind, to be integrated into blood, flesh and individual internal responses. The verb "to assimilate" goes further than the meaning "to absorb"; it includes conversion of extraneous material into fluids and tissues identical to those of the being in question. To assimilate means to convert another substance into ourselves. Hence the Small Intestine's link with the Heart, the core of our identity.

Common physical symptoms of poor assimilation are indigestion, low energy, anaemia, constipation and diarrhoea, all of which could be Spleen symptoms in the TCM system, where the Small Intestine works to the Spleen's orders. Emotionally, the manifestations are more complex. Shock is a major example of the bodymind's refusal to assimilate unacceptable information and Small Intestine is frequently diagnosed after a physical or emotional shock, while symptoms which remain sometimes for years after an accident (whiplash is a common example) often involve the Small Intestine meridian (see case history opposite). This is in contrast to the TCM diagnosis of shock, in which the Heart Protector absorbs the effects of shock in order to protect the Heart.

CASE HISTORY

A young woman presented with a consistent Small Intestine diagnosis over many treatments, which did not accord with any of her physical symptoms. She was, however, extremely nervous and anxious. On being questioned about the possibility of past shock, she revealed that her mother, while pregnant with her, had suffered from severe depression and had undergone a series of electroconvulsive treatments.

Shiatsu had a beneficial effect on her physical symptoms, but her nervousness and Hara diagnosis did not change until she herself became pregnant, when the Small Intestine diagnosis no longer appeared, perhaps as a result of the increased circulation in the abdomen which removed stagnation, perhaps because the emotional healing of a smooth and happy pregnancy removed old associations.

Emotional repression

Lack of assimilation can often manifest as an inability to acknowledge unpleasant memories or one's own unacceptable emotions; the information is not integrated or made available to consciousness. Since an area of the memory or personality is thus split off from conscious awareness, it must find expression elsewhere and often manifests as a split or disharmony between the top and bottom halves of the body. Chilling of the waist and legs accompanied by hotness of the face and weakness of the lower half of the body causing heaviness of the legs are symptoms noted by Masunaga as accompanying this condition. It is often visible as a disproportion between the size or development of the top in relation to the bottom of the body.

Linking Heart to Hara

The link between Heart and Small Intestine is recognized in Zen Shiatsu as the link between consciousness and Ki. Whereas in the upper body the Heart, as consciousness, integrates emotional and sensory input, the Small Intestine in the lower body integrates physical substance (nutrients) in order to make Blood and Ki. The Small Intestine thus provides a source of Ki in the Hara, while at the same time bringing the presence of the Heart down there to provide calmness and composure. Masunaga accordingly associates characteristics such as patience and determination with the Small Intestine. If the Small Intestine is out of balance, there is nervousness and anxiety.

Making the Blood

According to Zen Shiatsu, the Small Intestine works in tandem with the Heart, not only in integrating emotional and sensory input but in making the Blood. Masunaga was familiar with evidence from research over the last 20 years in Japan which shows that blood is manufactured in the small intestine under normal conditions and is only made in the bone marrow under conditions of physical stress, such as fasting or loss of blood*. Anaemia and low energy result from a failure in this function, which TCM ascribes to the Spleen.

Abdominal and pelvic circulation

Another important link between the Heart and the Small Intestine is via the abdominal circulation. We have already seen the function of the small intestine in assimilating nutrients and making the blood. It also influences, and is influenced by, the condition of the intestinal artery. Whereas the Large Intestine tends to be associated more with stagnation of Ki in the lower half of the body, the Small Intestine is on the whole connected more with Blood stagnation. Shock is physiologically connected with stagnation of blood in the abdomen, as the blood retreats to the vital organs in case of limb injury. Masunaga also associates appendicitis or problems following appendectomy with this meridian, as well as lower back pain, dysmenorrhoea and gynaecological problems. Often, in the TCM model, these would have been linked with the Liver, which tends to form stagnation of Ki, thus over time encouraging stagnation of Blood.

Revolution of Biology and Medicine, Kikuo Chichima, Neo-Haematological Press, GIFU, Japan. I am grateful to Paul Lundberg for this reference.

The ovaries

The diagnostic area for the Small Intestine lies over the ovaries in women, and ovarian and menstrual functions are closely associated with this meridian, linked with the Blood stagnation mentioned above. Small Intestine is often diagnosed around the time of a period when there are menstrual disorders, or after a difficult birth.

The meridian

Tension in the neck and shoulders is commonly associated with the Small intestine meridian and lower back pain can also manifest. Symptoms are likely to date from an accident, shock or emotional upheaval. Problems with hearing can also relate to the Small Intestine meridian, which ends in front of the ear, and this can be associated with inability to assimilate or integrate information received through the ears.

The Small Intestine meridian and how to treat it

The classical Small Intestine meridian runs from the ulnar side of the little fingernail along the edge of the hand and wrist and up the edge of the ulna, crossing over it to the medial part of the elbow. It then travels up the centre of the triceps muscle, "on the border of the red and the white skin", via the back of the axillary crease to the shoulder just below the acromion, then zigzags twice diagonally across the scapula. It then ascends to the vicinity of C7 before moving diagonally up the neck across the SCM muscle to the area behind the jaw, then up under the cheekbone, moving laterally to end in front of the ear.

Masunaga's version of the classical meridian has it very slightly radial to the edge of the ulna on the forearm, to accommodate the Zen Shiatsu Kidney which runs along the edge of the bone. The zigzag on the scapula is a sketchy and inaccurate affair on the Zen Shiatsu charts and the two points of the zigzag which classically lie above the scapular spine are treated in the Zen Shiatsu method by working in a line above the spine of the scapula, although the two points mentioned account for only the medial third of this line.

Masunaga extends the meridian down the back, down the lateral border of the iliocostalis muscle (which, according to the placement of the scapula on the ribs, is either just medial or just lateral to the inferior angle of the scapula) to the back diagnostic area, level with the first two lumbar vertebrae. There is a branch down the highest part of the buttock. The meridian then penetrates the body to re-emerge in the groin, whence it travels posterior to the Spleen meridian, down the groove between the vastus medialis and adductor magnus. On the lower leg it

runs down posterior to the Spleen meridian behind the tibia, posterior to the medial malleolus and under the foot to the border between heel-pad and instep (Fig. 9.7A).

The Hara diagnostic areas for the Small Intestine are two wide sausage shapes, bisecting the line from iliac crest to pubis and aiming diagonally up towards the navel (Fig 9.7B).

The back diagnostic area extends from the first two lumbar vertebrae outward across the back to connect with the meridian (Fig. 9.7C).

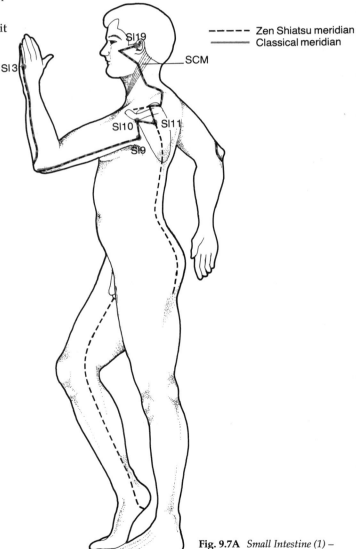

Fig. 9.7A *Small Intestine (1) – meridian and points.*

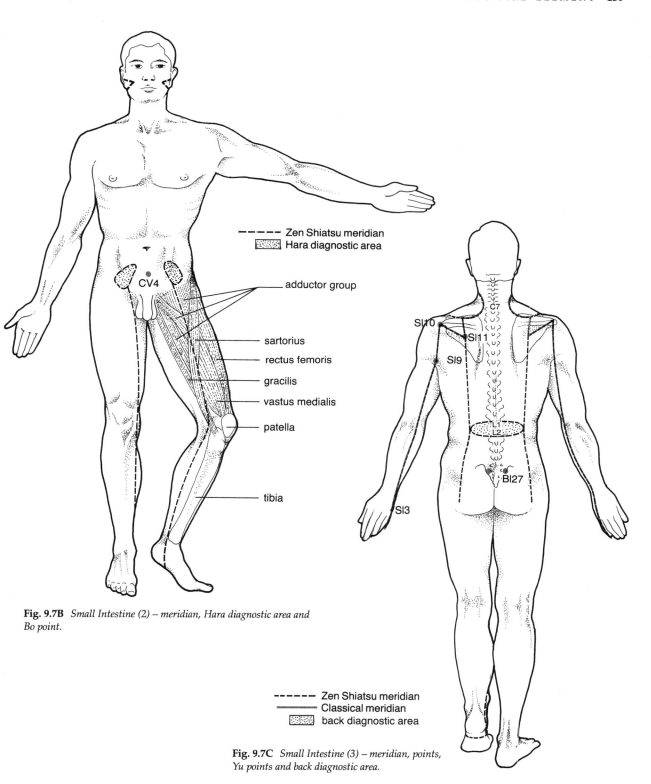

- - - - - Zen Shiatsu meridian
[...] Hara diagnostic area

adductor group

sartorius

rectus femoris

gracilis

vastus medialis

patella

tibia

CV4

Fig. 9.7B *Small Intestine (2) – meridian, Hara diagnostic area and Bo point.*

C7

SI10

SI11

SI9

L1
L2

BI27

SI3

- - - - - Zen Shiatsu meridian
———— Classical meridian
[...] back diagnostic area

Fig. 9.7C *Small Intestine (3) – meridian, points, Yu points and back diagnostic area.*

Treatment procedure

1. The Small Intestine in the neck runs in a straight line down from just under the earlobe, crossing to the posterior border of the SCM muscle. Where the neck meets the shoulders, it travels round the base of the neck to the side of the seventh cervical vertebra. The whole of this pathway can be reached with the thumb, with the receiver in side position, and with the giver's mother hand stretching down the shoulder slightly (Fig. 9.8A).

2. Alternatively, the same part of the meridian can be treated in supine, although it is not possible to reach to the back of the neck. A very effective treatment can be given to the accessible part of the meridian, however, by putting the neck into the stretch described on p. 48 in Chapter 4 and working it with the thumb while stretching the shoulder down with the mother hand (Fig. 9.8B).

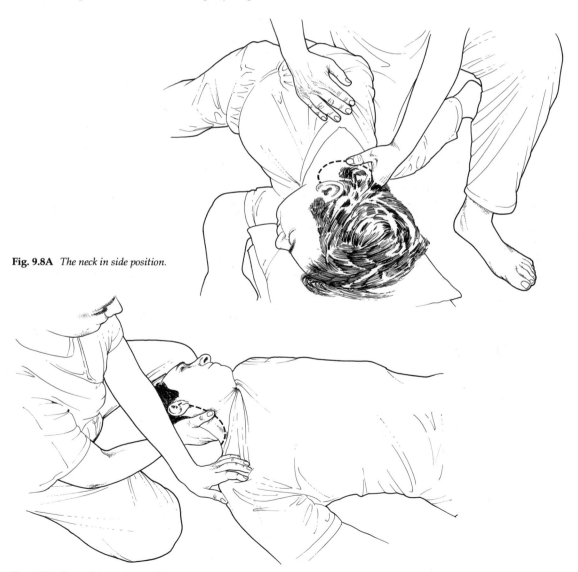

Fig. 9.8A *The neck in side position.*

Fig. 9.8B *The neck in supine position.*

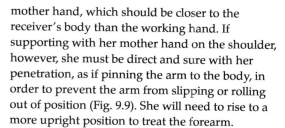

3. The meridian in the arm can be worked in all the treatment positions, providing the arm is placed in an appropriate stretch. The most commonly taught method is in supine, with the arm folded back over the clavicle. The giver can support the receiver's elbow, changing hands when she reaches it, but loses some of the effect of her mother hand, which should be closer to the receiver's body than the working hand. If supporting with her mother hand on the shoulder, however, she must be direct and sure with her penetration, as if pinning the arm to the body, in order to prevent the arm from slipping or rolling out of position (Fig. 9.9). She will need to rise to a more upright position to treat the forearm.

4. The shoulder, likewise, can be treated in side, sitting or prone position. Prone is shown here for ease of illustration. The giver is thumbing the line just above the scapular spine (Fig. 9.10). (The meridian accounts for only the medial third of this line (see above) but the whole area is worked for the sake of completeness of sensation.) Her mother hand is at the top of the spine and the child hand works outwards from it. Palming or elbowing are equally appropriate.

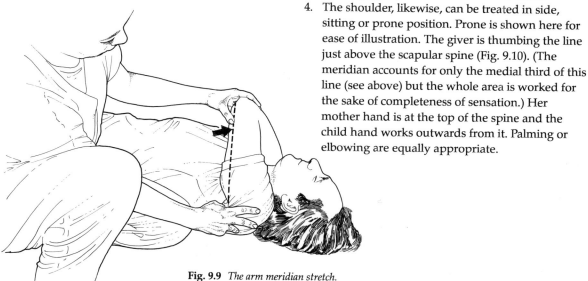

Fig. 9.9 *The arm meridian stretch.*

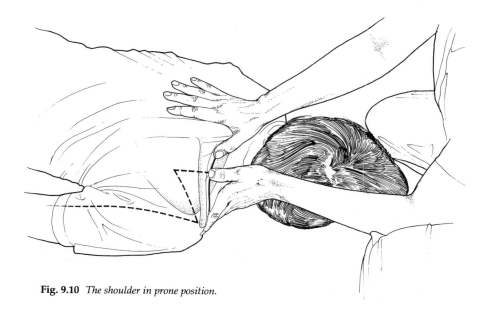

Fig. 9.10 *The shoulder in prone position.*

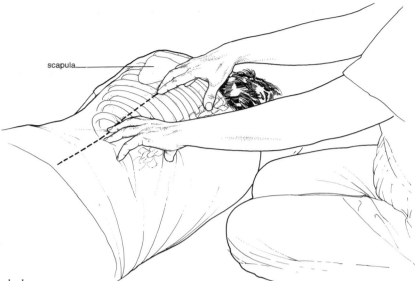

scapula

Fig. 9.11 *The back.*

5. In the back, the meridian is approximately halfway between the Bladder and the Triple Heater meridians. The groove on the lateral border of the iliocostalis muscle is usually palpable. Check to see whether it begins medially (more common) or laterally to the inferior angle of the scapula. Here the giver is working with fingertips (Fig. 9.11), but the meridian can be palmed, thumbed or elbowed in prone position.

6. The Small Intestine in the hip is on the highest point of the buttock, posterior to the Large Intestine and approximately halfway between the midline of the sacrum and the greater trochanter of the femur. It can be worked in prone position, as here, or in side position, with palm, thumb, elbow or fingertips (Fig. 9.12).

7. In the leg, the Small Intestine lies posterior to the Spleen. It is usually treated in supine position and the meridian stretch is effected by placing the heel to the opposite knee. A deep groove then appears between the quadriceps and the adductor muscles and the meridian is in the deepest part of this groove (Fig. 9.13)

8. The Small Intestine crosses under the medial malleolus to the junction of the heel and the instep. This area is treated with the receiver in prone, with the thumb (Fig. 9.14).

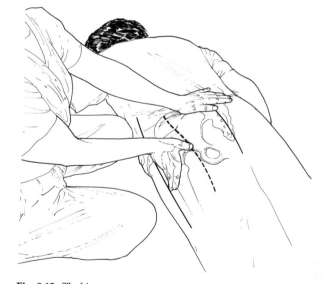

Fig. 9.12 *The hip.*

Major points on the Small Intestine meridian

Small Intestine 3

On the ulnar edge of the hand, just proximal to the head of the fifth metacarpal, on the border "between the red and the white skin".

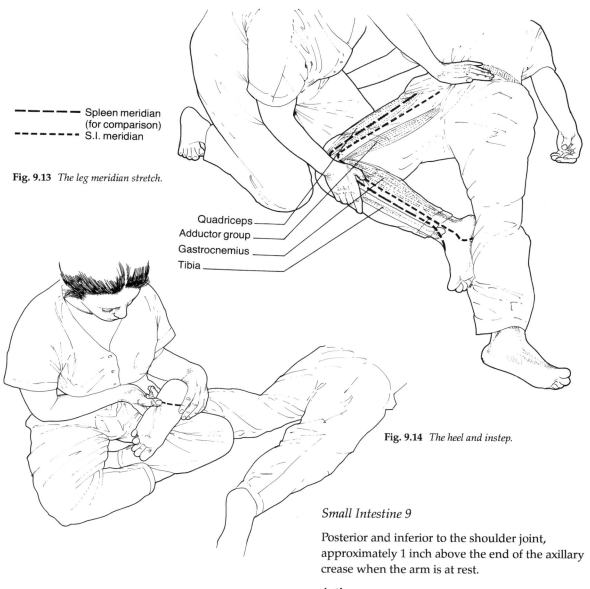

– – – – – Spleen meridian
(for comparison)
– – – – – S.I. meridian

Fig. 9.13 *The leg meridian stretch.*

Quadriceps
Adductor group
Gastrocnemius
Tibia

Fig. 9.14 *The heel and instep.*

Actions

- Opening point of the Governing Vessel, therefore benefits the back and the neck
- Eliminates Interior and Exterior wind (particularly when there are back and neck symptoms)
- confers clarity of mind

Small Intestine 9

Posterior and inferior to the shoulder joint, approximately 1 inch above the end of the axillary crease when the arm is at rest.

Actions

- Benefits the shoulder

Small Intestine 10

Directly above SI 9, in the depression inferior and lateral to the scapular spine.

Actions

- Benefits the shoulder

Small Intestine 11

At the junction of the upper and middle third of the distance between the lower border of the scapular spine and the inferior angle of the scapula (see above).

Actions

- Benefits the shoulder

Small Intestine 19

Between the temporomandibular joint and the tragus of the ear, in the depression formed when the mouth is open.

Actions

- Benefits the ear

Small Intestine Bo point

CV 4 – on the midline of the abdomen, four fingers' width below the umbilicus.

Small Intestine Yu point

Bl 27 – at the level of the first sacral foramen, two fingers' width lateral to the midline of the spine.

The Heart Protector in TCM

There are many names for this function. It is sometimes called the Pericardium, after the protective outer covering of the heart which, together with the deep blood vessels, is the physical structure to which the meridian is related; it is also called the Heart Constrictor, because it helps the Heart with its pumping action, and the Heart Governor (because it governs *for* the Heart, not because it governs the Heart). For the same reason it is sometimes called the Master of the Heart, where Master is used in the sense of minister or agent; and one school calls it Circulation-Sex. I prefer to call it the Heart Protector, because the name describes its functions with less possibility of confusion.

Mediates with the Source

Like the Triple Heater, the Heart Protector is often mentioned in the ancient texts as having "a name but no form", although it does indeed pertain to a form, the pericardium. However, "no- form", in Chinese metaphysics, refers to an indefinable energetic matrix which is the Source of all being. Both the Shen and the Source Ki derive from no-form. The Heart Protector and the Triple Heater both mediate between this energetic source and the meridians, the Triple Heater on the level of Ki, via its connection with Ming-Men and the Source Ki, the Heart Protector on the level of consciousness, via its connection with the Heart and the Shen*.

Because the Heart Protector has no form, it is a function, an avenue for awareness and information throughout the body. "The master of the heart is the master of the 12 meridians. If there is an empty space, then everything is permeated by the master of the heart" (ibid). Because it is primarily a function and not an organ, there are no patterns of disease associated with it and the meridian is used exclusively in TCM to treat problems of the Heart.

Protects the Heart

The physical structure of the pericardium protects the heart organ and one of the main tasks of the Heart Protector is to shield the Heart from injury, whether from external pernicious influences or from shock or emotional trauma. It does this by permeating and surrounding the Heart with its Ki, as well as by the physical protection of the pericardium, so that it forms a kind of energetic buffer zone surrounding the Heart[†].

Heat and Phlegm are the factors most likely to injure the Heart, and thus the Shen and the Heart Protector meridian are used in treating delirium, epilepsy, coma and other problems, such as tongue

---

* "The triple warmer manages the qi alchemical transformations....The master of the heart substitutes for the shen functions." Nangyo Tekkan by Sosen Hirooka, 1750, from *Hara Diagnosis: Reflections on the Sea*, p. 121.
[†]"If evil influences are present in the heart, they are always in the network enclosing the heart." Ting Chin, quoting from the Ling Shu in his commentary on Nan Jing 25 (Nan Jing, p. 314).

ulcers, caused by these external influences. High fevers, which affect the Heart through Heat, can also be treated through the Heart Protector.

Protects the Blood

Since this meridian protects the Heart, by association it also protects the Blood of the Heart. "The Triple Warmer is the father of the Qi, the Pericardium is the mother of the Blood" (Wang Shou He's commentary on Nan Jing 25, quoted in *Hara Diagnosis: Reflections on the Sea*, p. 121). The Heart Protector is related to the circulation of the Blood in the great vessels and thus influences the condition of the Blood. The meridian is therefore used to treat Heat in the Blood, causing excessive bleeding, and to move and regulate the Blood when there is Blood stagnation, especially in the chest, causing chest pain or discomfort.

Protects the Shen

Since the Shen is affected by the condition of the Heart and its Blood, the Heart Protector also ensures the stability of the Shen. Its meridian is therefore used for insomnia, mental agitation, incessant talking and manic behaviour. It also has a powerful calming action on anxiety and irritability. Any shock or emotional trauma which might scatter the Shen is to some extent absorbed and palliated by the Heart Protector.

The Heart Protector also spreads the influence of the Shen throughout the bodymind; it is known as "the ambassador... from it joy and happiness derive" (*Simple Questions* Ch. 8, quoted in *The Foundations of Chinese Medicine*, p. 103).

Assists the Heart

One of the ways in which the Heart Protector shields the Heart is by taking on some of its functions; it is sometimes called the Ministerial or Helping Fire (although many authorities take this as referring to Ming-Men, the Fire within the Kidneys) and is said to execute the will of the Sovereign Self, which resides in the Heart as Shen. The Heart stores the Shen; the Heart Protector carries out its intentions. It also works with the Heart in ensuring a smooth flow of Ki and Blood in the chest and throughout the body. The meridian can be used therefore to treat arrhythmias,

palpitations and chest pain and to regulate the action of the Heart in general.

The Heart Protector in Zen Shiatsu theory

The Heart Protector in Zen Shiatsu relates to the penultimate stage in the life cycle of the amoeba in which the amoeba, having learned to flee from predators, now takes further measures to protect itself from other outside influences. This necessarily involves constructing a defensive layer which will deflect or ward off unwanted encroachment. For us, the human animal, with our complicated social, psychological and emotional structures and interconnections, unwanted encroachment does not have to be from a declared enemy; any influence which comes too close to our emotional core may be perceived as a threat. The Triple Heater and the Heart Protector constitute our defensive shell or capsule. If we curl our bodies into the defensive position of the Makko-Ho exercise for these meridians (see p. 89), the Triple Heater meridian covers the exterior surface of the body while the Heart Protector is on all the inside surfaces. The Triple Heater, therefore, can be said to defend our physical and psychological surface, the Heart Protector to defend the zone closer to our emotional core.

The circulation

Masunaga equated the two zones of influence of the Heart Protector and Triple Heater meridians with the deep circulation of the great blood vessels and the peripheral circulation respectively. If the Heart Protector is out of balance, the central circulatory function will not work well. It is correspondingly associated with abnormal or fluctuating blood pressure and swelling or chilling of the extremities. If circulation in the chest is poor, there may be a feeling of obstruction in the chest which causes breathing difficulties and which is often accompanied by emotional distress. In TCM, this might be ascribed either to stagnation of Heart Blood or stagnation of Liver Ki in the chest; however, since the Heart Protector and Liver are associated in the Six

Divisions, the problem might well be treated via the Heart Protector meridian.

The heart and solar plexus

Heart problems such as angina or palpitations can manifest with a Heart Protector diagnosis. Chest pain in general, not necessarily associated with a heart problem, can also be a symptom. The Heart Protector diagnostic area is situated over the aorta, in the Middle Burning Space, so that painful conditions in this area, such as heartburn or gastric and duodenal ulcers, are also associated with the Heart Protector. Factors such as poor posture or a fixed working position, which may constrict the great blood vessels, have an adverse influence on the circulation and thence on the heart.

Quality of energy

The first half of the Masunaga life cycle is concerned with the obtaining and assimilation of Ki and nutrients. The second half is concerned with the various ways in which the Ki and nutrients are distributed around the body. The Heart Protector feeds the zone of the inner circulation with nutrients and energy from the blood and calm awareness from the emotional core. If the Heart Protector does not function well, this distribution does not take place and there is a tendency to be easily fatigued or totally exhausted. This may be complicated by the breathing difficulties mentioned above. When the Heart Protector is not distributing the Heart's calm, stress or tension result which cause restless and unsatisfying sleep (in TCM this would be due to lack of Heart Blood). The lack of distribution of energy may reflect the inability of the Heart Protector to execute the Heart's will, in a build-up of intention without the energy or power to carry it out; Masunaga calls it "great impatience without any ability to act" (*Zen Imagery Exercises*, p. 201).

Vulnerability and protection

The Heart Protector defends the zone directly surrounding our emotional core; "The heart-master, encircling the heart, basically constitutes something like walls encircling a royal residence" (Hsu Ta-ch'un's Commentary on Nan Jing 25; Nan Jing,

p. 312). If our sensitive inner emotional zone is threatened, the protective energy of the Heart Protector goes into defensive strategies. One, quoted by Masunaga, is overconcentration on work, so that personal issues are given less priority. Another is "abnormal emotions", in Masunaga's words, a category which covers a wide area. The emotions may manifest as hypersensitivity and extremely intense behaviour, so that the Heart's vulnerability is camouflaged by a demanding or aggressive stance, or they may be held in check, so that an apparent lack of emotion manifests. Absent-mindedness is another decoy strategy, fogging emotional reactions with vagueness. Often these protective mechanisms are confusing to the Shiatsu giver, who takes them for an emotional manifestation from another meridian, and the receiver with a Heart Protector imbalance is almost always unaware that the root of his behaviour is vulnerability and fear of contact.

The Heart Protector meridian and how to treat it

The classical Heart Protector meridian begins just lateral to the nipple and ascends the breast to the level of the axillary fold, from where it descends the Yin surface of the arm along the midline, between the heads of the biceps, across the midpoints of the elbow and wrist creases to the centre of the palm of the hand and thence to the radial side of the middle fingernail.

Masunaga's meridian begins in the solar plexus, on the Hara diagnostic area, rising in a straight line to CV 17, the midpoint between the nipples, before arching slightly over the breast on each side to the starting point of the classical meridian, lateral to the nipple. From CV 17, a tulip-shaped pathway curves outward and upward over the upper ribs, then back to the midline to ascend the throat on either side of the voicebox. There is also a branch of the meridian in the buttocks, which descends on a diagonal, following the outline of the sacrum but slightly lateral to it. The meridian pathway in the leg is just anterior to the gracilis muscle and thus to the Liver meridian in the thigh and runs between the Small Intestine and Kidney down the Yin side of the calf,

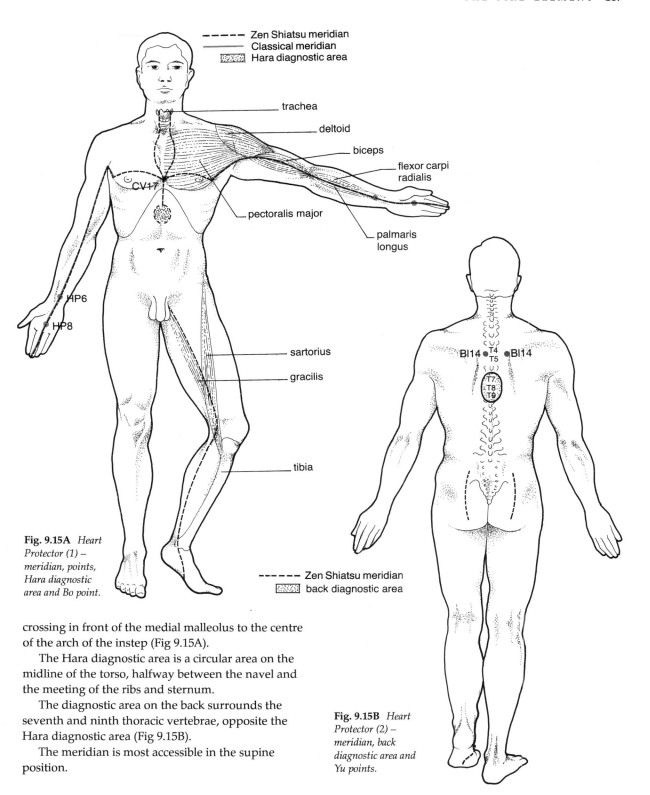

- – – – – Zen Shiatsu meridian
———— Classical meridian
▨▨▨ Hara diagnostic area

trachea

deltoid

biceps

flexor carpi
radialis

CV17

pectoralis major

palmaris
longus

HP6

HP8

sartorius

gracilis

tibia

Fig. 9.15A *Heart
Protector (1) –
meridian, points,
Hara diagnostic
area and Bo point.*

- – – – – Zen Shiatsu meridian
▨▨▨ back diagnostic area

Bl14 T4
       T5   Bl14

T7
T8
T9

Fig. 9.15B *Heart
Protector (2) –
meridian, back
diagnostic area and
Yu points.*

crossing in front of the medial malleolus to the centre
of the arch of the instep (Fig 9.15A).

The Hara diagnostic area is a circular area on the
midline of the torso, halfway between the navel and
the meeting of the ribs and sternum.

The diagnostic area on the back surrounds the
seventh and ninth thoracic vertebrae, opposite the
Hara diagnostic area (Fig 9.15B).

The meridian is most accessible in the supine
position.

Treatment procedure

1. The meridian stretch for working the arm in the supine position is palm up and at right angles to the body. In this stretch, the biceps rotates so that the groove between its heads can be felt on the midline of the upper arm. The meridian travels between the two central tendons on the forearm near the wrist. Palm, thumb or Dragon's Mouth can be used and gentle knee pressure is also effective (Fig. 9.16).

2. The meridian on the chest is treated in three parts. The first, from the Hara diagnostic area to CV 17 which lies on the midline of the sternum at the level of the nipples, is best worked by keeping your mother hand on the Hara diagnostic area and working up the midline of the sternum with the thumb (Fig. 9.17A).

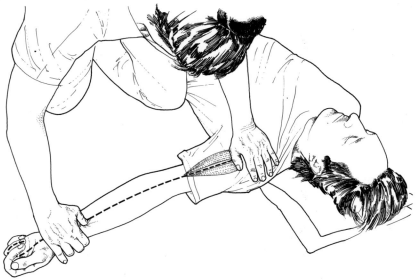

Fig. 9.16 *The arm meridian stretch.*

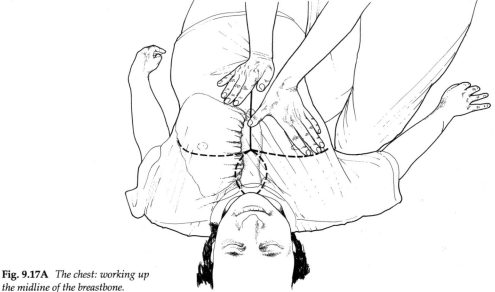

Fig. 9.17A *The chest: working up the midline of the breastbone.*

3. The second part is the branch which curves horizontally across the chest. It lies below the Heart meridian, between the third and fourth intercostal spaces, and follows the same curve. It is treated with fingertips, as shown, or with palms or thumbs. This part of the meridian crosses the breast on women and should therefore be worked with minimum pressure, but with focus and intention to aid penetration (Fig. 9.17B).

4. The third part of the meridian is the tulip-shaped curve up beside the upper sternum to the throat. It can be treated with the ulnar edge of cupped hands, as shown, or with thumbs or fingertips (Fig. 9.17C).

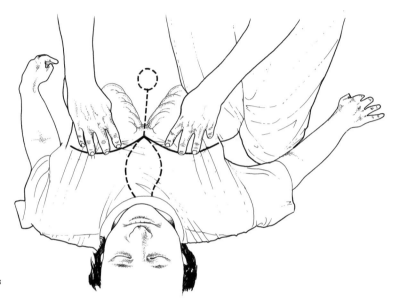

Fig. 9.17B *The chest: working across the chest with the fingertips.*

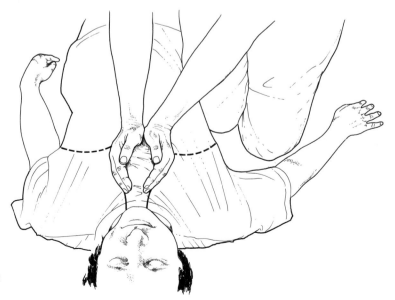

Fig. 9.17C *The chest: up the ribcage with the edge of the hands.*

5. The meridian in the throat lies alongside the trachea, on the carotid artery where the pulse is felt. It is treated from behind the receiver's head, with very gentle thumb pressure, one side at a time to avoid feelings of strangulation. The mother hand supports the back of the receiver's head or neck (Fig. 9.18).

6. In the buttock, the Heart Protector lies between the Kidney, which follows the outline of the sacrum, and the Small Intestine, which lies along the highest part of the buttock. It thus travels downward a couple of fingers' widths lateral to the sacrum. It is treated in prone or side position. Palm, thumb, elbow or knee can be used and the mother hand rests on the receiver's lumbar area (Fig. 9.19).

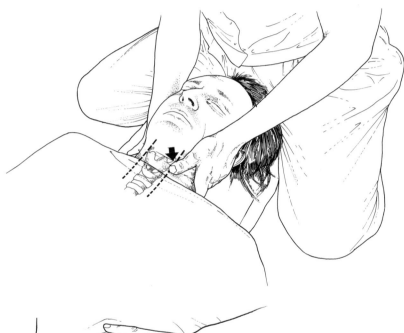

Fig. 9.18 *The throat.*

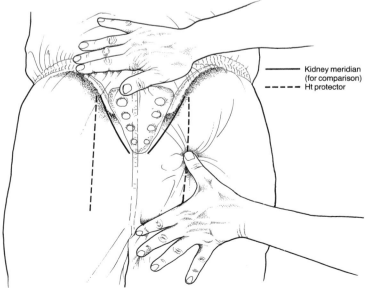

Kidney meridian (for comparison) ———
Ht protector - - - - -

Fig. 9.19 *The buttock.*

7. In the leg, the stretch for the Heart Protector is with the instep against the inside of the opposite knee. The meridian runs along the superior (in this position) border of the gracilis muscle, which is usually revealed as a tight band by this stretch, and follows the same line down the lower leg, between the Small Intestine and the Kidney. The giver may need to support the receiver's knee against her thighs as she palms and thumbs the meridian, with her mother hand on the lower Hara (Fig. 9.20).

8. The Heart Protector in the foot can be reached in the supine position with the thumb as a sequel to the procedure of point 7 above, but is shown in prone position for ease of illustration. The meridian crosses under the medial malleolus to the midline of the sole and runs up the arch to end just under Kidney 1 (Fig. 9.21).

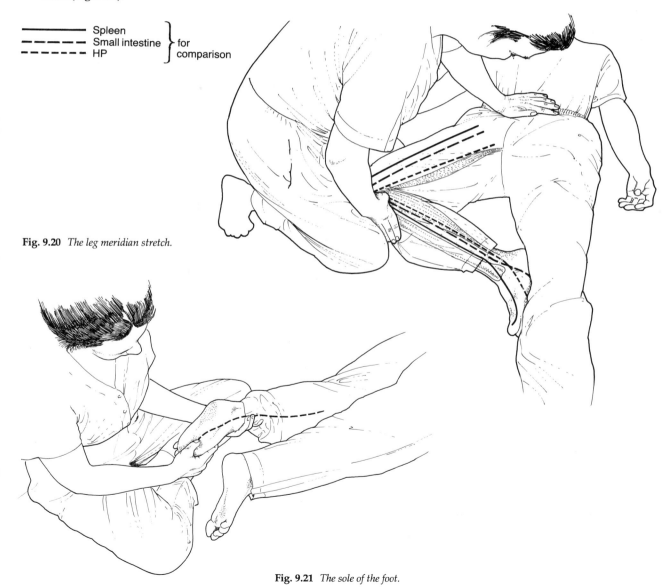

——————— Spleen
— — — — — Small intestine } for
— - — - — HP } comparison

Fig. 9.20 *The leg meridian stretch.*

Fig. 9.21 *The sole of the foot.*

Major points on the Heart Protector meridian

Heart Protector 3

On the elbow crease, on the ulnar side of the tendon of the biceps

Actions

- Clears Heat and Summer-Heat
- Cools the Blood
- Moves Blood stagnation
- Calms the Shen
- Resuscitation point
- Subdues Rebellious Stomach Ki

Heart Protector 6

Three fingers' width proximal to the transverse wrist crease, between the tendons of palmaris longus and flexor carpi radialis.

Actions

- Connects with the Triple Heater meridian
- Opens the chest and releases stagnation
- Calms the mind and promotes sleep
- Releases the diaphragm, harmonizes the Stomach and treats nausea and vomiting
- Regulates Heart Ki and Blood

Heart Protector 8

In the centre of the palm, between the second and third metacarpals.

Actions

- Clears Heart Fire and Heart-Heat
- Calms the Shen

Heart Protector Yu point

BL 14 – two fingers' width lateral to the midline of the spine, level with the lower border of the spinous process of T4.

Heart Protector Bo point

CV 17 – on the midline of the sternum, halfway between the nipples, level with the fourth intercostal space.

The Triple Heater in TCM

The Triple Heater, like the Heart Protector, represents a function rather than an organ; in fact, several functions. So many are its attributes that it is difficult to form a complete picture of the Triple Heater and many TCM texts will emphasize one or two functions, according to where the writer's interest lies. I must admit to a personal interest in justifying Masunaga's view of the Triple Heater's functions in terms of the various descriptions from classical sources.

Avenue for the Source Ki

The Triple Heater is named as an "avenue for the Source Ki" in the Nan Jing. It works with Ming-Men, the Fire within the Kidneys, to distribute the Source Ki*. Fire and Water, as the representatives of Yang and Yin respectively in the body, are both essential in helping Essence and Source Ki to function throughout the body and Ming-Men, as the Fire within the Kidneys, provides the essential link between Fire and Water; it has been described as the pilot light of a central heating system (Peter Deadman, lecture for JCM Seminars, January 1983). The Triple Heater, the avenue for the Source Ki, is the feed system which carries the ignition created by that pilot light to each organ of the body, via the Fire of each Burning Space, and to each meridian via the source point.

The Three Burning Spaces

Although many TCM texts associate the Triple Heater primarily with fluids, it is, as its name and its place

---

*Although originally associated with the right kidney, Ming-Men has for hundreds of years been identified with the point on the spine between the second and third lumbar vertebrae, between the Kidney Yu points and opposite the umbilicus. According to Japanese tradition, the developing fetus has two "umbilical" cords, the substantial one which is attached to the mother via the placenta and an insubstantial or energetic one which originates from Ming-Men and goes to the father (Kiiko Matsumoto, course notes, seminar at the Shiatsu College, London, 1991). This tradition illustrates the union of the Yin, female principle and the Yang, male principle in the creation of Source Ki and Essence, the foundations of life, in the Lower Burning Space.

within the Fire Element suggest, a warming force. The Three Burning Spaces are the areas of the body within which the Triple Heater exercises the transforming power of Fire and metabolic activity takes place. The Upper Burning Space, from the diaphragm upwards, deals with respiration and circulation and houses the Lungs and Heart. It receives and distributes. The Middle Burning Space, between the diaphragm and the navel, houses the Stomach, Spleen and Gall Bladder and the churning and transformation of the digestive process. The Lower Burning Space, from the navel downwards, includes the Large and Small Intestines, the Liver, Kidneys and Bladder. The Lower Burning Space has the most varied complex of actions. Its primary physiological function is to expel both the unnecessary, in the form of bodily waste, and the valuable, in the form of semen in men and the fully formed child in women: "There is an exit, but no entrance" (Nan Jing 31; 20); but it also assimilates, transforms and stores. Each organ brings its own Ki to the body processes but the Triple Heater contributes its Fire, its measure of Source Ki, to each Burning Space in order that they can proceed in harmony. Whenever a disorder seems to involve more than one organ and all in the same area, a malfunction of the whole Burning Space, and thus of the Triple Heater, can be suspected.

Protection

The Triple Heater has a defensive function and although it can be discerned by the primarily protective action of the points on the Triple Heater meridian, current TCM models do not stress this aspect of the theory. The Defensive Ki ruled by the Lungs protects the exterior of the body and works together with the Source Ki circulated by the Triple Heater, which protects by strengthening the surface from the inside.

■ *"The kidney belongs to water, ming men belongs to fire. The qi comes out from inside of the water-fire. The qi of the triple warmer starts there. Therefore, the source of the triple warmer is the shen that protects against evil. Breath reaches to the inside; the qi grows and then becomes solid. This protects the body against injury by evil. Protecting on the inside and defending on the outside, this is the qi." (Wang Shu He's Commentary on the Nan Jing, quoted in Hara Diagnosis: Reflections on the Sea, p. 113).*

It is interesting to note that the breath must reach deep into the body for this protection to occur, a good reason to practise Hara breathing.

Body thermostat

In some Western schools of Oriental medicine, it is taught that the Triple Heater is the "thermostat" which regulates body temperature. This is not a new idea; it appears in Japanese medical literature of the early nineteenth century. "In what way can we describe the triple warmer? The nature of the warmer is as heat ... this also is the regulator of the body temperature" (Kaitai Hatsumou Mitsutane, c. 1813, quoted in *Hara Diagnosis: Reflections on the Sea*, p. 115). Although this is primarily a Japanese development of the theory and does not appear in the current TCM model, it is easy to make the connection with TCM. The Source Ki, which the Triple Heater mediates to all the meridians, is the source of all the body's warming Yang. The Triple Heater also governs the environments in which all the vital substances, Ki which warms the body, Jing, Blood and Body Fluids which cool it, are made or stored. It follows that the body temperature will be dependent on the functioning of the Triple Heater, if not directly then through the other organs which depend on the Triple Heater for their working environment.

The surface

An eighteenth century Japanese commentary on the Nan Jing, when relating the Triple Heater to the Heart Protector, states: "The master of the heart controls the lining. The triple warmer controls the surface" (Nangyo Tekkan by Sosen Hirooka, 1750, from *Hara Diagnosis: Reflections on the Sea*, p.121). This refers to their Yin and Yang qualities, not only in terms of the placement of the meridians, but also their relationship with the Ki (Yang) and Blood (Yin). The Triple Heater, being the Yang part of the pair, is related more to Ki and the surface, while the Heart Protector pertains more to the Blood and the lining, or the inside of the body*. A Chinese commentary on the same text, from the same period, mentions that "The Triple Burner emits Qi in order to warm the flesh and fill the skin" (Ting Chin's Commentary on the Nan Jing, Nan Jing, p. 313).

Freeing and connecting

As well as providing separate environments for metabolic activity in the form of the Three Burning Spaces, the Triple Heater must also provide communication and connection between them, allowing free passage of Ki and fluids. One authority comments that the classical descriptions of the Triple Heater functions are all of "opening up" and "letting out" (*The Foundations of Chinese Medicine*, p. 118).

In current TCM theory, discussion of this function is often confined to the distribution of fluids, but the quality of the energy which opens up and connects is important in forming a picture of possible psychological functions of the Triple Heater. On the level of consciousness, which is the domain of the Fire Element, the Triple Heater allows us to open up and connect to awareness of our own inner processes and also awareness of our relationship with our environment and with other beings. Since the Triple Heater also protects, both on the physical and psychological levels, we can see the foundations of the possible interpretation of the Triple Heater as a socially adaptive function, which enables us to open

---

*A strong argument is presented by Matsumoto and Birch (op. cit.) that the Heart Protector and the Triple Heater govern the deep and superficial fasciae respectively. In view of modern theories suggesting that the fasciae are a unified system which carries information throughout the body and which regulates and harmonizes the activity of all the body tissues, this is a relevant and exciting hypothesis. It is also corroborated by the classical texts. Ting Chin, commenting on the Nan Jing in 1736, writes "...the heart-enclosing network (Heart Protector) is a small bag providing a network internally and an enclosure externally...The Triple Burner is a large bag supporting the organism from outside and holding it inside", and this seems to be a clear description of the pericardium's relationship to the superficial fasciae.

or close our energetic boundaries to others in an appropriate way.

The meridian

In spite of all the metaphysical discussion on the nature and functions of the Triple Heater, its meridian is used in TCM in a far more down-to-earth and specific way. Most of the points are used to clear Heat, Wind and obstruction, usually from the meridian pathway and particularly from the ears. It is used for ear infections, tinnitus and deafness, migraine headaches, swollen glands and tonsillitis, and stiff neck and shoulders. The only point which has a scope of action reflecting the influence of the Triple Heater is its source point, TH 4. The meridian does, however, reflect the Triple Heater's protective function.

The Triple Heater in Zen Shiatsu theory

Although Masunaga's version of the Triple Heater's functions may seem very different from the currently accepted view of the Triple Heater in TCM, it can be seen from the preceding section that his views have a historical context and are derived from the classics or from commentaries on the classics dating back centuries. The theory of Zen Shiatsu assigns more specific, individual functions to the Triple Heater than does TCM and the meridian can therefore be used to treat a wide variety of symptoms.

Circulation and protection

This is the catchword for the entire energetic phase embodied by the Heart Protector and Triple Heater in Zen Shiatsu, for both protect the body by means of the circulation. Masunaga associates the Triple Heater with the peripheral circulation of the blood and lymph. The peripheral circulation protects by oxygenating and nourishing the cells; the lymphatics protect by removing toxins and other harmful material. Poor circulation may result from a Triple Heater imbalance and poor lymphatic function may result in swollen glands or oedema.

Infections and allergies

The Triple Heater, which in TCM protects the body from the inside, here takes over a significant part of the Lungs' traditional role in protecting the body surface against external pernicious influences. The Triple Heater may be associated with constant colds, with clear mucus and watery eyes, or other infections. It is often diagnosed at the beginning of an illness of an Exterior nature. If it is overzealous in its protective function, allergies such as hayfever or urticaria, which result from a trigger-happy immune system, can occur.

The surface and adaptation

Via the peripheral circulation and the lymphatics, the Triple Heater is associated with the surface of the body, both the skin and the mucous membranes. The surface of the body is our interface with the environment but whereas the Metal Element allows us to exchange Ki with the environment, it is the Fire meridian of the Triple Heater which allows us to *communicate* with it and thereby to adapt. Failure in the Triple Heater function manifests as maladaptation to the environment which is often accompanied by some form of emotional response, however slight. Hypersensitive skin, ticklishness and oversensitive mucous membranes in the nose and throat are all conditions which precede the infections and allergies mentioned above. Abdominal pain can be caused by an oversensitive peritoneum. Inability to adapt body temperature to that of the environment is also common with a Triple Heater diagnosis and may result in feeling cold in hot weather or the reverse; or the receiver may find it hard to enter water which is slightly hot or cold. An emotional reaction to weather extremes is also likely. Since the Triple Heater meridian ends at the eye, the eyes may not adapt easily to extremes of light exposure, so that the receiver may be easily dazzled or experience night blindness. The eyes are likely to be sensitive and to tire easily.

The fasciae

Masunaga mentions the Triple Heater's connection with the mesentery, an important component of the abdominal fasciae (*Zen Imagery Exercises*, p. 71), but does not elaborate on its possible relationship to the fascial network as a whole. The current movement towards interpreting the Triple Heater as embodying the fascial connections will have to wait for more solid evidence on the role of the fasciae to become generally available. It seems likely, however, that the activity of the fasciae in distributing information between all the organ systems, which appears to be related to the cerebrospinal fluid, corresponds to the role of the Heart Protector and Triple Heater in spreading awareness and Source Ki throughout the body.

Emotional defence

The Triple Heater provides psychological as well as physical protection. There are similarities between the Triple Heater and the Lungs, since both deal with our physical surface and non-physical boundaries* but whereas the Metal Element deals with exchange through our boundaries on a basic and general level, in which consciousness is not necessarily implicated, the Triple Heater, as part of the Fire Element, involves us in emotional response to those processes. The Triple Heater therefore allows us to open up our boundaries and connect with people and situations outside our individual space (note that the nature of the Ki of the Triple Heater in TCM is to open up and connect – (see p. 174) or alternatively to close down our emotional boundaries.

Masunaga noted Triple Heater disharmony in receivers who were pampered as children and thus did not develop their own adaptive and protective mechanisms. The Shiatsu giver will often diagnose Triple Heater at a first Shiatsu session as the receiver involuntarily puts up an energetic shield, protecting himself from this potentially invasive experience. People with a long term Triple Heater imbalance are

---

*A graduate of the Shiatsu College, London, for her final year thesis analysed the Hara diagnoses of several AIDS patients over several weeks and found a strong preponderance of Lungs and Triple Heater over the other meridians. This result reflects the involvement on several levels of these two meridians; first, the general weakness of the protective function (immune system); second, the tendency for physical symptoms to appear on the skin or in the lungs; and third, feelings of isolation and untouchability experienced by these patients. (Jane Lyons, graduation thesis, 1989)

often highly cautious and self-protective, as a result of having opened up too much in the past. This is usually only apparent on closer acquaintance, however, since long experience of evading contact often gives a surface appearance of easy friendliness. As the receiver strains to maintain a safe distance, tension in the hands and forearms develops as the muscles involuntarily go into a pushing away mode. Deafness can also be related to a Triple Heater diagnosis, because of the defence which it provides. If we cannot hear what others are saying, we are less vulnerable to hurt.

The meridian

The Zen Shiatsu meridian, like the classical one, can be used to treat neck and shoulder problems; whiplash frequently manifests in the Triple Heater meridian, as the neck protects itself from impact. Ear infections are also connected with the Triple Heater, as well as deafness, since the meridian encircles the ear. Tonsillitis and swollen glands are also associated with the meridian pathway around the ear and neck.

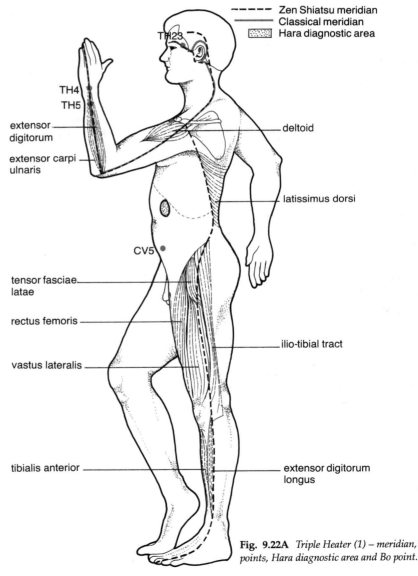

Fig. 9.22A *Triple Heater (1) – meridian, points, Hara diagnostic area and Bo point.*

The Triple Heater meridian and how to treat it

The classical Triple Heater meridian begins on the ulnar side of the ring finger and travels to the centre of the dorsal surface of the wrist joint, then up the midline of the forearm, over the wrist extensor muscles. It crosses the olecranon and travels in a straight line up the back of the arm to a point just posterior and inferior to the acromion, then crosses the shoulder above the scapula and up the groove between the trapezius and the sternocleidomastoid muscle to the mastoid process. From here it travels to the hollow under the earlobe, then follows the border of the ear up and around to the upper attachment of the ear, then ascends to finish on the lateral end of the eyebrow.

Masunaga's Triple Heater of the forearm is just to the ulnar side of the midline, which is occupied by the Gall Bladder meridian. The meridian is the neck appears to differ from the classical one, which is anterior to the Gall Bladder, while Masunaga's appears behind it. In practice, both meridians run in the groove between the trapezius and the sternocleidomastoid and there are no acupuncture points on this part of the neck meridian, so that its traditional position may be academic. The Zen Shiatsu meridian has a branch up the anterior as well as the posterior border of the ear and there is an extra branch which curves up the side of the head, between the two branches of the Gall Bladder meridian.

From the point posterior to the acromion, the Zen Shiatsu meridian travels down the lateral edge of the back, posterior to the Gall Bladder, crossing over at the waist to travel down the lateral edge of the front of the hip and leg, between the Stomach and the Gall Bladder. (This part of the meridian is a mirror image of the Large Intestine meridian, which travels down the lateral edge of the front of the torso and the lateral edge of the back of the hip and leg. The Gall Bladder meridian runs between them). The meridian then runs between the third and fourth metatarsals, to the third toe.

The meridian is most easily accessible in the side position.

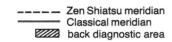
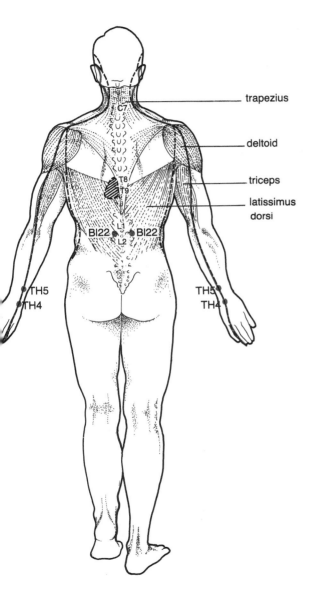

Fig. 9.22B *Triple Heater (2) – meridian, points, back diagnostic area and Yu points.*

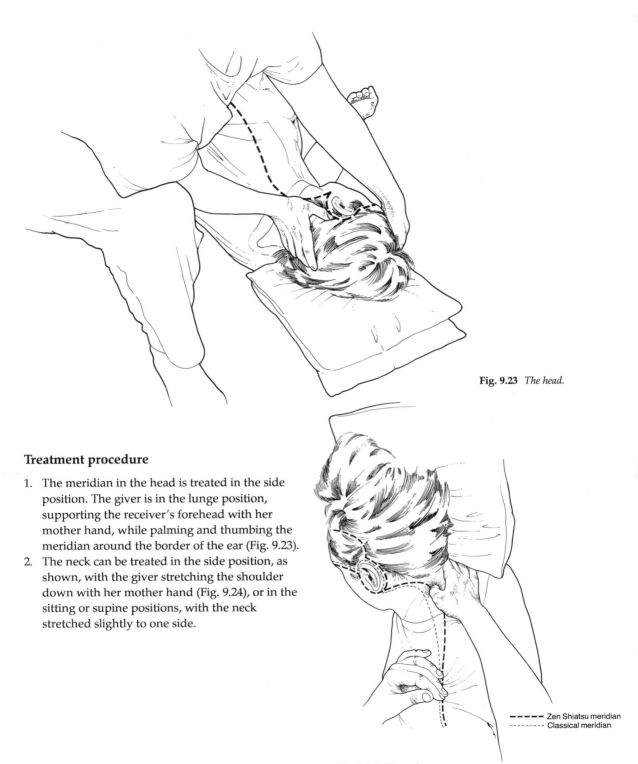

Fig. 9.23 *The head.*

Treatment procedure

1. The meridian in the head is treated in the side position. The giver is in the lunge position, supporting the receiver's forehead with her mother hand, while palming and thumbing the meridian around the border of the ear (Fig. 9.23).

2. The neck can be treated in the side position, as shown, with the giver stretching the shoulder down with her mother hand (Fig. 9.24), or in the sitting or supine positions, with the neck stretched slightly to one side.

- – – – – Zen Shiatsu meridian
- - - - - - Classical meridian

Fig. 9.24 *The neck.*

3. The meridian travels across the shoulder just posterior to the Gall Bladder meridian, which runs across the top surface. It can be treated in the prone position, as shown here, or the side or sitting positions, with the palms, thumbs or elbows (Fig. 9.25).

4. Likewise, the arm can be treated in the side or sitting positions, as described in Chapter 4, but the most effective meridian stretch is in the supine position, which is demonstrated here. The arm is laid across the diaphragm (one of the divisions between the Three Burning Spaces), supported by the mother hand at the shoulder. The hollow posterior to the acromion can easily be located in this stretch and the meridian worked straight down to the elbow, then around to the Yang surface of the forearm down to the ring finger (Fig. 9.26). The giver will need to rise to a higher position to achieve perpendicular penetration on the forearm.

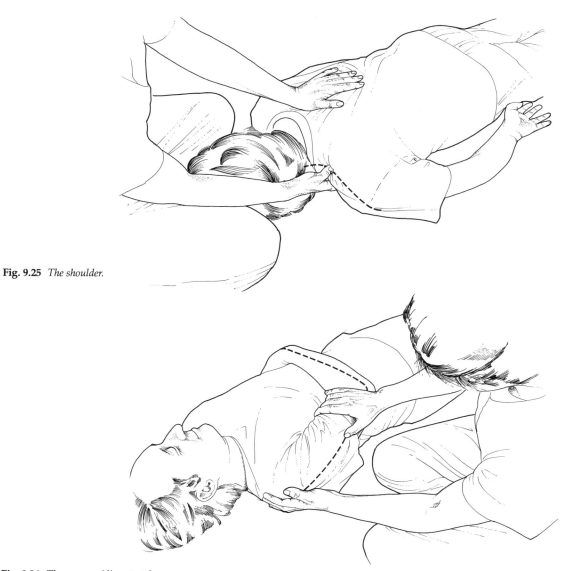

Fig. 9.25 *The shoulder.*

Fig. 9.26 *The arm meridian stretch.*

5. The meridian on the back is on the edge of the posterior surface of the torso. It can be treated in the side position, as shown, with the thumb, elbow or fingertips (Fig. 9.27). It can also be treated in prone with the palm, thumb or, most effectively, the knee (very gently).

6. The Triple Heater in the leg runs between the Stomach and the Gall Bladder. It can be treated most easily in the side position, but can also be reached in prone if the leg is flexed and moved up as high as possible, close to the receiver's torso. A more effective meridian stretch, however, is in the supine position, as shown. The receiver's foot is placed with toes next to the opposite ankle, as for the Spleen meridian stretch, but the Yang (lateral) side of the leg is exposed by rolling the leg over to the opposite side. The leg can be supported in this position if the giver places her knee under the

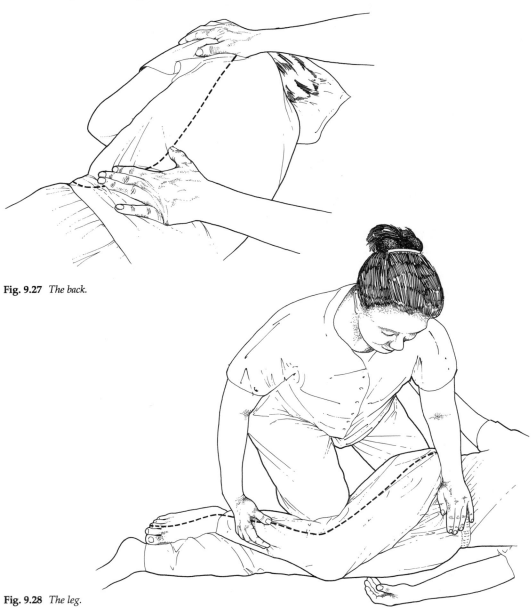

Fig. 9.27 *The back.*

Fig. 9.28 *The leg.*

receiver's bent knee, leaving both hands free, one as mother hand on the Hara and one to treat the meridian with palm and thumb (Fig. 9.28).

Major points on the Triple Heater meridian

Triple Heater 4

On the dorsum of the wrist joint, at the junction of the ulna and the carpal bones, in the depression on the ulnar side of the tendon of extensor digitorum.

Actions

- Source point – tonifies Source Ki of the whole body via the Source Ki of the Triple Heater
- Connects with the Conception Vessel and Chong Mai via Source Ki and regulates menstruation
- Transforms fluids and removes Dampness from Lower Burning Space
- Tonifies the Stomach

Triple Heater 5

Three fingers' width above TH 4, between the radius and ulna.

Actions

- Releases the Exterior
- Expels Wind-Heat
- Benefits the ear
- Subdues Liver Yang

Triple Heater 23

In the depression at the lateral end of the eyebrow.

Actions

- Expels Wind
- Brightens the eyes
- Stops pain (temporal headaches)

Triple Heater Yu point

Bl 22 – two fingers' width lateral to the midline of the spine, level with the lower border of the spinous process of L1.

Triple Heater Bo point

CV 5 – three fingers' width below the umbilicus.

10

The Earth Element – The Spleen and Stomach

■ *"We are part of the earth, and it is part of us...we love this earth as the newborn loves its mother's heartbeat."*

CHIEF SEATTLE,
FROM A SPEECH, 1854

Element associations: stability, support, fertility, receptivity, nourishment

The Earth Element is the foundation of our physical existence. Although we now know, through quantum physics, that all material phenomena consist of moving energy patterns, it is the Earth quality in those patterns which, for millions of years, has given us the sense of a stable, dependable reality. The earth itself is solid, supportive and apparently immovable, which is why earthquakes are so terrifying; we are used to taking the solidity of the earth for granted. In the same way, whatever represents stability and support in our lives, or in the shifting kaleidoscope of our perceptions, represents Earth for us, our security. It could be a place, a relationship, an intellectual structure like a belief or principle, a physical process like eating; something we find reassuring or dependable.

In the earliest days of life, unless we are truly unlucky, the constant, dependable and ever-present object is Mother. No doubt it is for this reason that nearly all cultures have called the Earth "Mother" – it is always there. A healthy Earth Element in the human character gives the capacity to support and comfort in the same way and we call someone who manifests this characteristic strongly an earth-mother.

Our relationship with the person who represents mother for us powerfully affects the Earth meridians within us.

But the association with "mother" goes beyond this for the word which we use to characterize the earth also describes a woman who can bear children. The earth is "fertile", a matrix from which come the plants which nourish us, the streams from which we drink, the minerals and metals which enrich our lives. This ability of the soil to contain and encourage abundance and variety within itself is the capacity of the Earth Element. "Earth permits sowing, growing and reaping" (from the Shang Shu, quoted in *The Foundations of Chinese Medicine*, p. 17). It is the Earth Element in the human body which supports a tiny cluster of cells as it grows into a baby; it is the Earth Element in the human mind which allows intellectual concepts to grow from the germ of an idea. Earth has within itself the potential for endless richness of manifestation.

Fertility, both of body and of mind, is the gift of the Earth Element and is derived from its Yin quality of receptivity. Earth absorbs lightning and grounds electricity; it soaks up the rain and whatever liquid is poured upon it. It also absorbs and transforms into itself all dead, rotten and waste material and this then becomes the basis for new growth and life, since the newly fertilized soil receives seeds and nourishes them. The ability to receive is crucial to the continued fertility of the earth. We will remember this later when we consider the Earth meridians of Stomach and Spleen.

Through receiving, then, the earth nourishes itself. It thus becomes fertile and produces new growth to nourish all the life forms which inhabit it. The theme of nourishment is central to the interpretation of the Earth Element and the Stomach and Spleen meridians; it embodies our ability to receive, process and give out again not only physical but also emotional and intellectual nourishment.

Spiritual capacity of the Element: intellect

The spiritual capacity of the Earth Element is Yi, whose Chinese character has two basic component parts, one which means "verbally expressed thoughts" and one which means "heart–mind" (*Hara Diagnosis: Reflections on the Sea*, p. 37). The Yi, therefore, puts the heart and mind into our verbally expressed thoughts, so that some authorities translate it as "purpose", but it is more commonly translated as ideas or intellect. It is worth remembering the "purpose" factor, however, since our intellect is a spiritual capacity only when it serves the purpose of our heart–mind, which is the full flowering of our human potential. According to Ted Kaptchuk (lecture at Imperial College, London, November 1989) the Yi or intellect offers us the possibilities or options for transformation, reflecting the Earth's potential for richness of manifestation. However, when a basic sense of physical security is lacking, as in the case of a deficient Earth Element, many of us seek a more reassuring reality in intellectual concepts and structures; hence the traditional association in TCM of "thinking too much" with Stomach and Spleen. The increasing emphasis in the modern world on the development of the intellect at the expense of other abilities tends to deplete the physical effectiveness of the Spleen and Stomach.

Movement of Element energy: stillness

In the same way that the earth itself is seemingly solid and unmoving, so the Earth Element has the quality of stillness. Whereas the other four Elements have their own characteristic movements and directions, the Earth Element provides the calm of the centre. Yet it is a stillness which allows for transition and movement; the earth's stability and the pull of its gravity influence our movements on its surface. A balanced Earth Element allows us to be "grounded" and centred; out of balance, it causes lethargy or purposeless overactivity, particularly of the mind.

Element emotion: reflective thought/empathy

The emotion of Earth has been variously translated as worry, concern, sympathy, reminiscence and overthinking. The ideogram for Si, the emotion ascribed to Earth, contains the radicals for heart and brain, so that it is neither completely emotion nor completely thought but links the two. "Reflective thought" is a fair translation of the character but fails to convey another potential dimension of its meaning, that of the intellect functioning in the world with compassionate, heartfelt motivation.

There is another emotion which is so often seen in connection with the Earth Element that it must be mentioned, though it is ignored by the texts. Since the earth's capacity is both to receive and to give, we can imagine that the Earth emotion would be both inwardly and outwardly directed. A balanced Earth Element in the human psyche will receive and give in equal measure, receiving emotional signals and communication from others and giving out support and nourishment, but also taking nourishment for itself. I have borrowed Iona Marsaa Teeguarden's word "empathy" (*The Joy of Feeling*, p. 91) to describe this double process. An Earth which is out of balance, however, may tend towards either the one or the other pole, with too much giving out and an inability to receive, or with great neediness and a lack of resources to give out.

Element colour: yellow

The soil of much of China is yellow and yellow is therefore traditionally a colour symbolic of peace and abundance, the qualities of Earth. Yellow only shows on the face, however, if the Stomach or Spleen energies are out of balance, when it appears as a yellow hue around the mouth or eyes. Look for a hue which comes and goes, not the facial skin tone. If the overall skin tone is orange or yellow, it usually indicates Dampness.

Element sound: singing

The characteristic sound which the Earth Element imparts to the voice is melodious resonance. When the Ki of the Stomach or Spleen is out of balance, the singing sound in the voice may become noticeable as a soothing, up-and-down singsong, like a lullaby. It conveys the message of empathy, no matter what the content of the words. The singing voice is appropriate when we need to soothe or comfort someone, but if we have an imbalance in Earth, we may have the singing voice as a permanent feature, emphasizing that empathy is our most comfortable mode of self-expression.

Element odour: fragrant

Among all the unpleasant-sounding smells of the Element imbalances, "fragrant" seems the most appealing. But the smells are only perceptible when there is disharmony and none of them are pleasant. The smell of an Earth disharmony has a sickly-sweet quality.

Element sense organ: the mouth

We connect with each of the Elements through one of our sense organs. In the case of the Earth Element, it is the mouth (as distinct from the tongue, which is governed by Fire). Western psychology has a model of the "oral" personality, which relates to the world primarily through the mouth, and this type embodies many of the themes suggested by Earth – neediness and craving, an issue around nourishment and the ability to receive it and a need for others as a source of security. As infants we receive our sense of security primarily through the feeding process. If this process is incomplete, we may remain attached to many substitute forms of oral satisfaction, such as eating, smoking or kissing. A disharmony in the Earth Element may produce mouth problems, such as a sticky mouth, bleeding gums, mouth ulcers or cold sores. There may also be an inability to taste food.

Element taste: sweet

If our palates were not conditioned early on by the intense sweetness of refined sugar, we would perceive the taste of grains and root vegetables as sweet. When thoroughly chewed and processed by salivary enzymes, these release natural sugars which burn at a slow rate to provide long-lasting physical energy. This is the balanced, reliable sweetness of Earth. Fruits also provide natural sugars, with a more intensely sweet flavour. When our Earth meridians of Stomach or Spleen are in disharmony, the functions of receiving and transforming nourishment are impaired and we crave the sweet taste. Refined sugars are actually instrumental in creating that disharmony, since the body burns them much more quickly and they set up a pattern of craving more sweetness. The addiction to sugar is similar to, though not as serious as, the addiction to alcohol, which contains large quantities of sugar and which is also related to imbalance in the Stomach or Spleen energy.

Element season: the last days of each season

Some schools of thought have late summer as the season associated with the Earth element. In some earlier traditions, however, the last 10 days of all the other seasons were the Earth season, since they constituted periods of stillness in preparation for change. The end of each season is a time of completion; the seasonal qualities of Ki have manifested and it is time for a new season to begin. In the stillness of the Earth period, the energies of this new season are incubating.

Element climate: dampness

As a Yin Element, Earth has the propensity to become damp rather than dry; because of its receptivity, it absorbs moisture. External conditions of dampness can penetrate the body, to affect the function of the Spleen meridian in particular. Conversely if the Spleen is not transforming and transporting fluids adequately, a condition of internal Dampness can result (see Chapter 5, p. 74).

Element time of day: 7–11 am

The time of day when the Stomach meridian has its energy peak is from 7 to 9 am, while the time of the Spleen is from 9 to 11 am. This implies that our digestive capacity is greatest in the morning, although most people with an imbalance in Earth will find it hard to muster an appetite until after mid-morning. It is common in rural communities, where people work with the earth and its cycles, for breakfast to be the heartiest meal of the day, after several hours of work in the fields. In many Westernized, urban societies, where long sedentary hours of mental work already put a strain on the Earth Element, the Earth time of day often passes with nothing but a cup of black coffee for the digestion to work on. People with a Spleen or Stomach imbalance need to be encouraged to eat breakfast!

---

*It is common, however, for a deficient Spleen to coexist with a hyperactive Stomach, which is constantly trying to compensate for the Spleen's inability to nourish the body; this can cause excessive appetite which further weakens the Spleen by overloading it with food. The stagnation of food in the Stomach causes Heat. Since Stomach Heat increases appetite, a feedback cycle is created. In Zen Shiatsu diagnosis, this situation would manifest as a Stomach very much more Jitsu than the Spleen.

The Spleen in TCM

In TCM, the entire digestive process, from appetite to elimination, is under the overall control of the Spleen, which is sometimes called the Spleen-Pancreas to indicate its wider variety of function. The Spleen is the source of all our Ki derived from food, in the same way that the Lungs are the source of our Ki from the air. These two give us Ki from Earth and Ki from Heaven, together forming our True Ki (see p. 65). The Spleen's connection with the Blood in TCM also arises from this function, since the Food Essence which the Spleen extracts from food is the basis for the production of Blood. The Spleen is also one of the main organs connected with the processing of fluids, the others being the Lungs and the Kidneys.

Transforming and transporting

This term describes the main function of the Spleen in processing food and fluids and in distributing the products of that process around the body. It transforms the purest part of the food which it receives from the Stomach into Food Ki, a kind of Ki which is not immediately usable by the body but which is sent up to the chest to combine with the Ki of air to make usable body Ki. At the same time, the Spleen helps the Stomach to extract the more substantial Essence from the food, which is processed in the Heart to form Blood. Another step in the same process is the extraction of pure fluids from the food and these are sent up to moisten the Lungs, which then distribute them further to the skin. The residues from these processes are sent down to the Intestines for further separation (see p. 70). The Spleen is thus responsible for the transformation of food into Ki, Blood and pure fluids; it is also responsible, with the Stomach, for transporting these substances throughout the body. For this reason it is described as the Root of Postnatal Ki. A healthy Spleen and Stomach are the foundation, therefore, not only of a good digestion but of abundant physical energy.

Digestion

In Japan and China, the first sign of a weak Spleen is lack of appetite, since the Spleen confers the ability to taste and enjoy food*. Inability of the Spleen to transform food results in such symptoms as tiredness after eating, a feeling of fullness or discomfort after meals, abdominal pain or distension and variable bowel habits. Traditionally, loose stools with undigested food show that the Spleen does not have the energy to process the food properly and remove the fluid from it, but constipation is a common sign of Spleen Deficiency in the West, often connected with a sedentary lifestyle and mental overwork.

Fluids, Damp and Phlegm

Failure of the Spleen to transform fluids efficiently will manifest in symptoms such as thirst, water retention and urinary problems. When fluids are not processed properly they can remain in the body tissues in the form of internal Dampness, which is a common accompaniment of Spleen Deficiency. Overweight is "dampness under the skin"; stiffness and swelling in the joints is Dampness; vaginal discharge is Dampness in the Lower Burning Space; difficulty in urination is due to Dampness obstructing the Bladder; diarrhoea is Dampness in the Intestines, and so on. When Dampness has been present for a considerable time, it may become Phlegm, which can be either "substantial" or "insubstantial" (see p. 74). Substantial Phlegm produced by the Spleen manifests not only as Phlegm in the Lungs but also as fatty lumps or swellings. Insubstantial Phlegm obstructs the meridians, causing numbness or paralysis, and can obstruct the function of the Heart, disturbing the Shen, as in epilepsy; hallucinations or delirium can also result.

Physical energy

When the Spleen does not transform the food we eat into Ki, we feel fatigue. A malfunction in any of the meridians can result in tiredness, but Spleen fatigue is particularly physical in nature, since Ki is not being transported to the muscles. The Chinese call this type of tiredness "weakness of the four limbs, desires to lie down", and people with a deficient Spleen are usually relieved to adopt a horizontal position.

The flesh

Since the Spleen provides the Food Ki and Essence which builds our physical being from birth onwards,

it is natural that it should be seen as governing our ground-substance, our flesh. When we say that the Spleen governs the muscles, we are referring to the fleshy part of the muscles, the "meat" of the body, rather than the sinews which are ruled by the Liver and determine the muscles' elasticity. The Spleen gives us the "earth" of our bodies, the flesh and its characteristic texture and tone. Resilient, firm, well-circulated flesh, neither too fat nor too lean, denotes a healthy Spleen. Loose, flabby or wasted flesh is not sufficiently nourished by Ki and Blood and its opposite, lumpy, fatty or congested flesh, may be due to Dampness obstructing the circulation of Ki.

The Blood

The Blood is made in the Heart from Food Essence and pure fluids extracted from food by the Stomach and Spleen. If the Spleen is not transforming and transporting Food Essence and fluids, there will be symptoms of Blood Deficiency such as scanty menstruation, dizziness, insomnia and depression (see p. 68). The Spleen is also said to "contain" the Blood. This function follows on from that of providing good quality flesh within which the Blood can flow. Our flesh, our ground-substance, is like the earth banks surrounding a waterway. Any weakness in the banks will lead to some leakage of the water. In the same way, failure of the Spleen to contain the Blood will mean some leakage of blood, such as blood in the stools, sputum or urine, nosebleeds, broken capillaries, varicose veins and excessive or prolonged menstruation.

Governs the raising of Ki

The Spleen belongs to the Earth Element and the Ki of the Spleen supports us like the Earth. Spleen Ki "holds up" the body and if it is deficient, the body tissues and structures will sag downwards and ultimately prolapse. Haemorrhoids are a common result of the failure of this function, as are prolapses of any internal organ, such as the stomach, bladder, vagina and uterus, transverse colon or rectum. Varicose veins are another example of the Spleen's failure both to raise the Ki and to contain the Blood. External structures can sag too, particularly around the path of the Stomach or Spleen meridian – cheeks, jaw and chin, breasts and belly. This Spleen function also influences the springiness of our feet and ankles. When it is deficient, our energy may sag too and we need to lie down (see Physical Energy).

The mouth

The Spleen opens into the mouth and the condition of the mouth and lips are an indication of its health. A dry or sticky mouth, thirst or inability to taste show a Spleen malfunction. Some mouth problems, however, traditionally belong to the Stomach (see p. 194).

The intellect

The Spleen governs our capacity for abstract thought. In the same way that we physically digest food, breaking it down through various complex processes into its component substances, so we are also able to analyse experience, forming it into concepts which can be reassembled in different logical patterns to form a basis for intellectual speculation. The Spleen governs both these processes, so that we can talk about "chewing over an idea" or "mentally digesting a concept". All the meridians govern a different aspect of the human mind, and the province of ideas, of logical thought and the ability to play with it belongs to the Spleen. When the Spleen is in harmony, our intellect can both help us solve the practical problems of life and give us aesthetic enjoyment. Through perceiving contrasts, too, the intellect is the source of our sense of humour. When the Spleen is overburdened, thoughts go round and round without producing any positive result and are the source of worry.

The Spleen in Zen Shiatsu theory

In Zen Shiatsu, as in TCM, the functions of the Spleen and Stomach are two aspects of the same process, the transformation and distribution of nutrients. But there is a difference in emphasis. In physical terms, while the Stomach refers to the digestive tubes, the Spleen refers to the digestive juices which act upon the food and break it down into its component parts. Psychologically, whereas the Stomach in Zen Shiatsu is associated with hunger or the acquisitive urge, the principal characteristic of the Spleen is the capacity to contain, digest and analyse; the Stomach energy is outward-directed, while the Spleen's is more internalized.

The digestive juices and nourishment

The Spleen ensures that we receive nourishment, not only from our food but from all aspects of our lives. The Zen Shiatsu diagnostic area for the Spleen is around the umbilicus, which is the primary avenue for nourishment from the mother before birth. The ability to digest food with the digestive juices secreted by the Spleen subsequently brings us physical nourishment. On the mental level, the ability to analyse and process information and life experience allows these, too, to nourish us. On the emotional level, we are nourished by our capacity to render acceptable love and support from ourselves, as well as from others.

Eating habits

The Spleen and Stomach in Zen Shiatsu have important links with the sensations surrounding the process of eating and drinking – thirst, sticky mouth, preference for foods with high liquid content and for a lot of liquids with a meal, poor salivation – these are all signs pointing to a low supply of digestive juices and thus involving the Spleen as primary cause. No appetite, overeating or constantly nibbling, eating too quickly, craving for sweets, no appreciation of taste; these are all dysfunctions deriving from the traditional association of the Spleen with the sense of taste and the appetite. The Ki of the Spleen and Stomach manifests strongly in the quality of food desired and the eating habits. In their turn, eating habits strongly influence the Ki of the Spleen and Stomach. According to both TCM and Zen Shiatsu, irregular eating, eating with the mind elsewhere or when emotionally upset, overeating or undereating, and eating too quickly all damage the Spleen Ki and hence the digestive capacity. Most women in Western countries weaken their Spleen energy from adolescence onward by dieting and bingeing. Eating disorders such as anorexia nervosa and bulimia are manifesting increasingly frequently in the West and are often linked with a Stomach or Spleen diagnosis.

Digestion

Whereas, according to TCM, all digestive disturbances are likely to involve the Spleen in some way, Zen Shiatsu diagnosis is more likely to point to the meridian of the actual digestive organ affected. In clinical practice, a Spleen diagnosis can indicate overweight, irritable bowel syndrome, colitis, gas and bloating, diarrhoea, constipation and general abdominal discomfort. These conditions could also manifest with any other meridian diagnosis, but if the Spleen is diagnosed, they will be connected with worry and overthinking, as well as with poor secretion of digestive juices.

Overuse of the brain

While Masunaga observes that mental fatigue adversely affects the Spleen, the symptom is an effect as well as a cause of the imbalance. One aspect of the Spleen's function is the process of information breakdown and mental analysis, and overactivity in this area will lead to mental fatigue. In its turn, mental fatigue will deplete the Spleen Ki and thus affect its physical function. A hyperactive Spleen is often associated with the intellectual type of person whose life experience is only acceptable when thoroughly conceptualized and contained within the logical mind; this bias towards the intellect tends to create further disharmony in the functioning of the Spleen.

Lack of exercise

The Spleen, together with the Stomach and the Large Intestine, is associated with lack of exercise both as a cause and as an effect of imbalance. "Overuse of the mind and underuse of the body" (*Zen Imagery Exercises*, p. 198) sums up the problem. Enjoyable exercise can restore the balance and is always a good recommendation for a condition rooted in the Spleen.

Fatigue

Since the Spleen prepares food for assimilation by the body by secreting digestive juices, a deficient Spleen is likely to lead to fatigue and physical weakness resulting from lack of Ki, which is another reason for reluctance to exercise. Masunaga also associates anaemia with this condition, since the body cannot make blood from poorly digested food.

Reproductive hormones

The Spleen and Stomach are associated with the hormonal changes of the menstrual cycle and pregnancy. Masunaga writes of "reproductive hormones related to the breast and ovaries" and the Stomach and Spleen meridians both pass through these areas. Premenstrual syndrome can involve many of the meridians, but where it is associated with breast tenderness and tiredness it is often associated with the Spleen. If the Spleen is not functioning well, there is likely to be an irregular menstrual cycle.

The Spleen meridian and how to treat it

The traditional Spleen meridian starts at the medial edge of the big toe and travels up the medial aspect of the instep and over the medial malleolus to ascend the inner surface of the leg, in the groove posterior to the shinbone. It moves on up the inside edge of the kneecap, then up the medial edge of rectus femoris, just medial to the midline of the thigh. It moves up the groin briefly before ascending the abdomen, lateral to the Stomach meridian, along the outside border of rectus abdominis, then ascends the ribcage diagonally and laterally, then up the lateral edge of the breast to the second intercostal space, then descends to its last point, halfway down the side of the ribcage.

Masunaga's extended Spleen meridian has a branch which moves from the second intercostal space down the inner surface of the arm just medial to the Lung meridian, to end at the ulnar edge of the index finger. It ascends higher than the traditional Spleen, moving up across the clavicle to the origin of the posterior head of the sternocleidomastoid. It then ascends the neck, deep to that muscle, to the angle of the jawbone, and then moves up the side of the face to finish at the corner of the hairline. This facial

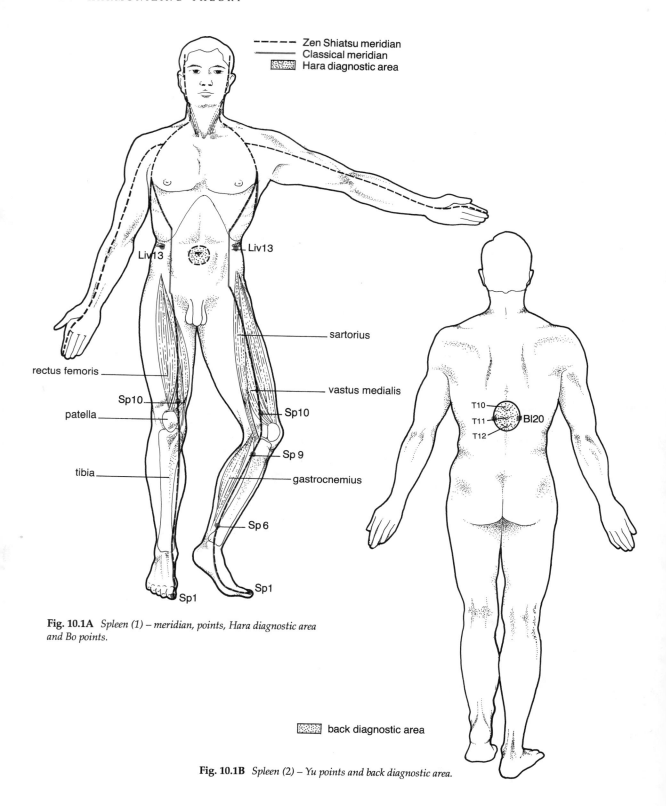

- - - - Zen Shiatsu meridian
———— Classical meridian
▦ Hara diagnostic area

Liv13

Liv13

sartorius

rectus femoris

vastus medialis

Sp10

Sp10

patella

Sp 9

tibia

gastrocnemius

Sp 6

Sp1

Sp1

Fig. 10.1A *Spleen (1) – meridian, points, Hara diagnostic area and Bo points.*

T10

T11

Bl20

T12

▦ back diagnostic area

Fig. 10.1B *Spleen (2) – Yu points and back diagnostic area.*

portion of the Zen Shiatsu Spleen meridian is a branch of the classical Stomach pathway (Fig. 10.1A).

The diagnostic area for the Spleen on the Hara is a small circle around the navel.

The back diagnostic area surrounds the tenth, eleventh and twelfth vertebrae (Fig. 10.1B).

Like the Stomach meridian, the Spleen is most accessible in the supine position.

Treatment procedure

1. The Spleen in the leg is treated in supine position, with the receiver's leg crooked slightly outwards, toe to opposite ankle. With her mother hand resting on the receiver's Hara, the giver works the meridian with palm or thumb. It may be necessary to support the receiver's leg between the giver's knees (Fig. 10.2).

2. Where the meridian ascends the ribcage, curving from navel to shoulder, it is best worked with the fingertips, both hands alternating, angling the pressure in towards the centre of the body. On women, it may be necessary to slide the fingertips under the breast tissue before applying pressure along the side of the breast (Fig. 10.3).

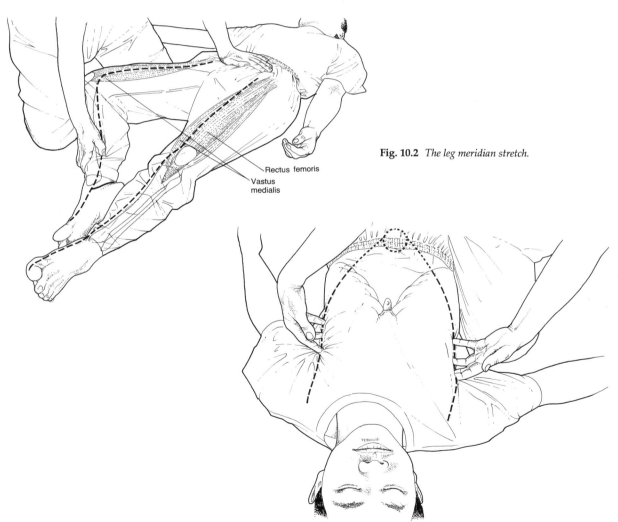

Rectus femoris
Vastus medialis

Fig. 10.2 *The leg meridian stretch.*

Fig. 10.3 *Up the sides of the chest.*

3. Masunaga's Spleen meridian on the arm is just medial to the traditional Lung meridian and is worked similarly, with palm or thumb, and mother hand resting on the same shoulder (Fig. 10.4).

4. The meridian in the neck lies just underneath and slightly lateral to the Stomach meridian, under the sternocleidomastoid. The giver kneels behind the receiver's head, supporting it with one hand under the occipital ridge, and works down the anterior border of the muscle, applying a "hooking" movement with the tip of the thumb to move the muscle out of the way and reach under it to the meridian (Fig. 10.5).

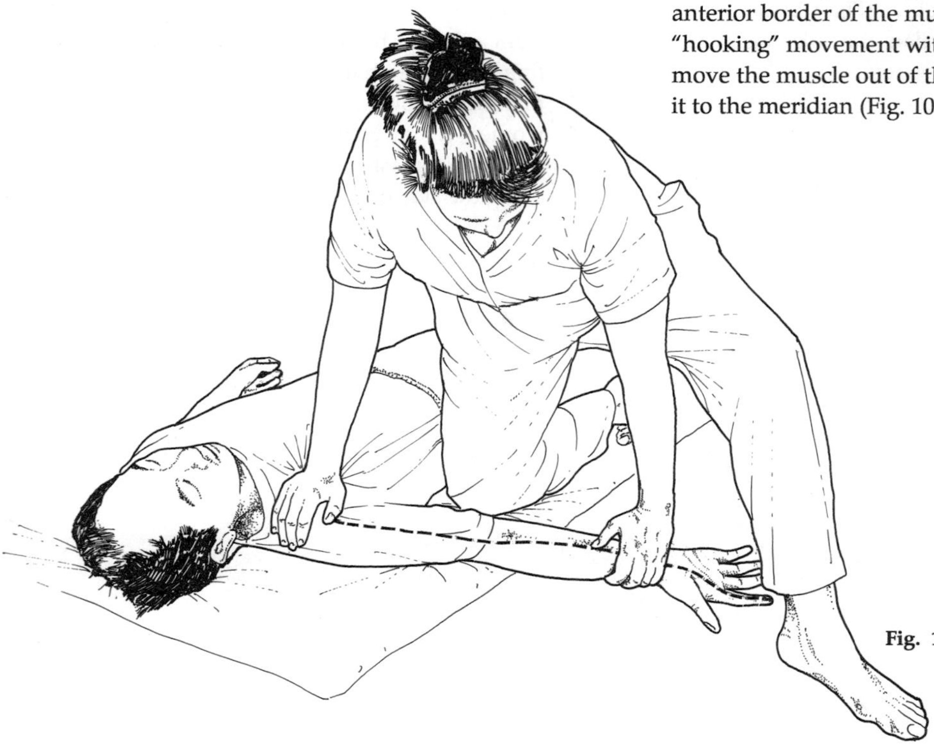

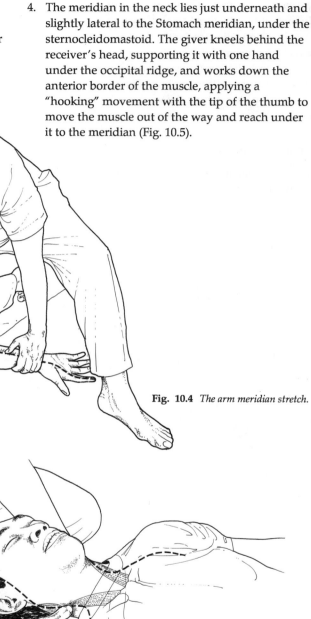

Fig. 10.4 *The arm meridian stretch.*

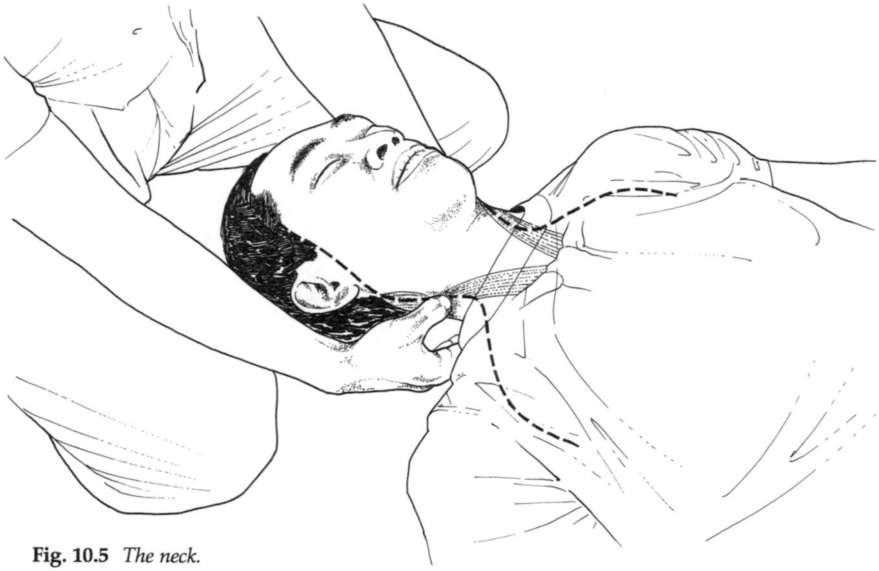

Fig. 10.5 *The neck.*

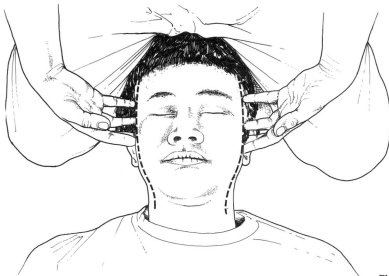

Fig. 10.6 *The face.*

5. Where Masunaga's Spleen meridian runs up the side of the face, it can be treated as above, turning the receiver's head to the side and working with the thumb or, as shown, using the fingertips of both hands horizontally (Fig. 10.6).

Major points on the Spleen meridian

Spleen 1

On the medial side of the big toe, about 1/10" medial to the corner of the nail.

Actions

- Removes Blood stagnation
- Helps contain the Blood
- Calms the mind

Spleen 6

Four fingers' width directly above the tip of the medial malleolus, in the groove posterior to the tibia.

DO NOT USE DURING PREGNANCY

Actions

- Moves, cools and nourishes the Blood
- Removes Dampness
- Nourishes Yin, calms the Shen and promotes sleep
- Benefits the Spleen, Liver and Kidneys

Spleen 9

On the lower border of the medial condyle of the tibia, in the depression between the posterior border of the tibia and the gastrocnemius.

Action

- Removes Dampness, especially from the Lower Burning Space

Spleen 10

Three fingers' width above the medial edge of the superior border of the patella, on the bulge of vastus intermedius.

Action

- Cools, moves and nourishes the Blood

Spleen Yu point

Bl 20 – two fingers' width lateral to the midline of the spine, parallel with the lower border of the spinous process of the eleventh thoracic vertebra.

Spleen Bo point

Liv 13 – on the lateral side of the abdomen, below the free end of the eleventh floating rib.

The Stomach in TCM

The Stomach in TCM is considered to be one of the most important of the Yang organs. Together with the Spleen, it forms the basis for our Postnatal Ki, the Ki which we derive from breathing and eating, and which is supplied by the Stomach and Spleen to the other organs and the rest of the body. If the Stomach is weak, all the other organs are weak. It is often used to treat Spleen problems in TCM, in accordance with the tradition of treating the Yin organ via the Yang one.

Rotting and ripening

This is an approximate translation for the Chinese term for the first part of the digestive process, in which the Stomach breaks food down into a more usable form so that it can be more easily transformed by the Spleen into Food Ki. This process begins in the mouth with chewing and the predigestion of food and continues in the Stomach itself. If the Stomach fails to do this properly, it weakens the Spleen and produces the characteristic signs of Spleen Yang Deficiency, specifically loose stools with undigested food. Conversely, if the Spleen is weak, the Stomach has to work harder to provide it with prepared food. A hyperactive Stomach (particularly when combined with worry, overwork or emotional problems and Hot energy food or drink) develops Stomach Fire, whose typical symptoms are bad breath, bleeding or painful gums, constipation, excessive appetite and insomnia.

Transportation of Food Essence

The Stomach is equally responsible with the Spleen for extracting the nourishing Essence from food and for transporting it around the body. In this function, which is nominally the Spleen's, the Stomach, being the more energetic Yang force, is perhaps more important. If it fails, fatigue, especially in the morning (Earth time), will result.

Descending of food and Food Ki

The Stomach is the principal force behind the downward movement of food and Food Ki through the digestive system. If the Ki of the Stomach is weak, food may tend to remain in the stomach, leading to a sensation of fullness or bloating after eating; or the Ki may rise upward in the form of belching, hiccuping, nausea or vomiting (this is known as Rebellious Ki).

Association with fluids

Like the Spleen, the Stomach is responsible for the digestive process which makes the fluid part of food and drink available and transports fluids throughout the body. Unlike the Spleen, which "loathes dampness", the Stomach needs large quantities of fluids available to it for the process of digestion. The Kidneys supply these fluids and the Kidneys are hence sometimes called "the Gateway to the Stomach". The Yin capacity of the Stomach to retain these fluids is delicate and easily damaged, especially by irregular eating or by indulging in mental work while eating. When Stomach Yin is thus damaged, a form of Empty Heat (see p. 79) develops in the Stomach, characterized by gastric pain, constipation and a dry mouth.

The mouth

Since the sense organ of the Earth Element is the mouth, many Stomach problems produce symptoms there, such as cold sores and mouth ulcers, which show Heat in the Stomach. Bleeding, swollen or painful gums and bad breath are signs of Stomach Fire (see above).

Association with the mind

The Stomach, with the Spleen, is in charge of the process of logical thought, the Yi or intellect. It also assists the Spleen in the proper processing of food and fluids so that they so not cause Dampness or Phlegm. If the Stomach or Spleen fails in this function, Phlegm can cloud the mind, leading to a feeling of fuzziness and disorientation. If the mental aspect of the Stomach energy is out of balance, logical thought patterns can become obsessive and destructive neuroses. In certain conditions, such as Phlegm-Fire in the Stomach in which Fire also disturbs the Shen, all factors may combine to create serious mental derangement, manifesting as delirium, confusion or hallucinations.

The meridian

The Stomach meridian is one of the three long Yang meridians chiefly responsible for keeping us upright (the others being the Bladder and Gall Bladder) and supports the entire front of the body, neck and head. Problems in the face, jaw, throat, breasts, abdomen, thighs, knees and feet can all be treated via the Stomach meridian.

The Stomach in Zen Shiatsu theory

The Stomach and Spleen together represent the second stage of the Zen Shiatsu life cycle. The physical expression of this stage is the obtaining and breakdown of food and the energy picture is one of attraction and forward movement, followed by enfolding and containing. The energetic movement of this phase of the life cycle provides a further connection between the Earth meridians and the female reproductive system, since it represents the capacity of the female to accept the male seed and then to contain the developing embryo. The Stomach embodies the first part of the energetic process, that of attraction and movement towards a desired object. On the physical level, the Stomach governs the tubes and organs of the digestive system, the structures which transport our food from outside to inside in the "acquiring" stage. On the psychological level, the Stomach represents our hungers and needs, the steps we take to fulfil them and our capacity to accept the results.

Digestive tubes

This is how Masunaga referred to the physical domain of the Stomach. The entire digestive tract consists of structures designed either to convey food into our bodies or to allow nutrients to be absorbed; they all embody the "acquiring" function of the Stomach meridian. Problems with any part of the upper digestive tract, such as the oesophagus and duodenum, may relate to a Stomach diagnosis. Occasionally a Stomach malfunction may also cause problems in the small intestine or colon.

Appetite

The Stomach function represents our quest for nourishment. It encompasses all our appetites or hungers, including the hunger for security, the hunger for knowledge and the hunger for love. Wherever there is frustration of a primary need, the Stomach meridian will attempt to compensate, for its primary aim is fulfilment. Whenever Stomach appears consistently in the diagnosis, look for an area of life where the receiver's needs are not being met. Compensation eating is a common effect of frustration, also associated with the Stomach. Zen Shiatsu connects Stomach and Spleen problems with overeating or eating too quickly.

Acceptance

The Stomach also represents our ability to accept nourishment on all levels. When the Stomach meridian is affected very early in life, by either physical or emotional malnourishment, the individual's capacity to accept nourishment thereafter may be permanently impaired; the organism never learns to accept and may reject instead. Physically, this could manifest as poor appetite or as nausea, in which the body reacts to nourishment with a rejection pattern. When the mind rejects food, eating disorders such as anorexia nervosa or bulimia appear and these then lead to an impaired digestive function. A common emotional manifestation of a Stomach diagnosis is the inability to accept support or appreciation from others.

The front and the need to please

The above pattern often disguises itself as a propensity for giving, since constant giving hides the fact that we are unable to receive. Pleasing others is also a way of fulfilling our own need for love and appreciation. The motherly woman who wears herself out helping others or the kind, jolly man who is always on call are obvious examples of this pattern, although it can manifest in a myriad other personalities. There is usually considerable investment of energy in the outward behaviour and great efforts may be made to be entertaining, humorous, expressive or just plain "nice". The Stomach and Spleen meridians run down the front of the body and a disharmony in either may manifest as a "front" of behaviour designed to please, behind which are hidden the patterns of need and rejection. Physical symptoms and signs of a Stomach imbalance are often in the front of the body.

Overthinking

This is a characteristic result of Stomach and Spleen disharmony, in both TCM and Zen Shiatsu. A healthy Stomach energy gives us mental curiosity and an ability to take in new information. If the Stomach is hyperactive, more information is taken in than can be usefully assimilated. A long term imbalance of this sort may lead to an insatiable appetite for mental input, as seen in the kind of person with a mentally stressful job who takes 20 paperbacks to read on holiday. If the Stomach is low in energy, there may be an inability to accept new ideas and a tendency to "chew over" old memories. Worry is another Stomach manifestation, in which the mind churns an idea round and round without being able either to accept or reject it. In either case, a Stomach imbalance brings an inability to rest the mind. Lack of exercise is often another facet of the problem, since as the mind is given greater priority, less and less attention is paid to the body.

Menstrual cycle

Although Western physiology does not link the Stomach with female hormones, there is an undoubted connection between nourishment, exercise and the menstrual cycle. The proportion of fat to muscle in women affects the regularity of the periods, which often cease altogether in athletes and anorexics. This connection has long been known in TCM and is retained in Zen Shiatsu theory, in which irregularity of the menstrual cycle and "malfunctioning of the female organs" often accompany a Stomach diagnosis.

The meridian

Many of the symptoms ascribed to Stomach dysfunction in Zen Shiatsu relate to the meridian pathway, as in TCM. Jaw and neck tension often combine to produce a stiff and painful neck. Eyestrain from too much reading is linked to the beginning of the meridian under the eye. Nasal congestion and sneezing relate to the junction between the Large Intestine and Stomach meridians, between the nose and the eye. Tension and pain in the mid-to-low back often accompany weak abdominal muscles and pain or discomfort in the solar plexus and abdomen are also common. Heavy thighs or legs, knee problems and weak feet and ankles also relate to the Stomach meridian. The meridian runs through the nipple and breast problems may accompany a Stomach imbalance.

The Stomach meridian and how to treat it

The traditional Stomach meridian is one of the longest in the body. It is one of the three great Yang "postural" meridians and supports the front of the body in the same way that the Bladder supports the back and the Gall Bladder supports the sides. It begins under the eye and runs down the cheek past the corner of the mouth to the jawline, where a secondary line branches out to the angle of the jaw and up to a point just within the corner of the hairline. The meridian then descends on either side of the oesophagus to run horizontally along the superior edge of the clavicle to its midpoint, whence it descends to the nipple. It then runs down the ribcage and narrows to descend the abdomen in a straight line to just above the pubic bone, whence it moves diagonally across the groin to the outside of the thigh. It descends the lateral border of rectus femoris (just outside the midline of the thigh) to the lateral border of the kneecap, thence down tibialis anterior, just lateral to the dorsum of the foot between the second and third metatarsals to the lateral edge of the nail of the second toe.

Masunaga divided off the branch of the classical meridian which runs from jaw to hairline, assigning it to the Spleen rather than to the Stomach. There is an extra branch to his extended Stomach meridian which runs under the mouth, between the lower lip and the chin. He also traced the Stomach meridian from the midpoint of the clavicle around to the meeting point of the Yang meridians, GV 14, just below C 7 at the back of the neck, and thence along the upper border of the scapula (not the scapular

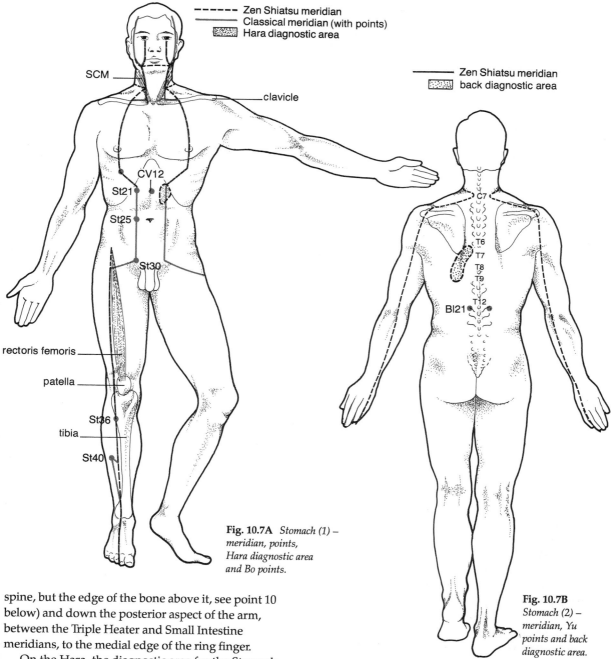

Fig. 10.7A *Stomach (1) – meridian, points, Hara diagnostic area and Bo points.*

Fig. 10.7B *Stomach (2) – meridian, Yu points and back diagnostic area.*

spine, but the edge of the bone above it, see point 10 below) and down the posterior aspect of the arm, between the Triple Heater and Small Intestine meridians, to the medial edge of the ring finger.

On the Hara, the diagnostic area for the Stomach is next to the border of the upper part of the ribcage, on the left-hand side, over the actual Stomach organ (Fig. 10.7A).

The Stomach diagnostic area on the back lies to the left of the spine, roughly from the seventh to the tenth thoracic vertebrae, sloping laterally out under the inferior angle of the left scapula, towards the Small Intestine meridian (Fig. 10.7B).

The Stomach meridian is usually treated in the supine position, as it is on the front of the body.

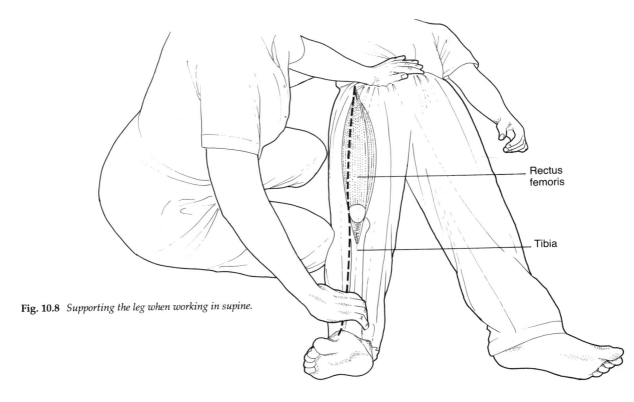

Rectus femoris

Tibia

Fig. 10.8 *Supporting the leg when working in supine.*

Treatment procedure

1. The Stomach in the leg is most easily treated in the supine position. Since it lies just lateral to the midline, it is important, if the leg has a tendency to roll outwards, to support it in order to apply perpendicular pressure; this can be done with the giver's knee or foot, while the meridian is worked with thumb or palm, angling straight downwards, with the mother hand on the receiver's Hara (Fig. 10.8).

2. The Stomach meridian on the foot can often be reached from the previous position as a continuation of the meridian on the leg; however, if the receiver's legs are long or the giver's arms are short, it may be treated as part of a complete front-of-foot sequence (Fig. 10.9).

3. The meridian as it runs the length of the torso along the nipple line can be treated with thumbs or fingertips, kneeling beside the receiver's Hara for the area below the breasts (A), and behind the receiver's head for the upper chest (B). Avoid working over the breast tissue on women (Figs 10.10A and B).

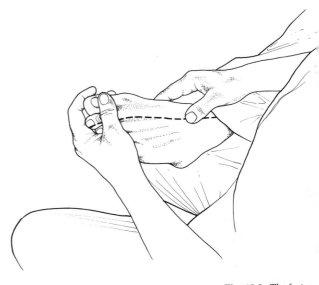

Fig. 10.9 *The foot.*

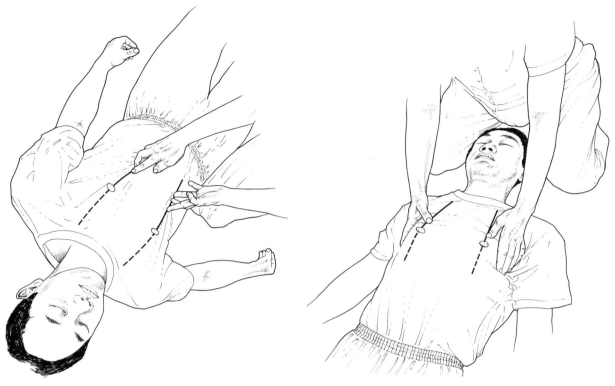

Fig. 10.10A *The lower ribcage.*

Fig. 10.10B *The upper chest.*

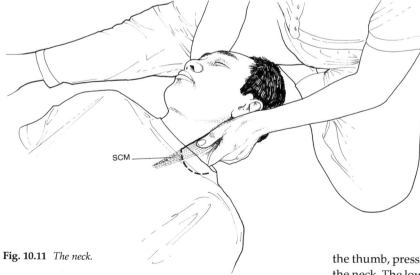

Fig. 10.11 *The neck.*

4. The Stomach in the neck runs along the anterior border of the sternocleidomastoid and is often a significant cause of neck stiffness. It is treated with the thumb, pressing gently towards the middle of the neck. The lower third of this part of the meridian should be avoided so as not to stimulate the cough reflex or the nerves supplying the arm (Fig. 10.11).

5. It is occasionally necessary to treat the Stomach meridian in the hollow above the collarbone when there is tension in the front of the neck. It should be worked deeply but gently, with the thumb, working into the groove between the bone and the soft tissue (Fig. 10.12).

6. The Stomach meridian in the jaw is also intimately connected with neck stiffness. It lies along the upper edge of the mandible and is worked with the thumbs, while the fingers support the lower edge. Work deeply but not too hard (Fig. 10.13).

7. The meridian in the face is usually included in the general face Shiatsu (see p. 50).

8. Working the Stomach meridian in the arm can be accomplished in one stage, but may be easier in two stages. The first stage is work on the upper arm, which is best reached in supine position by laying the receiver's arm over his torso with the forearm lying horizontally across the Stomach diagnostic area. The Stomach meridian lies between the Triple Heater and Small Intestine and is worked in the upper arm in a straight line from behind the posterior border of the deltoid to the

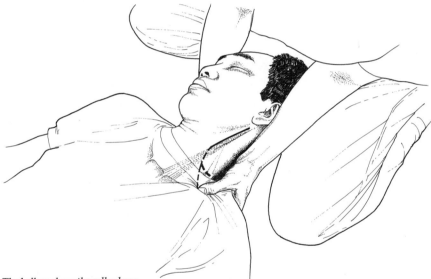

Fig. 10.12 *The hollow above the collar bone.*

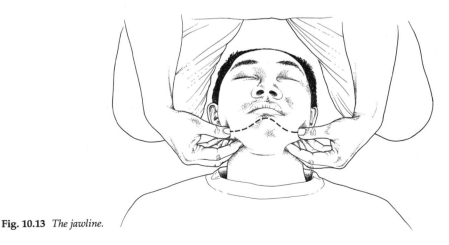

Fig. 10.13 *The jawline.*

hollow above the olecranon, with palm or thumb, with the mother hand supporting the receiver's shoulder and the knee supporting his elbow (Fig. 10.14A).

9. The second stage is working the forearm, for which the arm may be laid palm down by the receiver's side, and the Stomach meridian, which crosses the elbow to the upper surface of the forearm down to the wrist, between Small Intestine and Triple Heater, worked with palm, thumb or Dragon's Mouth (Fig. 10.14B). The final part, between the fourth and fifth metacarpals and down the fourth finger, is then worked with the thumb, while the other hand supports the wrist. The forearm can also be worked from the position in 8 above, but is not so accessible.

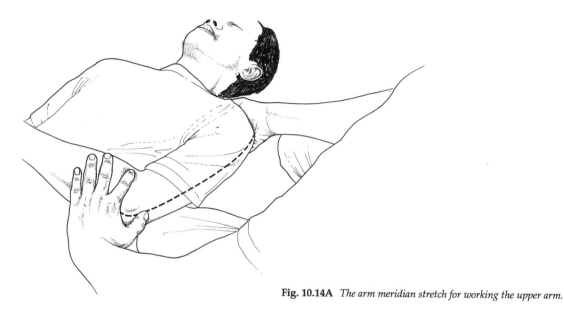

Fig. 10.14A *The arm meridian stretch for working the upper arm.*

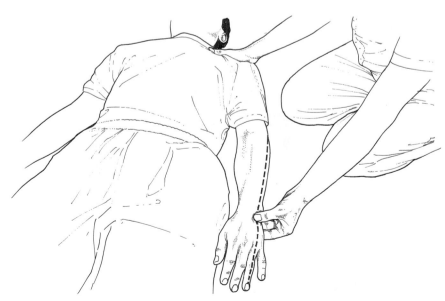

Fig. 10.14B *The forearm.*

10. The Stomach meridian in the shoulders lies along the upper edge of the scapula, not along the upper edge of the scapular spine, which is the Small Intestine meridian (see p. 161). The Stomach can be felt, on deeper palpation, as a parallel and superior groove. This can be worked with thumb or elbow in the sitting position (Fig. 10.15), angling straight down to the floor, either bilaterally or one side at a time, in which case the mother hand is on the same shoulder.

11. The shoulders can also be treated in the prone position, with the thumbs, either bilaterally, with alternating pressures, or one side at a time, with the mother hand on the opposite shoulder. The angle of penetration is towards the receiver's feet (Fig. 10.16).

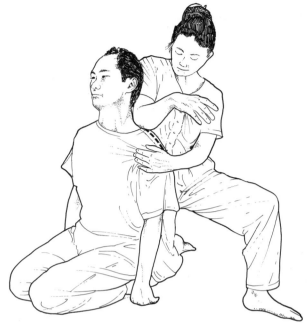

Fig. 10.15 *The shoulders in sitting position.*

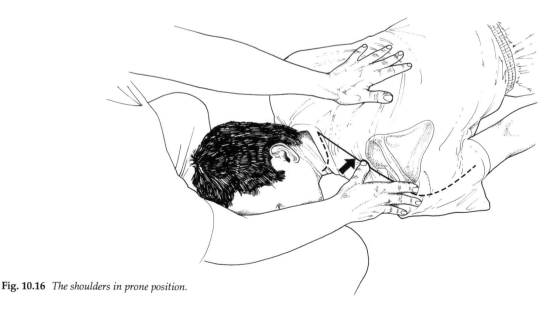

Fig. 10.16 *The shoulders in prone position.*

Major points on the Stomach meridian

Stomach 21

Approximately six fingers' width above the navel and three fingers' width lateral to the midline.

Actions

- Regulates the Stomach and stops pain
- Subdues Rebellious Ki

Stomach 25

Three fingers' width lateral to the centre of the umbilicus.

Actions

- Bo point of the Large Intestine
- Tonifies the Intestines
- Clears Heat

Stomach 30

On the upper border of the pubic bone, two thumbs' width lateral to the midline.

Actions

- Removes stagnation of Ki and Blood in the Lower Burner
- Nourishes Essence
- Stimulates the digestive action of Stomach and Spleen

Stomach 36

Four fingers' width below the lower border of the patella, one finger's width lateral to the crest of the tibia.

Actions

- Tonifies Ki and Blood and strengthens the body
- Raises Yang and expels Excess Cold
- Expels Wind and Damp
- Tonifies Stomach and Spleen and regulates the Intestines

Stomach 40

Half the distance between the lateral malleolus and the knee crease, one finger's width lateral to the tibia.

Actions

- Expels substantial and insubstantial Phlegm
- Calms and clears the mind
- Opens the chest

Stomach Yu point

B1 21 – two fingers' width lateral to the midline of the spine, level with the lower edge of the spinous process of T 12.

Stomach Bo point

CV 12 – on the midline of the upper abdomen, halfway between the navel and the meeting of the ribs (the xiphisternal joint).

11

The Metal Element – The Lungs and Large Intestine

■ *"If you can imagine an Ideal Human Container... that ideal energetic container would be infinitely expandable, infinitely contractible, infinitely diffusable, infinitely condensable, with boundaries ranging from steel-like rigidity to mist-like permeability. The miracle is how nearly we have access to that range."*

JULIE HENDERSON, "THE LOVER WITHIN", STATION HILL PRESS, 1986

Element associations: value, conductivity, strength, precision

The Chinese ideogram usually translated as "Metal" more properly means "gold", which adds an extra dimension to the meaning; it means something of great value, untarnishable, non-degradable. Metal, in the form of gold, has been a symbol for value since civilization began and in this capacity has always been a medium of exchange or barter between individuals, groups and nations. We can associate both the Metal meridians with this meaning, since the Lungs act to take in the purest, most valuable component of the world outside, the Ki of the universe, and the Large Intestine works to expel from the body and mind all that is no longer of any value to the individual's life process. In this way, both Metal meridians work together for exchange.

A further intrinsic capacity of metal is its ability to conduct – temperature changes, magnetism, electricity, when passed through metal, are all speedily transmitted to the metal itself and thence to any other receptive substance. The metal, in a sense,

acts as a medium through which messages pass, messages whose transmission necessitates a change of state. The Shang Shu speaks of Metal as "that which can be moulded, and can harden". This is the essential quality of Metal energy, that it can change its state and yet return to its former structure. So the Metal Element in our own energetic make-up implies our ability to receive and transmit messages, to communicate with the environment and yet to remain our own selves. It conducts and connects.

Further attributes of the Metal Element in nature are tensile strength, density and sharpness or precision. All these make it suitable for making structures or instruments which require precision of design. Metal provides accuracy in measurement and precision for construction. This is true also of Metal in the human bodymind – "The Lung has the charge of minister and assistant, from it stem well regulated rhythms" (Su Wen, Ch. 8).

The rhythm of the breath is the most dependable occurrence in our lives. With this steady rhythm as our point of departure, we can move on to recognize and create symmetry and predictability, to structure our reality. In psychological terms, the Metal energy gives the ability to form strong but flexible belief systems to support and regulate our lives; through order, to create harmony between our inner and outer environments.

When our Metal energy is healthy, we feel that we are individuals in a situation of exchange with the universe. Not only do we feel our own value, but we know instinctively that we are *connected* to everything of value outside our own boundaries. We have self-worth and the capacity to change while remaining in harmony with our environment.

Quality, worth, whatever we most prize, is "in here" in abundance as well as "out there" and we are secure in our ability to connect with it.

If, on the other hand, our Metal is out of balance, no such security exists. Perhaps we reinforce our boundaries, in order to clamp down on what little we feel we have and to avoid further loss. This impairs our capacity to take in or eliminate, leading to a state of physical and mental deprivation and constipation. Or we may seek outside our own boundaries for an ideal perfection which we constantly pursue because of our own intrinsic sense of emptiness and lack of worth.

Spiritual capacity of the Element: the corporeal soul

The Metal Element forms the boundaries of our life on earth, with our first and last breath. Between the drawing of the first and last breaths, our bodies are inhabited by the corporeal soul, or Po, ruled by Metal. This is a counterpart to the ethereal soul, or Hun, which pertains to the Wood Element and which corresponds to a kind of "soul personality". The corporeal soul, however, returns to the earth after our death, in the same way as our physical substance, and represents more a kind of instinctual bodily intelligence. Our innate ability to respond to the environment, and above all our ability to exchange Ki with the universe through breath, are the gift of the Po. The sense of smell and the sense of touch, which contacts the Metal Element via the skin, are examples of the way in which the Po receives experience; this experience is non-verbal, non-conceptual, but nonetheless extraordinarily vivid and vital, since through it we re-establish our connection with our own intrinsic Ki and with that of the universe. If we think of the immediacy with which touch can communicate with our inmost feelings or how a smell can call up a memory and seem to transport us directly into the reality of a past situation, we have an idea of the way in which the Po operates.

Movement of Element energy: inwards and downwards

In the cycle of the movement of energy represented by the Elements through the seasons, the Metal phase is linked with the autumn, when summer's Yang peak of energy begins to reverse. Leaves fall, vegetation dies down and Ki moves down and inwards in preparation for the winter storage period. The Lungs also, uppermost in the body, draw Ki inward and send it down to the Kidneys (Hara) for anchoring; only then can it be dispersed outwards to the rest of the organs and tissues. The Large Intestine, too, moves waste downwards for disposal.

The movement of the Metal phase of energy is sometimes called "decline" and in fact there does seem to be a decline in visible manifestations of Ki, as it moves inwards; but if there is an understanding of the regenerative, Yin power of this movement back towards the source, then allowance and acceptance of this seeming decline can take place.

Element emotion: grief

The emotion associated with Metal is grief. In the natural cycle of birth, growth, waning, death and rebirth which manifests in the seasons, Metal embodies the phase of waning in autumn, when it is natural to feel existential grief. Sadness is inevitable in human existence, for the loss of youth, of vigour, of relations and friends and eventually of life itself. However, a healthy and flexible Metal Element is built to encompass such changes and to allow loss to make room in our lives for new intake. Old people who have successfully navigated the autumn of their lives can show us what that new intake is: acceptance, the wisdom of experience, mature individuality, humor, lightness and a true enjoyment of life. Healthy Metal energy does not prevent the experience of grief, but it prevents us from being trapped in it; it keeps us open to new possibilities.

If the Metal Element is weak within us it is harder to let go of sadness and bereavement, and loss of any kind can cause a prevailing state of melancholy or depression, which may or may not be followed by physical illness. The Metal energy can also be weakened in childhood by overharsh upbringing, which can lead to sadness and a lack of self-worth. Or the imbalance may be inherited and present from birth onwards as a permanent sense of deprivation or isolation. Grief is a natural consequence of inability to connect with the universe around us and vice versa; if we grieve excessively, we feel isolated and cannot connect.

Harder to notice but equally out of balance is the inability to grieve. The discharge of grief is an essential part of the bodymind's capacity to renew itself, but is often unacceptable to the individual or to our culture; if feelings of grief threaten to overwhelm us, we can repress them completely. The repression of grief in this way is often coupled with the search for perfection in our lives, but it also cuts us off from an essential part of existence and some of the vital flow between ourselves and the universal Ki is lost.

Element sense organ: the nose

The Lungs are said to open into the nose, although it is the Large Intestine meridian which connects with it directly. Both work to take in and release through the nose via the breath, generating the balance between taking in and letting go which is characteristic of the Metal Element.

The nose is also the source of our sense of smell, one of our ways of connecting with our environment which is immediate, physical and non-intellectual. The olfactory epithelium, the small patch of smell receptors at the back of each nostril, is the only part of the brain complex directly exposed to the atmosphere and via the olfactory bulbs it connects to the limbic system in the brain, where immediate emotional and instinctual responses are generated*; this is an example of the workings of the Po, the corporeal soul, the bodily intelligence which responds to sense impressions.

The nose and nasal passages are obviously affected when the Lungs are in poor condition, whether the condition is acute, as in colds and flu, or chronic, as in hayfever or sinusitis. An itchy, tickly nose, sneezing and nasal catarrh are common signs of a Lung or Large Intestine meridian problem.

Element colour: white

Perhaps the association of white with the Metal Element comes from its use throughout the Far East as the colour of mourning or perhaps it refers to the shiny quality of metal. However, it has a clinical

application, which is the diagnostic significance of the white "hue" emanating from the face. A shiny white complexion in TCM is a sign of Ki Deficiency, since the Lungs rule Ki. However, the most olive-toned skin can radiate a white hue in less chronic Metal disturbances and even in temporary disharmonies within the Metal energy, such as a cold, there may be a transparent whiteness around the eyes. There may also be a preference for wearing white.

Element sound: weeping

Still linked with the emotion of grief is the sound of the Metal imbalance. Even when grief is unconscious or suppressed, the sound of weeping will surface in the individual's voice, often in the form of a plaintive fall at the end of each phrase; if we would instinctively describe a voice as "whining" or "complaining", it is often a Metal imbalance we are hearing.

Element smell: rotten

The smells are difficult to describe and not always a useful diagnostic tool. However, the Metal smell is often discerned and resembles the smell of stale cauliflower or rotting vegetation.

Element taste: pungent

Since one of the characteristics of a Metal imbalance is a sense of remoteness from life, it is understandable that the preferred taste would be one with a "bite" to reawaken the senses, such as garlic, strong cheese or the hot taste of cayenne or chilli. The pungent taste tends to disperse Ki, counteracting the inward movement of the Metal energy, with its tendency to become dense or sluggish; but if there is a lack of Ki because of poor Lung function, the pungent taste will deplete it further.

Element season: autumn

Autumn is the season of decline and loss, when life in agricultural societies slows down after the harvest and allows time for reflection and adjustment. "The three months of autumn are called the period of tranquillity of one's conduct" (Nei Ching, p. 102). In our urban societies, however, autumn usually marks

*Acknowledgement for this reference to John Steele, from a talk at the International Journal of Aromatherapy conference, Sussex University, July 1993.

the beginning of the academic year and an important commercial season and tension builds up as the workload increases. It is possible that the epidemics of influenza and similar Lung-related illnesses which so often occur later in the winter could be avoided, if autumn were given its due and life allowed to take a more leisurely pace.

Element climate: dryness

The association of autumn with dryness is not immediately clear to natives of Western countries, where autumn brings abundant rain. In China, where the connection was made, autumn is a dry season. However, the connection with the Lungs remains valid, since dryness is injurious to the Lungs.

Element time of day: 3–7 am

The time of day of the Lung meridian is 3–5 am and that of the Large Intestine is 5–7 am. This time period is around dawn, as is appropriate for the meridians which begin the cycle of the Chinese Clock (see p. 86). In the Far East, dawn is the time to get up and the first action of the day is usually some form of breathing exercise; in China it has always been the time to gather in the parks to do Tai Chi. Probably the second action of the day is defecation, in Large Intestine time. When the Metal energies are out of balance, however, symptoms may be at their worst during this time. Asthmatics may be woken by an attack during Lung time and a classic symptom of clinical depression is early waking, usually at around 5 am, with a feeling of despair which comes from the Metal emotion of grief.

The Lungs in TCM

In the traditional Chinese medical model, the Lungs include the entire respiratory system, the nasal passages and the throat. They are our primary sources of Postnatal Ki, since they take in the Ki of Heaven, which requires no processing. Together with the Heart, they form a part of the Zong Ki, or "Big Ki of the chest", which governs circulation of both Ki and Blood throughout the body. They are also the "tender organ", which means the most vulnerable to external pernicious influences, hence the old Chinese

saying that all externally caused diseases begin with the symptoms of a cold.

Respiration

The primary process for which the Lungs are responsible is the intake of Ki through respiration. In consequence, all respiratory disorders involve the Lungs in some way. This is not to say, however that all respiratory diseases have the Lungs as their root. Any of the other meridians or organs may be the primary cause of such disorders as, say, asthma, according to the different symptoms and signs.

Intake of Ki

The Lungs are responsible for the intake of Ki through breath and for the dispersal of Ki downwards and outwards. They therefore govern the Ki of the whole body. Fatigue or lack of vitality in any body system can be due to a Lung imbalance. Poor circulation is a common symptom if there is not sufficient Ki to bring warmth or blood to the extremities. Deficiency of Lung Ki often leads to pallor, weakness and shortness of breath.

Protective shield

As well as governing Ki and dispersing it outwards, the Lungs generate our Defensive Ki, which is classically said to circulate in the space between the skin and the muscles. We can imagine the Defensive Ki as a "forcefield" on and just above the entire body surface, which protects us from injurious external influences such as weather. Weak Lungs, and thus weak Defensive Ki, will result in lowered resistance to infection. The Defensive Ki is related to the opening and closing of the pores, which is how we can "sweat out" colds and fevers. If our Ki is weak, as for example after 'flu, we sweat spontaneously after the slightest exertion. Our Defensive Ki also protects us on the psychological level, although this aspect is not stressed in TCM. Shallow breathing or holding the breath is a form of psychological self-protection associated with the Lungs. Smoking (fire) depletes the Yin, receptive principle of the Lungs and thus creates a relative excess of the Yang, protective principle, helping us to feel less psychologically vulnerable.

Dispersing downward

The Lungs are often referred to in medical texts as a "canopy" or "lid" on the human body's energetic structure, because they are the uppermost organs, closest to the Ki of Heaven. Thus they "descend and disperse" Ki throughout the body: in other words, they send energy downwards and outwards. Constipation can occur when the Ki and downward movement of the Lungs are weak. On the psychological side, weak Lung energy can cause us to feel nervous and ungrounded, because our energy is "up". When the Lungs have been attacked by an external pernicious influence, as in a cold, the Ki will feel blocked throughout the body and the Lung Ki will go up, not down, manifesting in coughs and sneezes. The Lungs also disperse fluids downwards and often a chronic imbalance in the Lungs will result in retention of fluids in the upper part of the body, with puffy face or eyes, watery eyes and sinus congestion.

Regulating water

The Lungs receive refined fluids from the Spleen and disperse them throughout the body, as mentioned above. It is said that "the Lungs regulate the water passages", which means that often the patterns of urination or sweating are disturbed when the Lung Ki is weak or obstructed. When the Lungs are blocked by an attack of Wind-Cold (see Ch. 5) and not dispersing fluids to the skin, there is no sweating, as in 'flu. By the same token, a chronic Deficiency of the Lungs over time can lead to dry skin, dry hair, dry lips and so on.

The skin

The Lungs rule the skin which, because of its similar function of gas exchange, is known also in the West as "the third lung". Chronic skin diseases such as eczema or psoriasis are often part of a Lung disharmony. However, eruptive skin disorders such as boils or acne are more likely to be an attempt to eliminate and are therefore associated more with the Large Intestine function (see p. 216).

The nose

The Lungs open into the nose. A blocked or runny nose, sinus problems, sneezing and so on are usually treated as Lung-related, although these symptoms can also be due to overproduction of mucus by the Spleen or the Large Intestine's failure to eliminate the mucus. The Lungs also give us our sense of smell.

The throat

The throat, which is also affected by Lung disorders, giving rise to a sore or tickly throat and cough, is not a sense organ in TCM terms, but it is dignified by the title of "Gateway to the Lungs", so that the connection between throat and respiratory system is made. It is also the source of the voice, whose strength is determined by the strength of Lung Ki, so that loss of voice can occur in acute Lung disorders, and a quiet, weak voice in chronic Lung imbalance.

The corporeal soul

Since the Lungs govern the Ki, they account for the vitality of the body. The corporeal soul or Po, which is ruled by the Lungs, accounts for its responsiveness. This includes our response to our bodily sensations and to the sense impressions we receive from the environment. One of the bodily sensations received by the corporeal soul is pain, a necessary survival response to save us from injury. Anaesthetics, either general or local, which block the sensation of pain, are said to have an adverse effect on the Lungs through the corporeal soul.

The Lungs in Zen Shiatsu theory

In Zen Shiatsu theory, the essential role of the Lungs is to facilitate the process of exchange between the individual and the environment and this exchange can be either physical or psychological. In Western terms, the lungs provide an ultrathin internal surface where the life-giving process of the exchange of oxygen for carbon dioxide takes place. Masunaga made a connection between the Lungs' traditional relationship with the skin and with the Defensive Ki, in other words with the body surface and its surface "field", and the physiological fact of the Lungs' permeability: thus emerged a picture of the Lung Ki as forming a kind of energetic "border", external as well as internal, through which exchange can take place. It is the Lungs which both differentiate the individual from the environment, via the skin surface, and connect him or her to it, via the breath. Viewed from a broader perspective, our first breath and our last constitute the boundaries of our lifespan, so that even in the area of destiny, the Lungs are responsible for our "borders".

The permeable surface

The Lungs govern the skin (as in TCM), which is a surface capable of both absorption and exertion. The lungs themselves consist largely of epithelial surface in direct contact with the atmosphere, which is designed for absorption and excretion. The Large Intestine, which also opens directly to the exterior, has a large surface area and its main functions are absorption and excretion. Exchange through the different surface areas of the Metal Element is the essential key to an understanding of the Lungs and Large Intestine in Zen Shiatsu.

The gas exchange of the Lungs and the material exchange of the Large Intestine are aspects of the exchange of Ki through the borders which define and differentiate the individual from the rest of the universe.

Making a border

Psychologically, since the Lungs are related to our boundaries, an imbalance in Lung Ki will lead to feelings of isolation from others, either depression or a general feeling of alienation, as if "in a fish-tank". When the Lungs' function is impaired, we are cut off from the Ki of the universe and a feedback cycle of depression and feelings of unworthiness results. We learn to restrict our breathing to defend ourselves from painful feelings and thus further weaken our connection with the Ki of Heaven.

Intake of Ki

The act of taking in the Ki of the universe from outside our individual boundaries implies an ability also to take in new experiences, to be open. The new Ki represents the new vitality required for growth, on both the physical and the psychological level, and its intake is half of the process of exchange with the environment. The other half is the release of products which the organism no longer needs, so that the Lungs work in tandem with their partner, the Large Intestine, which lets go of unwanted materials, patterns, structures and emotions to make room for new intake. The two work together synergistically to bring "new breath" to our lives.

Respiration

Physiologically, Zen Shiatsu sees the Lungs as primarily concerned with the respiratory system, as in the Western model. Sighing, watery eyes, frequent colds and coughs, breathlessness or stuffiness in the chest and nasal congestion are obvious Lung symptoms. Stiffness and pain in the upper back are also commonly found when Lungs are diagnosed. Any respiratory disorder is likely to involve the Lung meridian, as in TCM.

Vitality but not immunity

In Zen Shiatsu, as in TCM, the Lungs govern the body's ability to create Ki. Pallor, fatigue, cold hands and feet are familiar from the TCM model, but Masunaga adds obesity as another possible Lung symptom, since low vitality can hinder the body from processing food properly.

In Masunaga's view, the body's system of self-defence was the province not so much of the Lungs as of the Triple Heater, by virtue of its connection with the surface circulation and thus, by extension, with the Ki of the body surface. Triple Heater is often diagnosed on the Hara at the beginning of a cold. Skin rashes, when they stem from an allergic sensitivity, are more likely to be a Triple Heater problem, but chronic skin disorders remain associated with the Lungs.

The Lung meridian and how to treat it

The traditional Lung meridian travels from the upper part of the chest down the lateral edge of the arm, to

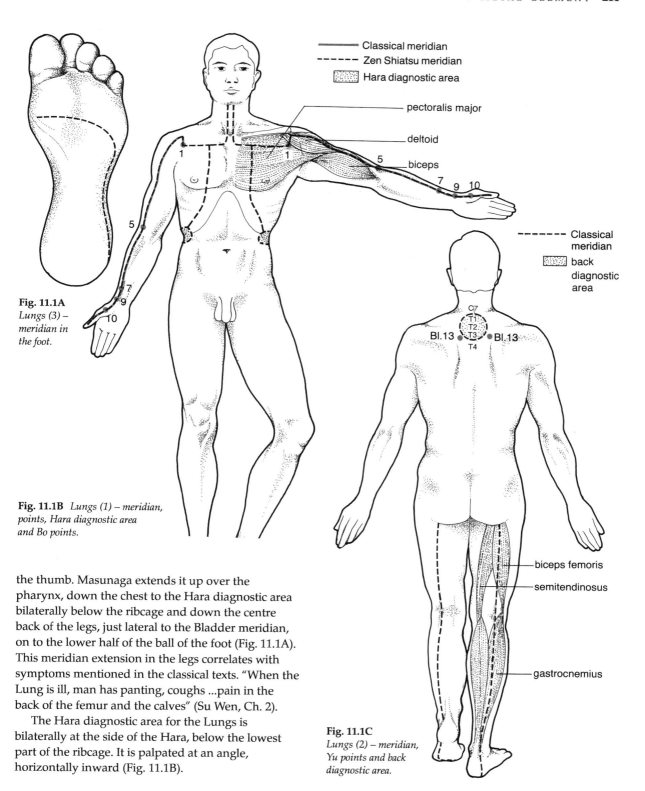

Classical meridian
Zen Shiatsu meridian
Hara diagnostic area

pectoralis major

deltoid

biceps

Fig. 11.1A
*Lungs (3) –
meridian in
the foot.*

Classical
meridian

back
diagnostic
area

Fig. 11.1B *Lungs (1) – meridian,
points, Hara diagnostic area
and Bo points.*

biceps femoris

semitendinosus

gastrocnemius

the thumb. Masunaga extends it up over the
pharynx, down the chest to the Hara diagnostic area
bilaterally below the ribcage and down the centre
back of the legs, just lateral to the Bladder meridian,
on to the lower half of the ball of the foot (Fig. 11.1A).
This meridian extension in the legs correlates with
symptoms mentioned in the classical texts. "When the
Lung is ill, man has panting, coughs ...pain in the
back of the femur and the calves" (Su Wen, Ch. 2).

The Hara diagnostic area for the Lungs is
bilaterally at the side of the Hara, below the lowest
part of the ribcage. It is palpated at an angle,
horizontally inward (Fig. 11.1B).

Fig. 11.1C
*Lungs (2) – meridian,
Yu points and back
diagnostic area.*

The back diagnostic area is around the first three thoracic vertebrae, close to the traditional Lung Yu points (Fig. 11.1C).

Treatment procedure

1. In the supine position, the Lung in the arm is best reached by downward pressure angled medially

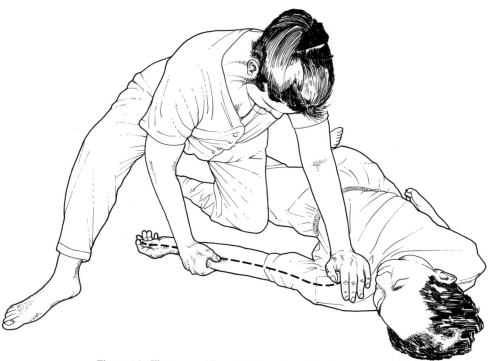

Fig. 11.2A *The arm meridian stretch (supine position).*

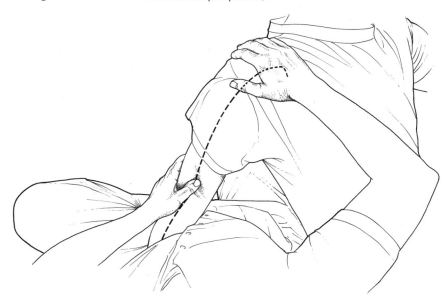

Fig. 11.2B *The arm meridian stretch (side position).*

toward the centre of the arm. The meridian stretch is achieved by laying the arm palm up at a 30° angle to the body (Fig. 11.2A).

2. In the side position, the arm can be abducted after a rotation and placed on the other side of the giver's body, in the stretch shown on p. 52, to expose the Lung meridian which can then be worked with palm, elbow or thumb, with the mother hand supporting the shoulder (Fig. 11.2B).

3. The Lungs benefit greatly from bilateral palm pressure on Lu 1, in the groove between chest and shoulder. This can be given from behind the head, as shown in chapter 4, or from a position beside the Hara, with the receiver in supine position (Fig. 11.3).

4. The Lung in the chest ascends from the diagnostic area up the front of the torso, between the Kidney and Stomach meridians to below the second rib, where it moves laterally to join Lu 1. It is usually treated from the position shown in point 3, one side at a time, with fingertips or thumb and with the giver's mother hand on the Hara diagnostic area. Go very lightly over the breast tissue on women (Fig. 11.4).

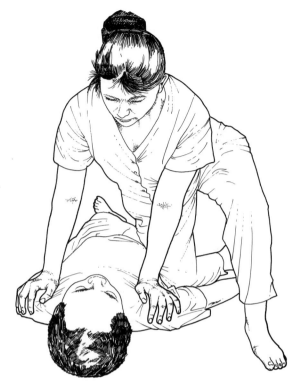

Fig. 11.3 *Leaning on Lung 1.*

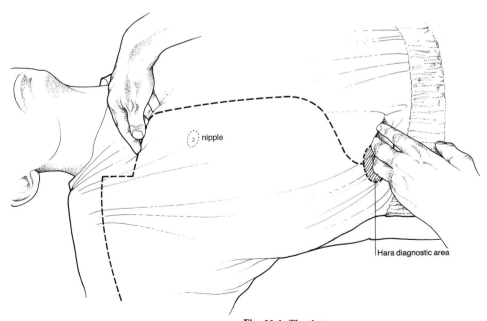

Fig. 11.4 *The chest.*

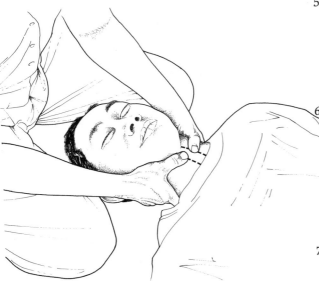

Fig. 11.5 *The throat.*

5. Masunaga's Lung meridian goes up the throat. With the receiver in supine, the giver behind the receiver's head, very gentle thumb pressure is given bilaterally just outside the midline of the throat, over the larynx. The thumbs should be alternated, to reduce feelings of vulnerability in the receiver (Fig. 11.5).

6. Masunaga's Lung meridian in the leg is down the centre of the back of the leg, just lateral to the Bladder meridian. It is worked with the receiver in prone position, with straight palm or thumb pressure downwards, with the mother hand on the sacrum, like the Bladder meridian (Fig. 11.6). The upper part of the leg can be worked with your knee, with the receiver supine, also like the Bladder meridian.

7. The Lung meridian in the foot runs horizontally across the lower part of the ball of the foot. It can be reached with the receiver prone from a position below the receiver's feet, as shown (Fig. 11.7), or can be worked with the receiver supine, foot supported on your thigh (see p. 45, Fig. 4.12).

Fig. 11.6 *The back of the leg.*

- - - - - - - Lung meridian
————— Bladder meridian
(for comparison)

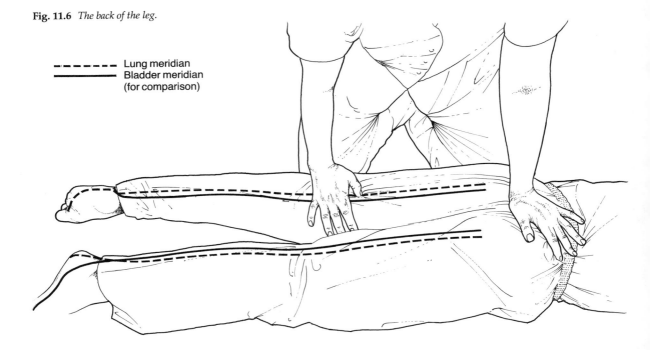

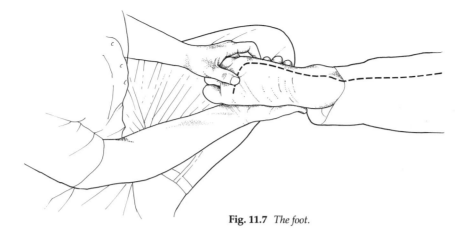

Fig. 11.7 *The foot.*

Major Points on the Lung meridian

Lung 1

Approximately 1 inch below the hollow under the lateral end of the clavicle.

Actions

- Bo point of the Lungs
- Clears fullness, Phlegm, fluids, etc. from the chest
- Helps pain in the chest and upper back

Lung 5

In the most lateral depression in the elbow crease.

Actions

- Clears Phlegm from the Lungs
- Clears Heat and Cold from the Lungs
- Helps Lungs descend Ki and fluids

Lung 7

On the lateral edge of the radius, proximal to the styloid process, in the depression approximately two fingers' width above the end of the wrist crease.

Actions

- Releases the Exterior (clears Wind-Heat or Wind-Cold in the early stages) ·
- Stimulates Defensive Ki and causes.sweating
- Helps the descending function of the Lungs
- Benefits the face and head
- Releases grief and tension

Lung 9

At the lateral end of the wrist crease, in the depression lateral to the radial artery.

Actions

- Source points of the Lungs
- Tonifies Lung Ki and Lung Yin
- Tonifies chest Ki and influences the circulation
- Resolves Phlegm

Lung 10

Halfway along the radial edge of the first metacarpal bone, "at the junction of the red and the white skin".

Actions

- Clears Heat
- Benefits the throat

Lung Yu point

B1 13 – two fingers' width lateral to the midline of the spine, parallel with the lower border of the spinous process of the third thoracic vertebra.

Lung Bo point

Lu 1 – see above

The Large Intestine in TCM

In TCM the meridian of the Large Intestine, like all the other Yang meridians, is regarded as the energetic or moving aspect of its coupled Yin meridian, in this case the Lungs. Although the organs themselves have different functions, the meridians do not always reflect this and the Yang meridian will often be used to shift the energy of the Yin organ.

Intestinal function

TCM ascribes the same functions to the Large Intestine organ as Western physiology, namely those of absorbing excess fluids from the faecal mass and propelling it towards the rectum for elimination. However, it carries out these functions under the direction of the Spleen, and the Spleen and Stomach meridians are usually employed to treat bowel problems, especially since these meridians are in the lower part of the body and thus have a more direct connection with the abdomen than the traditional Large Intestine meridian in the arm.

Elimination

The energetic function of the Large Intestine is elimination in all its aspects, through the skin, the bowel, the breath and the mind, and the meridian is used to help disperse external pathogenic influences at the beginning of an illness. It has a dispersing function related to that of the Lungs and by virtue of this is used to tonify Ki, since it disperses whatever obstructs free Ki flow. A point particularly used for this purpose is LI 4, named in ancient times "The Great Eliminator" – the strong dispersing action of this point means that it should not be used in pregnancy.

The nose and face

The Large Intestine meridian ends next to the nose and it is useful to treat it in cases of sinusitis and sinus headaches, hayfever or the common cold. It can also be used for eruptive skin problems such as acne and boils. Both these applications are also linked with the meridian's eliminatory function.

Meridian problems

Otherwise, the Large Intestine meridian is mainly used in TCM to treat local meridian problems, such as arm, shoulder and neck pain.

The Large Intestine in Zen Shiatsu theory

Masunaga extended the Large Intestine meridian, like all the others, throughout the body, according to his patients' sensations and reactions. The traditional Large Intestine meridian in the arm has on the whole a fairly weak effect on the lower part of the body, which is why its influence on actual bowel movement is relatively slight. Masunaga knew not only of the importance of the eliminatory function in the health of the bodymind and spirit, but also of the physiological importance of such a sizeable organ as the colon in the healthy functioning of the entire abdominal area. The Large Intestine meridian which he traced in the hips and legs reflects this importance. It is a meridian which produces powerful sensations in treatment and strongly affects the energetic workings of the lower part of the body.

Elimination

The same eliminatory function applies to the Large Intestine in Zen Shiatsu theory as in classical Chinese medicine. Nasal congestion and coughing result from poor elimination from the respiratory system; as in TCM, this may be a simple failure to eliminate mucus or an inability to eliminate external pathogenic influences, since one of the associated symptoms is a tendency to catch colds. The skin can also reflect a failure to eliminate, manifesting in itchy skin or skin prone to inflammation and pus, in other words, boils, acne and other eruptive skin problems. There is also, of course, elimination through the bowel, which is related to the following function.

Ki circulation in the lower Hara, back and legs

Masunaga noted that because of the size of the Large Intestine organ, sluggishness in its function will affect the entire abdomen and also the lower part of the body generally. For this reason, not only constipation and diarrhoea can derive from a Large Intestine disharmony. Other common symptoms are coldness or poor circulation in the lower Hara, which may affect the uterus, ovaries or Bladder as well as the intestines, and lower back pain resulting from congestion or stagnation. Lower back pain is often felt around the Large Intestine Yu point and diagnostic area and frequently accompanies a Large Intestine diagnosis in clinical Shiatsu practice, although TCM relates it only to the Kidney and Bladder. Another common symptom is coldness and poor circulation in the legs, resulting from general sluggishness of Ki in the lower part of the body.

Letting go

Most of the psychological traits associated with a Large Intestine diagnosis come from a failure in the letting go function, which is a crucial part of the process of exchange with the environment, discussed in the section on the Lungs (see p. 210). The mind as well as the body can become burdened with unwanted material in the form of old behaviour patterns which no longer serve their original purpose and which usually impose even greater limitations on new experience. For example, the inability to release disappointment can mean that the individual thereafter remains closed to the possibility of repeating the experience which led to the disappointment. Fear of failure, defensive pride and anticipation of rejection are all examples of patterns which limit new experience and leave the individual stuck in unwanted life structures. "I want to leave, but..." is the theme often heard with a Large Intestine diagnosis.

This inability to let go is the cause of much stagnation on both physical and psychological levels. Although in TCM it is the Liver whose poor functioning causes stagnation, a Zen Shiatsu diagnosis of Large Intestine often accompanies symptoms which have stagnation as a factor, such as constipation, menstrual pain, lower back stiffness or sinusitis.

Alienation and depression

Since expression of emotion is a vital part of the process of release, a Large Intestine disharmony commonly manifests as a lack of expression. This can be seen physically, as a lack of facial expressivity, or socially, as a lack of friends. Masunaga expresses the Large Intestine quandary as "perpetual dissatisfaction; no friend with whom he can confer". There is dissatisfaction with the unwanted life situations yet because of the isolation which the individual feels when cut off from exchange with the environment, his or her behaviour tends to be antisocial and there are no friends with whom to discuss the dissatisfaction. It is a vicious circle which is a major feature of depression.

Breathing and exercise

One of the features of Zen Shiatsu theory is that symptoms of an imbalance can also, in a circular way, be the causes of the imbalance. So it is with the Large Intestine. Because the individual is reluctant to initiate exchange with the environment, he or she will tend to have shallow or restricted breathing patterns. These patterns keep the exchange with the environment at a minimum level and maintain the original weakness of the Lung and Large Intestine functions. The same applies to exercise. Poor motivation for change means that those with a Large Intestine disharmony are reluctant to exercise; thus their breathing remains shallow and their intestinal function is not stimulated by physical movement, with the same result, that the Lung and Large Intestine energy remains out of balance. An excellent recommendation for someone with a Metal disharmony is gentle, regular exercise.

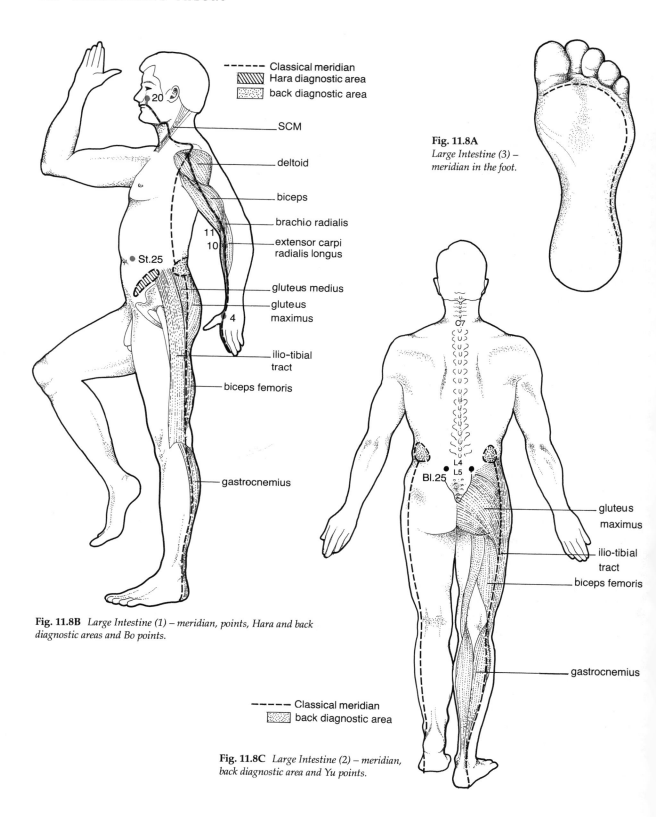

Classical meridian
Hara diagnostic area
back diagnostic area

20

SCM

deltoid

biceps

brachio radialis

extensor carpi
radialis longus

11
10

St.25

gluteus medius
gluteus
maximus

4

ilio-tibial
tract

biceps femoris

gastrocnemius

Fig. 11.8A
*Large Intestine (3) –
meridian in the foot.*

C7

L4
L5
Bl.25

gluteus
maximus

ilio-tibial
tract

biceps femoris

gastrocnemius

Fig. 11.8B *Large Intestine (1) – meridian, points, Hara and back
diagnostic areas and Bo points.*

Classical meridian
back diagnostic area

Fig. 11.8C *Large Intestine (2) – meridian,
back diagnostic area and Yu points.*

The Large Intestine meridian and how to treat it

The traditional Large Intestine meridian runs from the tip of the index finger up the anterior lateral aspect of the arm, crossing the acromioclavicular joint to the top of the shoulder and travelling diagonally over the front of the neck and jaw to the corner of the nose; it then crosses under the nose to terminate at the side of the other nostril. Masunaga's extended meridian travels down the anterolateral aspect of the torso from shoulder to hip, where it connects with both Hara and back diagnostic areas. From the back diagnostic area, above the iliac crest, it moves down the lateral posterior aspect of gluteus medius and maximus and thence follows the posterior border of the iliotibial tract down the lateral back of the thigh. It continues down the posterolateral aspect of the calf to run under the lateral edge of the foot to the ball of the foot, where it runs horizontally along the pad under the toes (Fig. 11.8A).

The diagnostic area in the Hara is bilaterally in a strip running diagonally just within the hipbones (Fig. 11.8B).

In the back, the diagnostic area is bilaterally on the sides of the body, just above the iliac crest (Fig. 11.8C).

Treatment procedure

1. The classical Large Intestine meridian runs across the anterior aspect of the shoulder and down the radial aspect of the arm, just posterior to "the border between the red and the white skin". It is worked in the supine position with the receiver's hand resting with LI 4 uppermost, with the giver's pressure angled slightly inward and the mother hand on the shoulder. Palm, thumb or Dragon's Mouth are used for treating (Fig. 11.9).
2. The LI in the arm can also be reached in the sitting position, when the giver raises her knee and lays the receiver's arm across it. The meridian can then be comfortably worked with the elbow (Fig. 11.10A).
3. The LI in the arm is also accessible in the side position, when the arm is abducted and rested on the other side of the giver's body, supported on

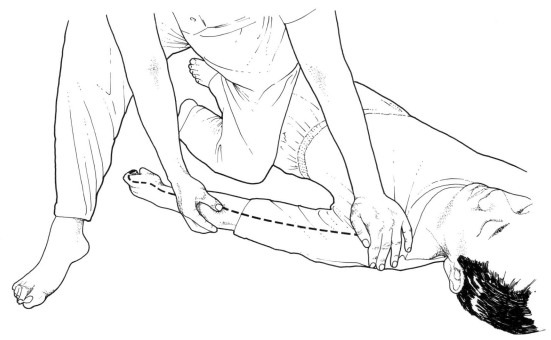

Fig. 11.9 *The shoulder and arm in supine.*

her thigh. It can then be worked with palm, thumb or elbow, with the mother hand exerting slight backward pressure on the shoulder (Fig. 11.10B).

4. The LI down the lateral front of the body, anterior to the Gall Bladder, can be worked in the same

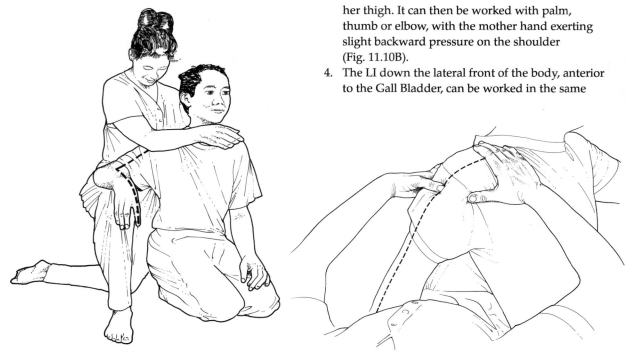

Fig. 11.10A *Treating the arm in sitting position.*

Fig. 11.10B *Treating the arm in side position.*

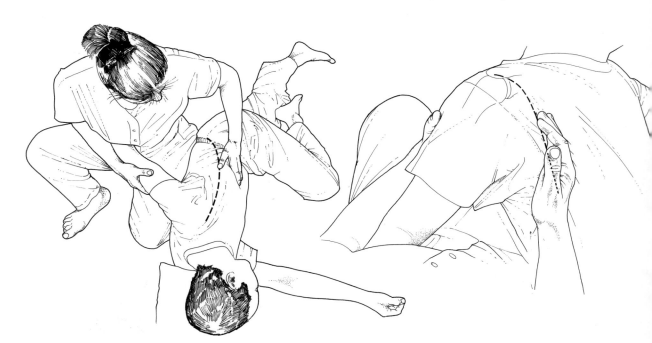

Fig. 11.11A *Treating the torso with the arm in the meridian stretch.*

Fig. 11.11B *Treating the shoulder with the arm in the meridian stretch.*

position with palm, thumb or fingertips, with the mother hand supporting the shoulder (Figs 11.11A and B).

5. The traditional LI in the neck can easily be worked in the side position, with *gentle* downward pressure on a diagonal line from the jaw across the sternocleidomastoid muscle. The mother hand should be supporting the shoulder (Fig. 11.12A).

6. Supine is also a good position for working the LI in the neck with the thumb. The receiver's head should be supported by the other hand and turned slightly sideways. Do not work the lowest third of the meridian in the neck (Fig. 11.12B).

7. Masunaga's LI in the hips is on neither the lateral nor the posterior aspect of the body but "on the corner", just posterior to the Gall Bladder. It can

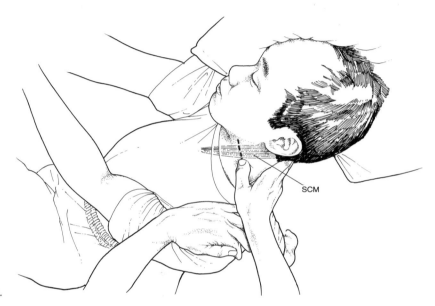

Fig. 11.12A *The neck (side position).*

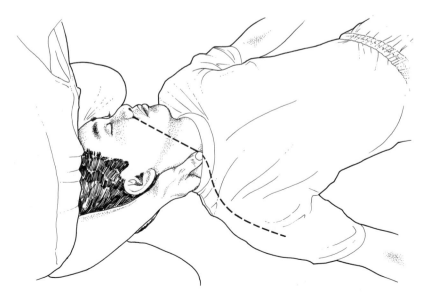

Fig. 11.12B *The neck (supine position).*

be reached in prone position and worked with thumb, knee, elbow, palm or fingertips, with the mother hand supporting the lumbar region. The angle of penetration should be horizontal (Fig. 11.13).

8. The LI in the leg follows on from the location in the hips, namely down the "corner" or posterolateral aspect of the thigh and calf. When working this part of the meridian in the prone position, it is useful to hook the receiver's nearest foot over the other, as shown. The meridian is then exposed and stable and can be worked as a continuation of the hips, using any of the methods from point 7 above, angling in to the centre of the leg (Fig. 11.14).

9. The LI in the hips and legs is also reached in the side position, when the thumbs can be used very precisely. The angle of pressure should be vertically downward (Fig. 11.15).

10. The LI in the thigh can be worked in the supine position. From a rotation, with your mother hand on the Hara and your other hand supporting the

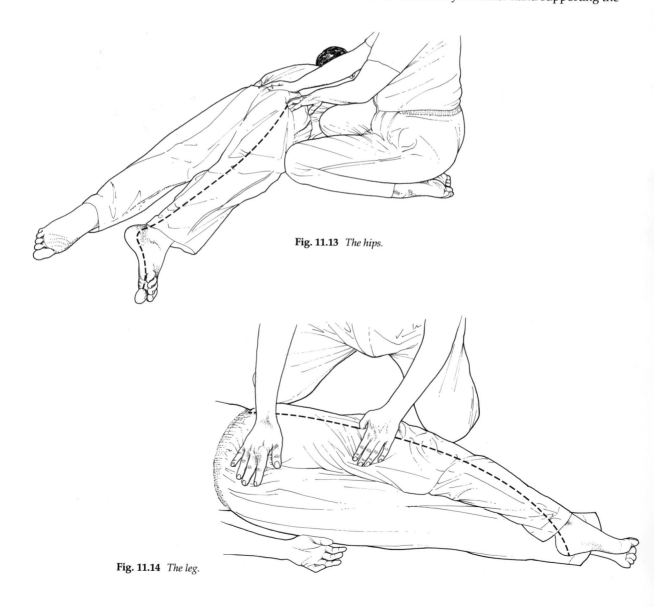

Fig. 11.13 *The hips.*

Fig. 11.14 *The leg.*

receiver's bent leg, place your knee on the Large Intestine in the thigh and bring the receiver's leg back towards you, thus exerting pressure with your knee on the meridian (Fig. 11.16).

11. The meridian runs down the lateral edge of the sole and horizontally along the pad under the toes. It is easiest to reach with the thumb, with the receiver in the prone position (Fig. 11.17).

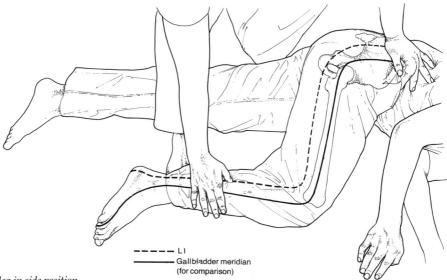

- - - - - L I
—— Gallbladder meridian
(for comparison)

Fig. 11.15 *Treating hip and leg in side position.*

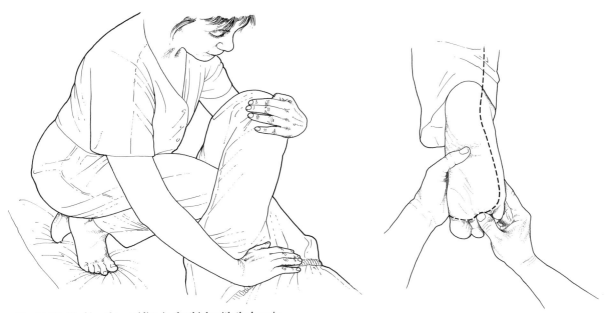

Fig. 11.16 *Working the meridian in the thigh with the knee in supine.*

Fig. 11.17 *The foot.*

Major points on the Large Intestine meridian

Large Intestine 4

On the highest point of the web of flesh between the first and second metacarpals.

Actions

- Source point of the Large Intestine
- Releases the Exterior and expels Exterior influences
- Main point for the face, e.g. sinusitis, toothache, frontal headache, etc.
- Stops pain

NOT TO BE USED IN PREGNANCY

Large Intestine 10

Three fingers' width below the elbow crease, just posterior to the border between "the red and the white skin", on the bulge of the brachioradialis muscle.

Actions

- Tonifies Ki and Blood
- Benefits the arm (major point for physical problems of any kind in the arm)

Large Intestine 11

At the lateral end of the elbow crease, halfway between Lu 5 and the lateral epicondyle of the humerus.

Actions

- Expels Heat, Wind and Dampness
- Cools the Blood

Large Intestine 20

In the nasolabial groove , at the level of the midpoint of ala nasi.

Actions

- Expels Exterior Wind (common cold, hayfever, facial paralysis)

Large Intestine Yu Point

Bl 25 – two fingers' width from the midline of the spine, level with the lower border of the spinous process of L 4.

Large Intestine Bo Point

St 25 – three fingers' width lateral to the centre of the navel.

Bringing theory and practice together

12

The Four Methods of diagnosis

There are four traditional ways of diagnosing in Far Eastern medicine, which in Japan are known as the Setsu-Shin ("Four Methods"); they are listening, observing, feeling and asking. When diagnosing TCM syndromes, we should not rely on only one method; at least three should point towards a particular diagnosis. When diagnosing according to Zen Shiatsu methods, "feeling" or palpation is the main method but any of the other methods can be used to confirm the feeling diagnosis and establish a possible aetiology and prognosis. Diagnosis can begin with the first moment of seeing or hearing the receiver. It is an ongoing procedure, which depends on detached, relaxed assessment of your own sensory impressions as well as on interpretation of the receiver's symptoms and signs.

Listening

In the listening diagnosis, the emphasis is not on listening to the receiver's story but on listening to the receiver.

The sound of the voice

The sound of the voice can, if it attracts your attention, be important in indicating a temporary or long term imbalance in one of the Five Elements. Not all imbalances manifest in the voice but enough do to make this a significant diagnostic tool. At a certain point in the taking of the case history, it can be useful to disassociate your attention voluntarily from what the receiver is saying, and to widen your aural focus

for a short time; in other words, to open your hearing field and hear the receiver's voice as if listening to music. It is then sometimes possible to hear one of the five sounds described in Section Three under the individual Elements.

The appropriateness of the voice

The appropriateness of the voice can be a clue to an imbalance. The giver accustomed to listening as described above will be able to hear the sound of the receiver's voice at the same time as listening to what he is saying. Many receivers will express themselves in a laughing voice when they are happy, a shouting voice when they are angry, a weeping voice when they are complaining about something and so on. But if the sound of the receiver's voice is not appropriate to what he is saying, there is an imbalance in the Element corresponding to the sound of his voice.

Listening between the lines

Listening between the lines is a technique to which some are more attuned than others. It has nothing to do with the sound of the voice, more with the quality of the receiver's expression, his use of pauses or his eagerness to gloss over a particular subject. These signs indicate that some issue is significant to the receiver and while they may not point immediately to a particular Element or meridian, they can be helpful in determining the cause of a condition or the date at which it commenced.

Note: It would be inappropriate to pursue the receiver on the hidden content of what he is saying.

227

Observing

There are four visible diagnostic signs which can easily be observed: the receiver's facial colour and hue, demeanour and presentation, tongue, and energy or postural patterns.

Facial colour and hue

Facial colour and hue are two different things. The receiver's facial colour is related to his skin tone and is unlikely to vary substantially in the short term, although it may change gradually over time if it was caused by a pattern of disharmony which is being eliminated. Facial colours can indicate specific disharmonies in TCM terms, as follows:

- *Bright pale or shiny white* – Ki Deficiency; if the skin is puffy and pasty, it is likely to be Spleen Ki which is Deficient, but otherwise the Lungs are usually involved.
- *Dull pale or "bloodless"* – Blood Deficiency. This appearance can often accompany the skin tone below.
- *Sallow skin, with a brown or olive tint* – Liver involvement, often Liver Blood Deficiency (unless this skin tone is a racial characteristic). Sometimes Liver imbalance is indicated by a brown or olive tone around the eye area.
- *Red skin tone* – Heat or Fire (pathogenic Fire, not the Fire Element meridians necessarily).
- *Red patches* on the cheekbones indicate Empty Heat (Yin Deficiency).
- *Blue-black circles under the eyes* are signs of Kidney Deficiency.

These skin tones are, of course, most easily seen on Caucasian faces and can be discerned only to a limited extent on Asian or African skins.

The facial hue, conversely, can be seen on any colour of skin, since it is not a part of the skin but a transparent overlay, like a reflection. The hues correspond to the colours of the Elements, as described in the chapters on the individual Elements and meridians. To recapitulate, they are:

- red – Fire
- blue-black – Water
- yellow – Earth
- green – Wood
- white – Metal

It is impossible to see a hue when focusing narrowly on the receiver's face. In the same way that the sounds of the Elements are most easily heard when "opening the ears" with relaxed attention, so the colours of the Elements are best seen when opening the visual focus wide. When the receiver's face is seen with this kind of openness and not with strict attention to detail, the colours manifest, sometimes as a flash, glimpsed out of the corner of the giver's eye. Element hues come and go and rarely cover the whole face; they are most likely to be perceived around the eyes and the mouth.

Demeanour

Demeanour is the receiver's Ki expressing itself in movement, facial expression and body language.

In TCM terms, the relevant aspects of demeanour are the strength of the receiver's movements, the quality of his attention, the energy and appropriateness of his behaviour and the strength of his voice:

- Strong movements, agitation and a loud voice are signs of Excess.
- Slow movements, lethargy, vacancy or absentmindedness and a weak voice are signs of Deficiency.
- Confusion, incessant talking and inappropriate behaviour are signs of disturbed Shen.

From the Western standpoint, considerably more subtle observations and interpretations can be made concerning both demeanour and presentation, especially if connections can be made to specific Elements or meridians. Underlying emotions can be perceived from the receiver's intonation, the expression in his eyes or simply from rigorous scrutiny of your own subjective reactions to him. Since the interaction with the Shiatsu giver, if the treatment course lasts more than one or two sessions, tends to include some measure of emotional contact, it can be useful to observe it, not in order to dwell upon it or discuss it, as in psychotherapy, but to use it as a diagnostic reference point for the receiver's emotional condition.

It is important, when using this kind of behavioural observation, that we do not base our entire diagnosis on it but rather use it to confirm a diagnosis made from other signs and symptoms. It is more useful in determining the best style of approach to treatment with a particular receiver than it is in diagnosis.

Presentation

Presentation includes the receiver's style of dress and grooming and his social manner; the veneer or appearance which, consciously or unconsciously, he presents to the world. All of these can be valuable diagnostic signs when viewed from a detached position.

This is not always easy, since almost without exception we have conditioned responses which can be triggered by any aspect of the receiver's presentation. The receiver who makes us nervous, the receiver who complains, the receiver who exhausts us with his demands, the receiver who confuses us, the receiver who doesn't wash; all are making statements with their presentation about the Element or meridian which is out of balance in them. What is required of us as givers is that we observe our own reaction to the receiver and find its cause.

If we are irritated by a receiver because he reminds us of our primary school teacher or because we are always irritated by people who wear cravats, we are being offered a valuable exercise in detachment. If we are irritated by a receiver because he is, for example, consistently late for his appointments, we need to look at the relevance of his continual lateness to his symptoms and signs. Does he simply have too much to do and if so, why can't he give himself this time? Is it Gall Bladder over-responsibility or Large Intestine lack of self-worth? Or is it general absentmindedness and poor memory, part of a Blood Deficiency picture?

These signs can be particularly useful in determining a receiver's motivation and orientation to life when he does not supply much information about his own psychological or emotional state, for whatever reason.

The tongue

Observing the tongue is one of the main points of TCM observation diagnosis and although some Shiatsu givers hesitate to ask a receiver to show his tongue, it is indispensable in establishing any TCM syndrome. For

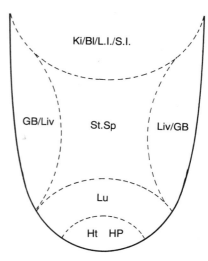

Fig. 12.1 *Tongue map.*

the hesitant, it can be an equalizing move if the giver accompanies the request by sticking her own tongue out, to show the receiver that it can be done!

The tongue should be observed, if possible, close to a good source of a natural light. The receiver should not have to keep his tongue out for more than a minute without a rest, as the tongue changes colour with the effort.

Since hot food or drinks such as tea and coffee can alter the colour of the tongue and coating, it is advisable to wait for half an hour to an hour after food or drink have been taken before inspecting the receiver's tongue.

As a general rule, the shape and colour of the tongue body is an indication of the condition of the receiver's basic Ki, Blood and internal organs; the thickness and colour of the coating show any Excess that may be present. It is possible to pinpoint specific organs through tongue diagnosis by using the map in Figure 12.1, which shows locations on the tongue which correspond to organs or areas of the body.

At the level of tongue diagnosis appropriate to Shiatsu, the giver needs to observe:

- the colour of the tongue body
- the shape and possible movement of the tongue body and the location of any cracks
- the thickness and colour of the tongue coating or its absence
- the moisture of the tongue and coating.

Colour of the tongue body

- A normal tongue is pale, fresh red, "like very fresh meat".
- A pale tongue indicates a Deficiency of Yang or Blood, which may be accompanied by internal Cold.
- A red tongue body is a sign of Heat.
- A purple tongue shows stagnation of Ki or Blood.
- A reddish-purple tongue shows stagnation with Heat.
- A bluish-purple tongue shows stagnation with Cold.
- Red spots in any area indicate Heat in that area.
- Pale or orange-tinted sides to the tongue indicate Liver Blood Deficiency.
- Any area of a particular colour corresponds to a condition affecting a specific area or body organ, e.g. a red tongue tip indicates Heat in the Heart.

The tongue body colour usually indicates a condition which has already lasted some time. It can, however, change over weeks or months, as the condition improves or deteriorates.

Shape of the tongue body

- A long tongue indicates Interior Excess Heat. Long tongues are usually pointed.
- A swollen (fat or puffy) tongue, when pale, usually indicates deficiency of Yang, which causes Dampness. If there are teethmarks around the edges of a swollen tongue, they are a sign of Spleen Yang Deficiency.
- A red and swollen tongue shows Heat accompanying general Dampness.
- A thin or flabby tongue indicates Blood Deficiency.

Tongue shapes usually accompany a constitutional tendency towards a certain condition. They are therefore unlikely to change greatly during the course of treatment.

Movement of the tongue body

- A pale and quivering tongue indicates Deficiency of Ki.
- A red and quivering tongue shows that Heat is generating Interior Wind.

- A tongue that moves slowly and involuntarily from side to side indicates Interior Wind.

Cracks in the tongue body

- Short cracks around the edges of the tongue are a sign of Spleen Yang Deficiency.
- Cracks on each side of the midline of the tongue, just behind the tip, indicate a Lung problem or can refer to a past Lung disease, such as whooping cough, which has permanently affected the Lungs.
- A central crack reaching right to the tip of the tongue indicates a constitutional imbalance in the Heart, although it may not imply any physical disease but instead a tendency to a Fire psychological picture.
- A wide central crack which does not reach to the tip of the tongue is a sign of Stomach Ki Deficiency. If there is yellow fur inside the crack it indicates Heat and Phlegm in the Stomach.
- Many small cracks all over the surface of the tongue, like cracked glass or ice, indicate Deficiency of Yin.

Cracks usually indicate a deep-seated and long-standing condition and do not often disappear, although they may become less marked.

The tongue coating

- A coating which is firmly rooted is a healthier sign than one which seems powdery and easily dislodged.
- A thin white coating is normal.
- A thick coating indicates that an excess pathogenic factor is present and the thicker the coating, the stronger the excess.
- A white coating indicates Cold in the body area or organ corresponding to the coating.
- A yellow coating indicates Heat in the body area or organ corresponding to the coating
- A dry, black coating indicates extreme Heat; a wet, grey or black coating indicates extreme Cold.
- A slippery or sticky coating indicates Dampness or Phlegm in the body area or organ corresponding to the coating.
- Absence of coating is a sign of Deficiency. A tongue that seems peeled, or peeled in patches,

indicates Yin Deficiency, either in the whole body (stemming from the Kidneys) or in the area corresponding to the peeled coating. A red, peeled tongue is a definite sign of Kidney Yin Deficiency.

The thickness of the tongue coating can vary from day to day and may indicate a more short-term or recent condition if the colour and shape of the tongue body are normal. Absence of tongue coating indicates a long-standing condition.

The moisture of the tongue

- A wet tongue is a sign of Yang Deficiency or Cold.
- A dry tongue indicates Yin Deficiency or Heat.

Energy and postural patterns

The ability to see the condition and movement of a receiver's Ki is surprisingly easy. Most of the students I have taught are able to see for themselves after being shown one or two examples and are quite proficient after one lesson. It is, however, easier to demonstrate in class than to explain on paper and, if possible, should be taught by an experienced teacher. (I was taught this technique by Pauline Sasaki, who made it both easy and fun.) It is advisable not to attempt to look at Ki before you have practised Shiatsu and developed your Hara for at least 1 year.

When learning the rudiments of looking at Ki, it is ideal if two or more receivers can be observed at the same time, since the differences highlighted by comparison make the perception of what we are looking for very much easier. This is not always possible, however, and so I shall proceed assuming that only one receiver is available.

How to look at Ki

Stand at the receiver's feet, if the receiver is in the prone or supine position, or sit or kneel behind him if he is in the sitting position. If possible, the light should be evenly diffused over the receiver's body, without strongly emphasizing one side or the other.

Make sure that you are grounded, relaxed and breathing into the Hara. Then open your visual focus

wide, as when observing the skin hue, and survey the receiver from that wide focus, without detailed scrutiny but with relaxed attention.

1. Begin with the question, "Is the receiver's energy up or down?". If the answer is not immediately apparent, avoid the temptation to scrutinize more closely but instead go to the window or door, take a few deep breaths into the Hara, relax again, tell yourself that it doesn't matter and mean it, and return for another wide, unfocused look. If you still cannot see whether the energy is up or down, it is possible that this receiver does not have a pronounced upper/lower discrepancy and you can proceed to the next step. If the answer is immediately apparent, but you then question it or doubt what you are seeing, in a word, *don't*. Proceed to the next step.

2. Now ask yourself, still keeping a wide, relaxed focus, "Is the receiver's Ki strong or weak?". It is a good idea, when asking this question, to maintain a feeling connection between your Hara, which is the source of your "seeing", and the receiver's Hara, which is the source of his Ki. (Do not focus visually upon the receiver's Hara at this stage!)

   If there is no answer immediately forthcoming (and it is difficult to assess relative strength of Ki without another receiver for comparison), move on to the next step.

3. Now ask yourself, "Is the receiver's Ki flowing or is it blocked?". Still from the wide, relaxed focus, the movement of Ki can appear like the flow of water over the body surface, transparent yet perceptible.

   - Blockages can be Jitsu, through concentration of Ki in an area, or Kyo, through weakness in an area which prevents flow.
   - Movement is not significant unless it is too strong, such as strong upward or downward movements. In a state of balance, the movement of Ki appears simply as a calm yet vibrant aliveness of the body or body part. Movement can also be perceived by comparison with an area of weakness or stagnation.

If there is no immediate answer to any of these questions, you will need to try again, either with another receiver or, preferably, with two receivers. If two or three tries still reveal nothing, there are three courses of action:

1. to study with a teacher;
2. to wait and work on the Hara, confidence and relaxation, reminding yourself that at least when you finally see the Ki, you will know you are not imagining it;
3. to forget about seeing Ki and concentrate on feeling it (see the section on Feeling, p. 233).

The advantages of looking at Ki

If you are clear about what you see, you can pick out significant imbalances in the receiver's Ki flow to act as indicators of the success or otherwise of your treatment. For example, you could say to yourself, "I would like to see the arms looking more connected to the body, and to reduce that fullness in the chest". Looking at the Ki again after the Shiatsu session will usually reveal that these indicators have changed to a greater or lesser extent, according to the receiver's response.

EXAMPLES

1. A female receiver has a flat sacrum and little Ki in the lower part of her body, except for a concentration in the front of her thighs, which appear blocked with Excess Ki. Her Hara diagnosis is Stomach Jitsu, Bladder Kyo. The giver tonifies the Bladder meridian in the back, sacrum and legs and disperses the Stomach in the thighs.
2. A male receiver seems to have a strong rush of Ki up the whole body and a concentration of Ki in the head, but a relative weakness in the upper chest. The diagnosis is Liver Jitsu, Lung Kyo. The giver concentrates on tonifying the Lung Yu points in the upper back and the Lu 1 area on the chest in order to strengthen that area, as well as the Lung meridian in the legs and feet to bring the Ki down. Since the Liver meridian does not go to the head, she disperses Gall Bladder in the head and shoulders, concentrating on sending Ki downwards, and disperses Liver in the shoulders while tonifying the Lu 1 area. She ends by holding the feet and concentrating on drawing Ki down to them.

Gaining an overall picture of the distribution of Ki in the receiver's body allows you to tailor your treatment to the receiver's needs. Working on the meridians indicated by the Hara diagnosis and using the tonification and sedation techniques described in Chapter 14, p. 254, you can concentrate on bringing Ki to areas of weakness, dispersing it in areas of blockage or Excess, and balancing its flow. (See examples below)

Postural patterns

These are so interconnected with Ki imbalances that it is hard to disassociate the two. Unless resulting from physical injury or handicap, most postural habits are the crystallization into form of a Ki imbalance and can be remedied by correcting the Ki flow in the meridians, which is one reason for Shiatsu's effectiveness in structural problems. It can be useful, however, to be able to see that a problem has begun to manifest on the physical as well as the energetic level, since the prognosis is for a longer course of treatment.

Common postural patterns are:

- misalignment of the hips
- an oblique left–right imbalance in which a shoulder compensates for the opposite hip
- sway back (lordosis)
- overcurvature of the thoracic area (kyphosis), coupled with a slump in the diaphragm or chest and extension of the neck.

When visually assessing postural imbalances which feature a left–right imbalance, it can be helpful to note which side of the receiver's body seems weaker. In line with the Zen Shiatsu focus on tonifying the Kyo, or Empty, before dispersing the Jitsu, or Full, it is always best to work on the weaker side first.

A further observation, which relates to postural distortion, can be made to assess the effect of the treatment, and this is to measure the receiver's leg length before and after treatment. While holding the receiver's ankles, with the edges of her thumbs resting on the tips of the medial malleoli, the giver brings the ankles together. Any misalignment of her thumbs will indicate that one leg is shorter than the other. This is almost always due to tension imbalance in the muscles of the pelvis, back or neck and can usually be corrected to some extent by the Shiatsu.

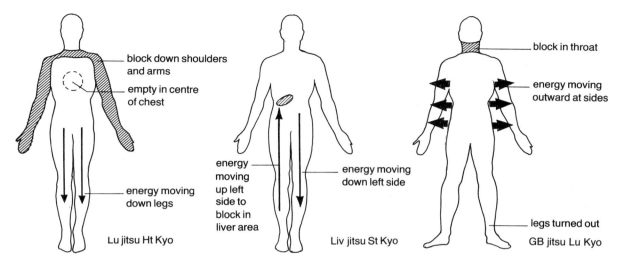

Fig. 12.2 *Examples of sketches of energy patterns.*

Postural distortions can easily be seen when focusing minutely on the receiver, whereas energetic distortions can only be viewed with a wide focus. Both can be noted in the case notes by drawing a simple sketch, using your own symbols to indicate movement or blockage. Some examples from my own case histories are shown in Figure 12.2.

Feeling

In modern TCM theory, feeling diagnosis is taken as referring simply to diagnosis from the pulse. However, in earlier times palpation of the whole of the receiver's body was such an important part of diagnosis that acupuncturists had to practise massage techniques as a preliminary to acupuncture training.

■ *"One has to examine the right and left, upper and lower ... feel and palpate the body to find something with your hands, then do some exercises and take the disease away with the points ..."*
  COMPENDIUM OF ACUPUNCTURE AND
  MOXIBUSTION, BY YANG JI ZHOU, 1601*.

*Quoted in *Extraordinary Vessels*, Matsumoto and Birch, Paradigm Publications, 1986, p. 60.

In fact, the whole of a Shiatsu treatment is a form of extended diagnosis, as we familiarize ourselves with the receiver's unique patterns of Ki and his particular areas of strength and weakness. For students of Shiatsu, this can be a fascinating process as their palpatory skills increase and they find more significance in their treatments. As a diagnostic form, however, it is too lengthy to be of any value to the professional, who must aim to find the most effective spot to treat on one or two meridians out of the 12 in order to rebalance the receiver's Ki.

Meridian diagnosis

Meridian diagnosis is a more focused form of the whole-body diagnosis which is the end result of a full treatment routine. Each time the giver begins to work on a limb or a body part such as the chest or back, she palms the whole area in order to find which meridians are the most distorted in that body part. The qualities of distortion she is seeking are those of Kyo and Jitsu.

Kyo qualities are those of emptiness:

- stiffness with a wooden quality (resistance without resilience)
- flaccidity
- lack of substance (the meridian feels like a deep trough)
- hollowness.

All these physical qualities are accompanied by the most basic quality of Kyo, which is *lack of response*. Kyo tends to feel inert.

Jitsu qualities are those of fullness:

- raised areas of tension
- rubbery and resilient areas of bunched-up muscle
- reactivity.

The response of a Jitsu area to penetration is palpable and often feels as if the receiver's Ki is "fighting back".

With practice and experience, and with knowledge of the meridian locations, the giver will be able to find the most Kyo and most Jitsu meridians in any area by palming it once and can then treat the most noticeably distorted meridian.

Meridian diagnosis can be used if the giver is not confident about her Hara diagnosis or when a receiver's problem is principally structural. Its disadvantage is that it is not appropriate for physically healthy and balanced receivers.

A variant of meridian diagnosis is when the giver "listens" down the length of a meridian from a particular point. The most usual ways of doing this are to "listen" down the spine or up the legs. To "listen" down the spine, hold the Bladder meridian at Bl 10 under the occiput and, while tuning in to this point, imagine or visualize the length of the receiver's spine. If there are any areas of distortion or blocked Ki in the spine, it is often possible to perceive them by this method. "Listening" up the legs is similar; hold both the receiver's feet at Ki 1 and use these points to tune in to the receiver's Ki. This technique can be used to determine which leg is more Kyo and to perceive distortions in the hips, but can often reveal problems further up the body.

Local diagnosis

Local diagnosis is another form of meridian diagnosis. When working on a body part which is causing pain or discomfort, perhaps as the result of a trauma or an accident, the giver will often perceive a meridian as out of balance locally but not in the rest of the body. The neck is also a particular area whose local meridian condition is often different from that of the body as a whole. In this situation, the giver treats the affected meridians in the individual body part with

tonification and sedation techniques as appropriate, returning to the general diagnosis on completion.

Hara diagnosis

The main form of palpatory diagnosis used in Japan is Hara diagnosis which is used not only by Shiatsu practitioners but also by acupuncturists to supplement their pulse diagnosis. There are many forms of Hara diagnosis, working on different models of the correspondence of Hara areas to meridians. Since each diagnostic model belongs to a particular treatment mode and since this book is interpreting the Zen Shiatsu treatment mode, I shall confine myself to the Zen Shiatsu model of Hara diagnosis, as taught by Pauline Sasaki, one of the leading teachers of this style. To the reader who is hoping to learn Hara diagnosis from this book, I must own that in my opinion this subtle and complex procedure can only be learned from a qualified teacher.

The basics of Hara diagnosis

Pressure. Hara diagnosis in this style of Zen Shiatsu is performed with relaxed fingertips and very light pressure. Your fingertips should barely indent the surface of the receiver's body, since you are contacting not the organs themselves but their Ki.

The Hara area. The Hara "map" is defined by the ribcage above, below by the oblique lines between the anterior superior iliac spines and the pubic bone and centrally by the navel. Since the proportions of this area vary from receiver to receiver, the inexperienced Shiatsu giver should familiarize herself first of all with these landmarks. She can then concentrate on locating the areas corresponding to specific meridians, which are outlined verbally in the chapters on the meridians and in diagrammatic from in Figure 12.3*.

The diagnostic areas. The Kidney and Bladder areas are not normally palpated in their entirety unless a preliminary palpation reveals the possibility of an imbalance. The Kidney is usually palpated at the two

---

*I am grateful to Pauline Sasaki and Clifford Andrews of the Shiatsu College, UK, who produced Figs 12.3–12.5.

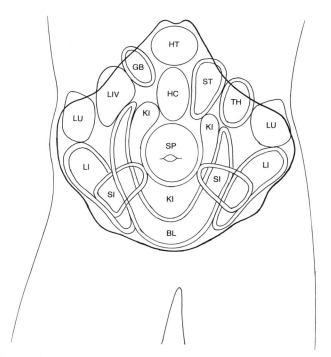

Fig. 12.3 *The Hara diagnostic areas.*

oblique ends of the area, just above the navel, and the belly of the horseshoe, just below the navel (corresponding to the energetic centre of the Hara). The Bladder is usually palpated level with the navel and lateral to the borders of rectus abdominis and also at its lowest point, just above the pubic bone.

One-handed palpation routine. While learning the location of the diagnostic areas, it is a good idea to acquire a routine order in which to palpate them. A numbered sequence for one-handed Hara palpation is given in Figure 12.4. When following this order with one hand, the other hand rests on one of the diagnostic areas as a mother hand; the mother hand and working hand can exchange functions for ease in working on both sides of the Hara. When diagnosing the upper Hara, the mother hand can rest on the Heart area; for the lower Hara, the Spleen area is more appropriate.

Two-handed palpation routine. Once the giver is proficient in locating the diagnostic areas, a two-handed palpation routine becomes possible. The

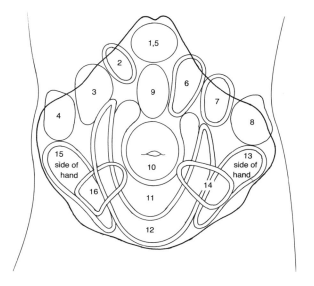

Fig. 12.4 *One-handed palpation routine.*

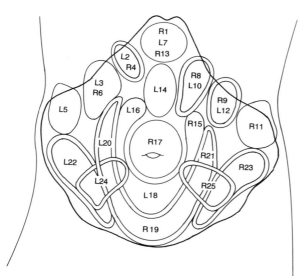

Fig. 12.5 *Two-handed palpation routine.*

advantage of a two-handed routine is that it can be performed quickly, without too much time to think (see below). In Figure 12.5 the numbered order is for both hands alternating, except for the sides of the upper Hara when the left hand palpates Gall Bladder and Liver in sequence and the right hand palpates Stomach and Triple Heater. The reason for this is simple technical ease of execution. If the giver is familiar with the location of the diagnostic areas, the new sequence can be practised on a medium-sized cushion as well as on real receivers.

How to diagnose

All the above steps are preliminaries to the art of diagnosis. It is impossible to begin to diagnose from the Hara unless the routine is utterly automatic; it should be performed from a state of relaxation and absence of thought.

Before beginning to diagnose, position yourself beside the receiver's Hara, relax, breathe into your own Hara and gently lay one hand on the receiver's abdomen. While sitting quietly in this way, it is helpful to observe the condition of your own Ki and mind. It does not matter whether you are agitated, calm, tired or nervous as long as you take a moment or two to experience how that state feels in your body. To do so will not make it worse or even necessarily better but it will allow you to make

contact with your own Ki and to establish the presence within yourself of an aware centre which is capable of observation.

Open your focus wide, as when seeing the colours and hearing the sounds of the Elements, but this time it is your sensate focus. Your whole body is to become a receptacle for the messages relayed by your fingertips from the receiver's Hara.

Looking for the most Jitsu meridian. Now ask yourself the question, "What is this receiver's most Jitsu meridian at this moment?". Having asked the question, return to a state of relaxed attentiveness and absence of thought to palpate the receiver's Hara, using the two-handed sequence and without pausing for deliberation. You are not consciously looking for anything and certainly not using your thinking mind to assess the qualities of the different diagnostic areas; you are simply waiting, with your awareness as attentive as you can make it without focusing, for the qualities of Jitsu to register.

The invariable qualities of Jitsu on the Hara are:

• obviousness
• energetic activity; the sensation of presence and movement
• resilience or reaction.

Many givers report different sensations in addition to those above, such as heat, pulsing, tingling in the fingers, a sensation of being pushed away (although a sensation of being strongly drawn in, if obvious enough, can also be Jitsu). Since these tend to be individual and subjective reactions, however, it is best to stay with the three invariable qualities if you are studying without a teacher.

The most Jitsu meridian will usually make itself known immediately, if you have confidence in your sensations. If you find yourself at a loss, relax further and ground yourself in your Hara before palpating once more. If two palpation sequences do not reveal a Jitsu, guess. Pauline Sasaki, one of the most respected living teachers of Zen Shiatsu, advises students to guess if they cannot reach a conclusive diagnosis. Far from reducing a Shiatsu treatment to a reckless hit-and-miss, this suggestion opens the door to a reliable form of sixth sense.

■ *"A syndrome called blindsight has been discovered, which can arise with lesions to the occipital lobe of the brain. In this condition the patient can remain completely unaware of visual stimuli presented within a certain part of the field of vision. Yet if asked to "guess", the patient can point very accurately to where a faint light has been flashed, or to discriminate a cross from a circle. One patient, when pressed, described the experience as a "feeling" that it was "smooth" (the O) or "jagged" (the X), yet he stressed that he did not **see** anything at all."*

WEISKRANTZ *ET AL.,*
FROM AN ARTICLE IN *BRAIN,* 1974*

Finding the most Kyo meridian. The Jitsu is the easiest quality to find, since it is a messenger for the Kyo. To look for the Kyo on its own is more difficult, since its very nature is that it is hidden and resists detection. Thus a diagnostic area on the Hara may manifest Kyo qualities such as:

- hollowness
- inactivity
- passive resistance (stiffness)

*Quoted in *A Lexicon of Psychology, Psychiatry and Psychoanalysis*, J.Cooper. Routledge, 1988, p. 94.

and still not be the most Kyo. The most Kyo area on the Hara is the area which palpably connects with the most Jitsu area. The quickest way to find it is thus to hold the Jitsu area lightly with the fingertips and to palpate around the Hara with the other hand until a connection is felt. The connection between the most Kyo and the most Jitsu areas occurs as a subjective sensation on the part of the giver and that sensation is highly individual. Givers have variously reported:

- a sensation like a "blip" passing between the two hands
- a sensation of the Jitsu area diminishing
- a sensation of the Kyo area swelling
- a buzzing in the giver's head
- a sensation of completion felt deep within the giver

and there are certainly many more possible sensations which may occur. If you observe yourself, however, rather than focusing on the receiver, you will find your own yardstick for knowing when the connection, which has been described as "the echo of life", is made.

Not remaining in doubt

It is difficult for some Western Shiatsu givers to abandon the scientific approach and to trust their own sensations. For successful diagnosis, however, it is essential to do so. The scientific approach in this case is the objective observation of your own subjective sensations. For this to take place, it is important to:

1. observe your own state before beginning the diagnosis, so as to establish a starting point;
2. maintain a state of relaxation and wide-focused awareness throughout the procedure, so as not to compromise your receptivity;
3. avoid questioning your responses, if they are clear, and if the previous two requirements have been satisfied.

You will probably confuse the diagnosis if you overpalpate, since the receiver's Hara will begin to respond, and you will confuse yourself by questioning your reactions or trying for another Kyo–Jitsu response after the first has manifested.

Back diagnosis

Diagnosis can equally well be made from the back, which also has diagnostic areas corresponding to the meridians. These are shown in Figure 12.6.

Palpation of the back is performed with both hands and usually with the receiver in the sitting position, which ensures that the shoulders are relaxed and the spine straight. The touch is not quite so light as in Hara diagnosis and different parts of the hand

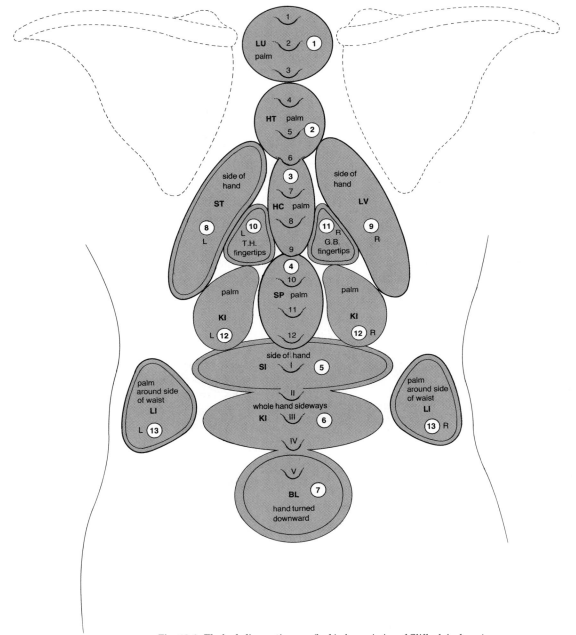

Fig. 12.6 *The back diagnostic areas (by kind permission of Clifford Andrews).*

are used as well as the fingertips; otherwise, the methodology is similar.

Since the back has the nature of a Yang, protective, supporting structure, it is likely to reflect long-standing imbalances which have influenced the receiver's spinal alignment or posture, as well as the current energy picture. For this reason it may not correspond to the Hara diagnosis on the same receiver and you should choose one or the other as a focus from which to work.

Diagnosis from the Yu points

The Yu points can be useful indicators of the condition of the organs, whether in TCM terms or according to Zen Shiatsu. They are, however, likely to indicate either long-standing imbalance or acute

conditions which affect the internal organs, rather than the temporary energetic changes which can be picked up on Hara diagnosis. Traditionally, it is the tenderness of the points on palpation which is the diagnostic sign, but you may well find that relevant Yu points "feel different" in some way. The locations of the Yu points are described in the individual chapters of Section Three, but a comprehensive chart is given in Figure 12.7.

Diagnosis from the Bo points

The Bo points, whose locations are given in the individual chapters of Section Three, are also considered to be diagnostic aids. In the TCM tradition, if a Bo point is tender on pressure, it indicates a pathological condition of the

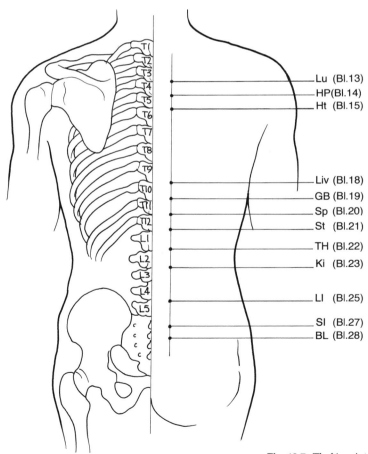

Fig. 12.7 *The Yu points.*

corresponding organ. Since some of the Bo points tend to be sensitive to standard Shiatsu pressure on most receivers, their diagnostic significance should be confined to extreme tenderness on relatively light pressure. The Bo points are not usually used for primary diagnosis in Shiatsu, but may give helpful confirmatory signs.

Asking

We now come to the fourth classical diagnostic tool of Oriental medicine, the taking of the case history. Case-taking technique is a skill which marks out the experienced Shiatsu giver and although many students feel trepidation at the thought of asking a receiver about his lifestyle and bodily processes, it is a worthwhile skill to master. Different givers have different styles of case-taking. Many feel that a questionnaire is too impersonal, and prefer to sketch out a broad case-history, filling in the details over time or as necessary. Others prefer a more formal and detailed approach. Clifford Andrews, a leading Zen Shiatsu practitioner in the UK, usually gives his receivers a questionnaire, but on occasions uses the two-question format, the two questions being:

1. What is happening for you at the moment?
2. Is there anything from the past you would like to tell me?
   If time is limited, these two questions are designed to elicit maximum information.

The purpose of the asking diagnosis is threefold:

1. to provide background information on the receiver's lifestyle and its possible contribution to his present condition;
2. to assess the receiver's general state of health, in order to ascertain his constitution and detect any longstanding imbalances;
3. to collect detailed information which may be relevant to the receiver's current health problem, if any such problem exists, both in the past, in terms of possible causes, and the present.

In general, to obtain full information on lifestyle and general health requires the format of a questionnaire, which may be given or sent to the receiver before treatment in order to save time. The questioning on the current condition is more specifically geared to the particular receiver and his particular condition and should be done verbally before treatment.

Questions about lifestyle

You should discover:

- the amount of exercise the receiver takes
- a rough idea of his diet and fluid intake
- whether he smokes and how much
- the extent of his alcohol, tea and coffee consumption.

Questions about general health

- It is usual to take details of major illnesses, operations and hospitalizations.
- You need to know if the receiver takes medication of any kind.
- Sleep patterns are important; if the receiver is wakeful, the time is significant. Light sleep or unrefreshing sleep, difficulty getting to sleep or constant waking all point to an imbalance (see Sections Two and Three for information about syndromes).
- You need to know about the receiver's urination patterns and how often he opens his bowels. If the answers to these questions reveal some deviation from the norm (urination 3–5 times a day but not at night, unless the receiver is elderly, and one or two bowel movements a day are normal) or if the receiver has come for some problem specifically connected with these functions, you may need to question further as to colour, smell, quantity or consistency.
- The receiver's energy level is significant, whether it is normal, consistently low or dips at a specific time of day.
- You should know the receiver's basic temperature; whether he tends to feel cold or hot or dislikes any extreme of temperature or if he feels cold or hot in specific body areas.
- Sweating can be important; day or night, after exertion or not and areas of the body.
- Pains anywhere from head to feet should be checked out for frequency, possible cause, the

nature of the pain, the precise area and whether it is better for pressure, heat, cold, movement or rest.

- In women, menstrual function should be checked for regularity, possible pain, specific PMS symptoms, duration and quantity. The quality and colour of the blood may be important if there is a dysfunction.
- Also for women, the circumstances surrounding pregnancies and births are significant. You should also know about IUDs, the Pill or hormone replacement therapy.
- It is useful to know what is the most common form of sickness for the receiver, such as colds, migraines, stomach upsets, for example.

Questions about the current condition

You need to ascertain the following:

- What are the precise symptoms of the condition as experienced by this particular receiver? A Western medical label such as "arthritis" or "PMS" is insufficient, since symptoms can vary widely within the spectrum of the condition.
- What makes the condition worse or better?

- What is the duration of the condition and what were the circumstances surrounding the initial onset?
- What has been the treatment so far and what have been the results?

These three categories provide a basic outline of the information necessary to form a clear picture of a physical disorder in terms of TCM and Zen Shiatsu. A case history is obviously not necessary in some circumstances, for example if a healthy receiver has been given a Shiatsu treatment as a present. On many other occasions, as when a receiver is coming for relaxation or for preventative reasons, a shorter and less comprehensive history can be taken.

The initial case history can form the basis for a file containing details of that receiver's treatments. On subsequent occasions, a 5-minute chat is usually enough to establish what changes have taken place. It is in your interest, if practising professionally, to keep as full a record as possible of the receiver's condition before and after each treatment, together with the Hara diagnosis and a summary of what was done. This establishes your professional approach in case of exceptional circumstances which might necessitate an enquiry into your records.

13

Interpreting the diagnosis

The interpretation of the material gathered through the Four Methods of diagnosis involves a combination of intuitive sensitivity and logical deduction. Each receiver manifests a unique combination of symptoms, signs, presentation and behaviour and the giver's own responses are an additional factor which may either clarify or confuse the issue. At the beginning, it can seem almost impossible to bring everything together, but interpretation is a skill which improves with exprience and as you progress in Shiatsu practice you find yourself, if not always certain, at least more flexible and more comfortable with different possibilities for interpretation.

In Zen Shiatsu, the key form of diagnosis is the palpation of the Hara or back. This is what will pinpoint the two meridians which are the focus of the session, the most Kyo and the most Jitsu meridians at the time of treatment. These two meridians provide the most effective Shiatsu treatment for the receiver's immediate condition. If you are clear which these two meridians are but cannot fit them into the general picture which you have put together from the asking, observing and listening diagnosis, it is not a crucial issue. After giving a treatment based on the most Kyo and most Jitsu meridians, you may find that a second Hara or back diagnosis reveals a more recognizable pattern. It is better to be open to uncertainty than to impose a preconceived or theoretical view on the situation and since human beings are complex by nature, new information tends to arrive little by little during the course of treatment which gradually amplifies your understanding of the diagnosis.

Understanding as much as possible at the outset is nonetheless the goal of diagnostic interpretation,

since understanding increases the giver's confidence and consequently that of the receiver. This fosters a good rapport between giver and receiver, with beneficial results for treatment.

The objectives in interpreting the diagnostic material are:

- to establish the receiver's immediate condition
- to establish the receiver's long term condition, which includes the strength of his basic Ki and constitution, as well as his imbalances
- to ascertain a possible cause for both current and long term problems
- to determine an appropriate treament approach.

In order to do this, the sum of the diagnostic material which is the product of your observation and intuitive responses must be integrated as much as possible with your theoretical knowledge of both the Zen Shiatsu and the TCM models (as well as any other systems with which you are familiar). It is important to be clear about which model you are using to draw any one diagnostic conclusion, and not to mix information from different systems.

Interpreting the Hara diagnosis

The Hara (or back) diagnosis is the axis of the Zen Shiatsu treatment mode. It can be used in an entirely pragmatic way, to focus the giver on two meridians out of the 12 which most need treatment at the time of the session, but it can also be interpreted on a wide range of levels, from the structural to the spiritual.

One way of interpreting the Hara diagnosis is on the level of current physical symptoms, for example:

- Stomach Jitsu – bleeding gums
- Lung Kyo – cough.

This works well only if there are actual physical symptoms. Also on the physical level are the features of the receiver's body type. If one or both of the meridians in the diagnosis can be connected with some aspect of the receiver's physical structure, it usually indicates that the diagnosis is a fairly long term one. Examples would be:

- Stomach Jitsu – heavy thighs, large stomach
- Lung Kyo – stooped shoulders.

A long term diagnosis of this type may be corroborated by the past health history, for example:

- Stomach Jitsu – duodenal ulcer 6 years ago
- Lung Kyo – colds as a child.

The above are illustrative examples. It is unlikely that both meridians in a diagnosis would refer to past problems alone, without reference to the current condition or to a continuing long term imbalance.

Finally, on the physical level, the meridians in the diagnosis can be related to lifestyle and habits, if they are known. For example:

- Stomach Jitsu – always eating
- Lung Kyo – just given up smoking.

It is possible to base the interpretation of a diagnosis solely on physical symptoms but to do so is to ignore the wider significance of Ki which encompasses all aspects of the receiver, the psychological as well as the physical, and thus to underestimate the deeper potential of Shiatsu treatment. It is not necessary to go into profound investigation of the receiver's psychological state; observation or information provided by the receiver can provide enough material to confirm the diagnosis. The following are examples of the kind of basic psychological observation which can be made:

- Stomach Jitsu – always worrying about others
- Lung Kyo – depressed.

The interpretation of Zen Shiatsu diagnosis at the highest level rests on an understanding of the meridians as expressions of a particular phase of

activity of Ki, as represented in the cycle described in Chapter 6. The catch phrases which capture the essence of each phase in the cycle can be applied to the condition of the receiver's Ki at this moment and interpreted according to our own understanding, in the light of the receiver's physical and psychological state. In this way, we can avoid relying on lists of symptoms or typecasting the receiver; instead, the receiver's condition is seen as an expression of the Ki in the meridians. Putting together the diagnosis and symptoms above, the giver might make the following mental notes to herself:

Stomach Jitsu

- *Hunger and satisfaction*; need is emphasized;
- Always eating – heavy thighs, large stomach; long term need has influenced physical shape.
- Always worrying; worry plus overeating led to duodenal ulcer?
- Some physical problem with Stomach meridian still – bleeding gums;
- Needs a comforting treatment.

Lung Kyo

- *Vitality through exchange*; intake of new Ki is neglected; depressed;
- Stooped shoulders and had colds as a child – long term problem (compensates with eating?);
- Has just given up smoking; lungs extra vulnerable at the moment, currently has cough;
- Needs to focus on breathing in new Ki – give simple breathing exercise?

The above example shows two long term imbalances manifesting in the Hara diagnosis, but either or both meridians could reflect a more recent situation or even a very temporary one resulting from feelings to do with the session itself. It is wise to bear the factor of duration in mind when interpreting the Hara diagnosis, since it can change in minutes. On the whole, the healthier and more balanced the receiver, the more variable the Hara diagnosis, since it is in the nature of Ki to move and change. The longer a receiver manifests a fixed pattern of Ki, the more likely he is to develop symptoms of disharmony.

There is only one situation in which the Hara diagnosis is likely to be wrong and that is when the most Kyo and the most Jitsu meridians are the two sides of a pair; for example, Large Intestine Jitsu, Lung Kyo. Since the Element pairs work together, such a diagnostic situation is impossible in all but the rarest circumstances. It is quite possible, however, that in the example above the Large Intestine is much *more* Jitsu than the Lung; but if the Large Intestine is the *most* Jitsu meridian, then the Lung cannot be the most Kyo. This situation is unlikely to arise if the diagnostic procedure described in Chapter 12 is followed.

Enlarging the diagnostic picture

For the giver trained in pure Zen Shiatsu, the Hara diagnosis and the symptom picture are all that is required for interpretation purposes. If she has some knowledge of TCM, however, she can extend the scope of her treatment and recommendations, using the material acquired by the Four Methods. It is important, however, not to mix TCM and Zen Shiatsu. When interpreting the Hara diagnosis of Stomach Jitsu, Lung Kyo above, she is working with the Zen Shiatsu diagnostic method and should adhere as closely as possible to the Zen Shiatsu model for interpretation; it would be confusing and counterproductive to insert TCM interpretations such as "Stomach supplying too much Food Essence to Lungs? Lungs not vaporizing fluids to Stomach?" which have no relevance to Zen Shiatsu treatment.

When is a TCM syndrome significant in the diagnosis?

The tongue is a reliable indicator of the receiver's condition in terms of TCM and the seriousness of a disorder can be seen from the appearance of the tongue. In general, the TCM syndrome is important in diagnosis and should be treated if:

- the tongue is peeled or has peeled patches, or is covered in small cracks indicating Deficiency of Yin;
- the tongue body is dark red, indicating extreme Heat, or noticeably purple, indicating stagnation

of Ki or more probably Blood, or blue, showing stagnation from Cold;
- there is a significant tongue coating, which shows accumulation of Dampness, Phlegm, Heat or Cold;
- the tongue is extremely swollen and pale, possibly quivering, indicating severe Deficiency of Ki and Yang;
- the tongue moves slowly from side to side, indicating Interior Wind.

The symptoms can indicate a TCM syndrome, if they fall into a recognizable pattern. Any acute disease pattern, such as the symptoms of a cold or flu or a stomach upset, will be represented among the TCM syndromes and can be treated effectively by TCM methods but other conditions besides acute disease may also be amenable to TCM interpretation and treatment.

Some examples of conditions are listed on page 246, one of which may be interpreted purely in Zen Shiatsu terms, three which invite a TCM interpretation as well and one where the TCM syndrome is not obvious but suspected.

Putting the diagnostic material together

The sum of the assembled diagnostic material to hand is:

1. The Hara or back diagnosis, which will indicate the receiver's most Kyo and most Jitsu meridians at the precise moment of diagnosing and which can be interpreted on either a physical or psychological basis or both, as described above.
2. The receiver's skin colour and the condition of his tongue, a product of the observation diagnosis, which will indicate a TCM interpretation of the receiver's current state and the probable length of its history.
3. The receiver's symptoms, signs, lifestyle and past health history, as revealed by the asking diagnosis. These will point to both Zen Shiatsu and TCM interpretations of both the receiver's current and long term conditions, as described above, and may help with deducing a possible cause.

EXAMPLES

Zen Shiatsu

Can't sleep, wakes unrefreshed, hip pain and neck tension, difficult decisions to make concerning relationship, represses feelings. Hara diagnosis: HP Jitsu, GB Kyo.

Here the symptoms accord completely with the Hara diagnosis and need no futher interpretation.

TCM

Dizzy, poor memory, spots in front of eyes, depressed, doesn't feel right since birth of her child, dry hair, dull pale skin, brittle nails. Hara diagnosis: Sp Jitsu, LI Kyo.

Here the symptoms suggest Blood Deficiency dating from the birth, and the receiver will need extra treatment, perhaps moxa and herbs.

Feels tired and lethargic, abdominal pain with diarrhoea (urgent, burning, with blood and mucus). Under medication for colitis due to stress. Hara diagnosis: SI Jitsu, LI Kyo.

In this case, the receiver has Damp-Heat in the Large Intestine and points to eliminate Damp and Heat are indicated.

Itchy red eczema in groin area, worse in summer, favourite food fish and chips, favourite drink beer (lots). Hara diagnosis: Liv Jitsu, Bl Kyo.

In this case the receiver has Heat in the Blood, probably coming from Heat in the Liver, caused by fatty food and alcohol. He needs points to cool the Blood. Dietary changes will supplement the effects of the Shiatsu and if that is not enough, he may need herbs.

Combination

Headaches from stress, very tired, can't relax, severe period pains, high achiever, difficult childhood. Hara diagnosis: BL Jitsu, SI Kyo.

In this case, there is a combination of symptoms which suggest Liver involvement, possibly Liver Yang rising (headaches) or stagnation of Liver Blood (severe period pains) or both. Shiatsu will certainly help the problem greatly, but further questioning to ascertain the TCM syndrome may suggest points for self-treatment in addition.

---

4. The predominant facial hue and the essential sound of the voice, which will point to the Element which is most out of balance.
5. The receiver's "Ki picture", the patterns of Ki flow and its relative accumulations and deficiencies revealed by observing the receiver's Ki, which indicates where Shiatsu treatment will have most effect. The energy picture may help to confirm a diagnosis but its primary use is practical, in determining an approach to treatment, and it is discussed further in Chapter 14.

You may also, depending on your training, have other material from methods such as facial diagnosis or pulse diagnosis which will contribute to your information on the receiver.

Your aim is to select what is relevant from all this material, in order to focus your treatment approach and recommendations specifically to the receiver's needs. These different inputs must be merged as much as possible into a cohesive whole, while respecting the differences between the TCM and Zen Shiatsu models.

1. The energy picture and the Hara or back diagnosis can be put together to indicate and the condition of the receiver's Ki at this precise moment in time: its relative strength, the most Kyo and most Jitsu meridians and the body areas where Ki is concentrated or lacking. This helps you to know which meridians to treat and in which areas, and determines your approach to the Shiatsu as a whole.
2. The symptoms and signs, lifestyle, presentation and behaviour can be used to confirm the Hara or back diagnosis, as outlined above.
3. The receiver's skin colour and the condition of his tongue can combine with his symptoms, signs and past health history to indicate a condition or combination of conditions in the TCM model, such as Spleen Yang Deficiency, Damp-Heat in the Intestines or stagnant Liver Ki. This may or may

not corroborate the Hara/back diagnosis (see below for contradictions between TCM syndrome and Zen Shiatsu diagnosis). TCM syndromes are not treated by Zen Shiatsu methods, but by pressure or moxa on specific points and via recommendations. This is discussed further in Chapter 14.

4. The facial hue and the sound of the voice merge with either the Hara/back diagnosis or the symptom/tongue picture to indicate which Element is the most imbalanced and serves to help the giver focus on the possible root cause of the receiver's problem.

In an ideal world, the Hara diagnosis, tongue, symptom picture, colour, sound, posture and hue would all corroborate each other and point to one or two meridians; of course, this is rarely the case. Even when working with a single medical system such as TCM, anomalies and seeming contradictions arise; when working with two different systems, there are many possibilities for confusion. Here is a list of the contradictions which most frequently arise, their probable causes and what to do.

Apparent contradictions and how to resolve them

The Hara diagnosis does not agree with the TCM symptom picture or tongue

This seeming contradiction occurs very frequently, since the two systems are dealing with different priorities and working from different principles. The following problems may occur.

A Deficient organ may appear as Jitsu on the Hara

Jitsu and Kyo are not the same as TCM Excess and Deficiency. This has been discussed at length in Section Two, Chapter 6, but bears repeating here since it confuses many students that Kidney Yin Deficiency or Spleen Yang Deficiency can manifest as Kidney or Spleen Jitsu on the Hara.

Kyo and Jitsu, like Yin and Yang, are variable and relative conditions. The meridian of an organ which is Deficient in TCM terms may manifest either as Kyo

or Jitsu; the Jitsu implies a greater investment of energy in the aspects of existence represented by the meridian. The Kyo represents a part of the bodymind which is neglected or ignored and therefore hidden.

The following case history illustrates a typical example.

EXAMPLE

A middle-aged women comes for treatment for insomnia. She also has scanty, dark, painful urination. She is extremely tense and anxious, always on the go, unable to relax and has a deep fear of water. Her cheeks are flushed and her tongue is red and completely peeled. All her symptoms and signs point in TCM terms to severe long term Deficiency of Kidney Yin, with resulting Empty Heat.

The Hara diagnosis, however, is commonly Kidney or Bladder Jitsu, Heat or Small Intestine Kyo, showing that her Ki activity is concentrated in the areas of expression of the Water meridians. Her main investment of energy is in impetus, or action, as a response to fear; she is thus in a constant state of stress. The neglected phase of energy in her life is assimilation into her emotional core; she is unable to process suggestions from those around her or from her own exhausted organs, to be peaceful or to relax.

The organs in the TCM syndrome may not appear in the Hara diagnosis

This may be for one of three reasons.

1. TCM and Zen Shiatsu offer different interpretations, in terms of specific meridian functions, of energetic or physiological patterns (see Section Three on the individual meridians). A simple example is the Triple Heater's association in Zen Shiatsu with the body's immune response, which in TCM is largely represented by the protective function of the Lungs and Defensive Ki. Another is the factor of stagnation of Blood, which is often represented by the Liver in TCM but by the Small Intestine in Zen Shiatsu.

2. Hara diagnosis is likely to pick up the specific body organ where an imbalance is occurring, whereas TCM will view the local problem as part

of a wider-reaching condition. This is especially true of problems which in TCM stem from the all-important Spleen and Kidneys, which supply Postnatal and Prenatal Essence and Source Ki.

For example, Spleen Yang Deficiency in TCM reflects a general inability to digest and metabolize food. Someone with Spleen Yang Deficiency is likely to have loose stools and copious urination, because the food and fluids are not being transformed. These symptoms may be picked up in the Hara diagnosis, but as distortions of the Large Intestine and Bladder meridians respectively, the areas where the symptoms are occurring.

3. The Hara diagnosis may represent a temporary psychological state, eclipsing the long term behavioural pattern associated with the physical symptoms. A typical example would be the case history below.

The facial hue and the sound of the voice do not agree with the Hara diagnosis and/or the TCM tongue/symptom picture

The Element associations of colour and sound will usually indicate either one of the Elements in the Hara diagnosis or the Element central to the TCM syndrome. If they confirm neither, they are probably pointing to an Element which is at the root cause of the receiver's condition and which may well surface in the Hara diagnosis later in the course of treatment.

The relationship between the Element manifesting in the Hara diagnosis or the symptom picture and the Element showing on the face or in the sound of the voice can usually be worked out via one of the Element cycles, the Creative or the Control (p. 81). For example, if a receiver with a Lungs Hara diagnosis and a phlegmy cough has a yellow hue or a singsong voice, then Earth may be involved in the

---

EXAMPLE

A middle-aged man has a long history of chronic lower back pain and asthma. His facial colour is white, with a bluish hue around the mouth and eyes, and his tongue is swollen, pale and wet, with hardly any coating. He has a sedentary job and mentions that he has been with the same firm for 20 years. He gives away very little else about his life and is quiet and reticent. For the first two treatments, the diagnosis is Stomach Jitsu, Gall Bladder Kyo; in subsequent treatments, the diagnosis is predominantly Lung and Large Intestine Jitsu, Kidney Kyo.

Later in the course of treatment, it transpires that, at the time of beginning his Shiatsu treatments, he had been refused promotion to a better position in his firm, and had been thinking of looking for another job. The diagnosis of Stomach Jitsu reflects his need for recognition and reward, the Gall Bladder Kyo his irresolution and repressed anger. After the dust has settled from this incident, he reverts to a more typical long term diagnosis.

The TCM syndrome is of Deficient Kidney Ki and Yang (lower backache, swollen, wet, pale tongue, bluish hue) failing to receive Ki from the Lungs (white

facial colour), which rises up again causing asthma. The long duration of the problem points either to a weak constitution (Kidneys), a difficult early family history (Kidneys – fear, perhaps of a rigid and authoritarian parent – Metal) or both.

The TCM syndrome does not conflict with the later Hara diagnoses, although the Zen Shiatsu interpretation of the receiver's symptoms and behaviour might be slightly different and might run like this. He has low motivation (Kidney Kyo – lack of impetus) and fear of change and failure (Lung/Large Intestine Jitsu – hanging on to boundaries, lack of exchange with the environment). These factors may have led to his long term sedentary employment, which has further contributed to his lower back pain and his asthma, symptoms which also stem from the Kidney and metal imbalance. As a result of lack of impetus and self-worth he has closed himself off further, becoming quiet and reticent and probably depressed (Metal – grief) problem, since it is not supplying enough nourishment to Metal along the Creative Cycle and may need to be treated, perhaps with regular moxa on St 36.

An alternative possibility might arise from a Control Cycle relationship between the Elements concerned, as in the following case history.

EXAMPLE

A young women comes for treatment for severe migraines along the pathway of the Gall Bladder meridian, which usually coincide with her period and are accompanied by visual disturbances. She often complains angrily about other people. Her facial hue is white and her voice alternates between weeping and shouting. Since she is going through a major life change, the Hara diagnoses often reflect passing emotional storms. Metal and Wood meridians figure frequently in the diagnosis, but in no permanent Kyo or Jitsu role.

In this case, although the symptoms are primarily in Wood, which is also highly active in the planning and decision-making going on in her life, the colour and sound suggest that Metal is also deeply implicated. Metal is too weak to control Wood and is severely strained in addition by the letting go process involved in her life change. As well as receiving Shiatsu on the meridians in the current Hara diagnosis, she needs to be taught how to tonify her Deficient Metal with breathing exercises and regular self-treatment of Lu 9 and LI 4.

■
14

The treatment

■ *"In the mind of the physician there should be no desires, only a receptive and accepting attitude, then the mind can become shen. The mind of the physician and the mind of the patient should be level and in harmony, following the movements..."*

ZHEN JIU DE CHENG, 1601 AD*

Now the case history has been taken and the diagnosis for this particular treatment has been made, you need to sketch out a rough plan for your treatment to follow . The meridians to treat have been chosen through the Hara diagnosis; it now remains to decide:

- what treatment position to choose
- what body areas to concentrate on
- the strength and type of treatment appropriate to the receiver.

Choice of treatment position

This will be influenced by the following considerations:

The receiver's body structure and symptoms

The receiver's comfort is paramount in treatment. Elderly people and pregnant women in particular need attention paid to the comfort of the treatment position and some ingenuity may be required in adapting techniques so that, for example, an old person can be treated sitting in a chair or a pregnant woman can be supported in a kneeling semi-prone sprawl by a pile of cushions. In general, the side position is the most comfortable of the classical positions and most receivers can manage it, though support from cushions may be needed.

The meridians to be treated

Your focus during treatment will be to bring the receiver's Ki into the Kyo meridian and away from the Jitsu. Both meridians therefore need to be treated, but you will be concentrating on the Kyo; the main position chosen should therefore allow maximum access to the Kyo meridian and as much access to the Jitsu meridian as possible. Examples of diagnoses and treatment positions are as follows:

- TH Jitsu, LI Kyo – side position
- St Jitsu, GB Kyo – side position, then supine
- B1 Jitsu, LI Kyo – side position, then prone
- Liv Jitsu, Lu Kyo – supine position, then side
- SI Jitsu, Ki Kyo – prone position, then side

Note: The sitting position can be used, when the receiver's symptoms and body structure indicate it, for loosening and releasing the upper torso, shoulders, arms and neck.

---

*Quoted in *Hara Diagnosis: Reflections on the Sea*, p. 38.

The body areas on which to focus

These will be determined by:

The receiver's energy picture

The focal point for the treatment will be the area which appears most deficient in Ki in the looking diagnosis. For example, a common pattern in Western receivers is a weak Hara area and lower body; in this case, the focus of treatment will be to encourage Ki to flow into this area by holding the Hara and tonifying (see p. 254) the lower back and hips, using the meridians in the Hara diagnosis or their Element pairs.

It may also be necessary to disperse (see p. 255) Ki from areas where it seems overfull and stagnant. With experience, it is possible to distinguish this type of Jitsu blockage from areas where Ki is excessive but mobile; these areas do not need much dispersing, since their Ki will move easily to a deficient body part as it is tonified. Occasionally, areas of blockage will monopolize the Ki and keep it from flowing into deficient areas and on these occasions the blocked Ki will need to be dispersed before the deficient area is tonified.

The receiver's symptoms and needs

The average receiver will come for Shiatsu treatment with a particular aim in mind; to get rid of a knee pain or to ease chronic shoulder tension, for instance. In most of these cases, the receiver will want the affected part to be given attention and it is wise to do so, even if you can see from your looking diagnosis that the knee pain is a direct result of a distortion in the neck or that the shoulders will relax by themselves once the Ki in the Hara is strengthened. The receiver's awareness of his own body is part of his Ki pattern and you can work with it to soothe when dispersing or encourage when tonifying, as necessary. You should therefore allow some time for working on the body parts which are important to the receiver, as well as the ones whose significance you perceive yourself.

The strength and type of treatment approach

There are surprising variations in the tolerance of individual receivers which make it hard to generalize on treatment approach. It is common to find receivers of the Deficient type who crave deep and powerful techniques and robust and vigorous receivers who are extremely sensitive.

It is wise, however, to start with a gentle approach on:

- extremely thin, frail or old receivers
- overweight receivers who are fluid-retentive rather than muscular
- receivers with osteoporosis or high blood pressure
- receivers who complain of permanent exhaustion
- receivers whose Ki appears deficient in the looking diagnosis
- receivers who seem emotionally distressed.

A gentle approach implies more emphasis on Ki penetration than physical pressure and a minimum of vigorous techniques such as rotations and stretches, together with increased attention to palming and holding, especially in deficient areas. You can often compensate for the lack of the physical pressure by the length of time spent in penetrating and holding points, since weak Ki needs time to respond. The session should be kept as short as possible, however, in order not to tire the receiver.

When treating such a receiver for the first time, you should ask for feedback every so often in order to establish the degree of pressure which is comfortable.

If the receiver's Ki picture suggests some particular quality of Ki, you may also determine what type of approach will best suit it and bear that intention in mind throughout the treatment, for example:

- loosening compacted Ki
- supporting debilitated Ki
- connecting a disjointed Ki picture
- calming agitated Ki.

At this point the treatment can begin and you ask the receiver to assume the chosen position, making him comfortable as necessary with cushions. Since many receivers quickly become cold when receiving Shiatsu, it is wise to have a blanket handy and to ask periodically if the receiver is warm enough.

Treatment routine and direction of Ki flow

The treatment will usually begin on the most Kyo meridian, on the most Kyo side of the body.

The order of the treatment routine will, however, be determined to some extent by your treatment focus. For example, if the receiver's diagnosis is Gall Bladder Jitsu, Bladder Kyo and the characteristics of the Ki picture are a stagnated accumulation of Ki around the shoulders and deficiency in the lower body and legs, you may wish to have the receiver in the sitting position to unblock the shoulder area as a whole, and particularly the Gall Bladder meridian, with rotations and dispersing techniques before laying him down in the prone position to tonify the Bladder in the lower back and legs.

Often, however, a pronounced indication of this kind does not arise or you may prefer to treat according to a routine, dealing with distortions as you feel them during the course of the treatment. As a general rule, in Zen Shiatsu, the body is treated in a downward direction and the limbs are treated from the torso out to the extremities. It is not necessary to start at any one place, however, and you can put together your own routine sequence. One example would be to start with the Hara diagnosis, then treat down the legs in the supine position, starting with the most Kyo meridian on the most Kyo leg, then work the chest and down the arms to the hands, then the neck and head; on changing from the supine to the side or prone position, you can work from the head down to the feet along the chosen meridians or their Element pairs.

A logical sequence for treating the meridians in any body part would be to start with the most Kyo meridian from the Hara diagnosis, or its Element pair, and to follow with the most Jitsu meridian from the Hara diagnosis, or its Element pair, in the same body part. If there is a local meridian distortion (see p. 234), this will also need to be treated. However, giving Shiatsu is not always a logical procedure and you will often find yourself following a different sequence. As long as you are aware of what you are doing and have not drifted into a trance, working according to intuitive promptings in this way can only be beneficial.

In the macrobiotic tradition of Shiatsu, the meridians are worked according to the direction of Ki flow within each Yin or Yang meridian, so that the Spleen would be treated from the foot up to the groin, whereas the Stomach would be worked down the leg to the foot. This technique is designed for work with the classical meridians, whose direction of Ki flow has been established by tradition; in the Zen Shiatsu meridian extensions, however, the direction of Ki flow is not formally indicated, so that the meridian flow cannot be followed in the same way.

No matter which meridians are indicated by the Hara diagnosis, every Shiatsu treatment should include:

- general work on the hands and feet
- a routine for face and head
- work down the spine (Bladder meridian, if Kidney or Bladder is not indicated in the Hara diagnosis)
- occipital balancing and/or work on the neck.

These can be thorough without being lengthy; however, at least 10 minutes of each session should be spent on the neck and back. The only exceptions to this general approach would be if the receiver's condition were extremely weak or the treatment time very short, for whatever reason.

Different qualities of touch

■ *"When rubbing, be very attentive and careful, as though one were holding a tiger by the tail. Do not be tense, keep one's hand relaxed."*

ZHEN JIU DA CHENG, 1601 AD*

From the diagnostic palpation which, as already described, is extremely light in the Zen Shiatsu style

*Quoted in *Hara Diagnosis: Reflections on the Sea.*

described here, the change to treatment mode is signalled with:

Preliminary contact

Once the receiver is comfortable and in the right position, lay your hands on the receiver on an accessible area, preferably a non-threatening area, between the shoulderblades or the feet, for example, to establish contact.

The quality of the preliminary contact with the receiver is important in establishing the "tone" of the treatment to come, and several seconds of attention should be allowed for it.

For some givers, the first contact will be one of "listening". Extend your sensory perceptions out from your still centre of awareness established at the beginning of the Hara diagnosis (see p. 236) to make a feeling connection with the receiver's Ki. For many receivers, this in itself is a relaxing and opening sensation, since they feel completely acknowledged.

For other givers, the diagnostic procedure will have provided enough information on the state of the receiver's Ki and the preliminary contact will aim to set the feeling for the Shiatsu treatment. In this case, while yourself remaining centred in the Hara, extend a particular quality of feeling towards the receiver; calm support is universally acceptable but an experienced giver will be able to imbue that support with a quality of nurturing, stability or incisiveness, according to how she perceives the receiver's Ki. The qualities extended in her touch do not come from mental willpower, but from an aware response to the receiver's needs.

The even touch

When a meridian is diagnosed as Kyo or Jitsu on the Hara, it will not be Kyo or Jitsu for its entire length. It is even possible that a meridian diagnosed as Kyo on the Hara may be relatively Jitsu for much of its length and Kyo only in one small but highly significant area. For this reason, each meridian is tonified only in its Kyo areas and dispersed in its Jitsu areas and much of the Shiatsu treatment is given with the even touch, that is, neither tonifying nor dispersing.

The even touch is simple pressure to the level where you can sense the Ki in the meridian, with

awareness but no intention; a readiness to respond but not a response. It may carry the characteristics of the preliminary contact, those of calmness and support, with whatever additional necessary characteristics your intention can confer. It is also essential to "listen" through the even touch for distortions of Ki flow which will require tonification or dispersing. The use of the mother hand is basic to the application of the even touch, as it is to all the other qualities; your awareness should be as much in your mother hand as in your working hand, since it is often through the mother hand that the signal of a distortion in the meridian is felt.

In a sense, the even touch is the beginner's "crawling" technique taken to a higher level of Ki interaction; in the same way that the beginner will crawl over the receiver's body in an exploratory way until she finds a spot where she feels comfortable in resting her weight, so the experienced giver will use the even touch until she finds an empty or overfull spot in the meridian, where she can bring her Ki into play to tonify or to disperse.

Tonification touch and techniques

Tonification is the process of bringing Ki to a Kyo meridian or body part. The word Kyo means empty and emptiness is the prevailing sensation when touching Kyo in a meridian. The part may be empty of Ki response, wooden; or empty of physical resilience, flaccid; it often feels like a deep and empty trough or hole. The aim of tonification is to bring responsiveness, resilience and tone back to the area. When you feel a Kyo area, allow your touch to penetrate as deeply as the area will allow. It is essential not to press or use force, since both meridian and receiver will close up against this invasion of a vulnerable area, rather, the penetration should be like a plumb line sinking to the bottom of a well. Sometimes you will begin to feel a response before you have reached the bottom; sometimes you must penetrate to the deepest level and wait some time for a response, according to the degree of Kyo. If a spot or area is extremely Kyo and the wait is long, it can be very helpful to ask the receiver to breathe into the spot.

In order for tonification to take place, maintain a relaxed and steady presence, with no conscious thought or intention but with absolute awareness invested in both your mother hand and in the thumb or elbow which is penetrating the receiver's Kyo spot. This awareness is different from the "listening" awareness of the even touch and the difference is in the way your Ki si focused. In the even touch, the attitude of Ki might be compared to the gesture of a finger held in the air to feel which way the wind is blowing. When tonifying, the attitude of Ki is similar to that of someone pointing her finger in the air to show a traveller the path up a mountain. The gestures are very similar but the attitudes of Ki are very different. Whereas the first will not affect the receiver much, the second is designed to focus his awareness on his Kyo spot; it is showing him the way that his Ki wants to go (Fig. 14.1).

Although your awareness is focused in your mother hand and the penetrating hand, you are not consciously transferring Ki to the Kyo spot; you are allowing the receiver to send his own Ki there. Your aim is to attract the Yang qualities of Ki, warmth, movement and responsiveness, to the Kyo area and, since Yang is attracted to Yin, the quality of your penetration must be Yin, still and receptive. Imposing will upon the Kyo spot, even the well-intentioned will to bring Ki there, will have the opposite effect.

The response as Ki begins to flow into the Kyo area may be felt in either or both hands. It is your signal to move on immediately a response is felt; there is no point in waiting around, since the change has already taken place.

On extremely painful areas, tonification may be accomplished by intention alone, without the aid of penetration. The procedure is exactly as described above except that, instead of penetrating physically to the level of the meridian, the giver rests her working hand lightly on the receiver's body surface, or even above it, and connects her Hara and mother hand with the Kyo area of the meridian by means of visualization, breathing or intention. This technique, which can elicit as clear a response from the receiver's Ki as physical penetration, still requires attunement to the mother hand, which remains firmly supporting the Hara or another suitable area.

Tonification touch does not have to be slow, as long as absolute stillness is achieved at the deepest point of penetration. Calmness, non-invasiveness and focus are its essential qualifications.

Since movement tends to disperse Ki rather than

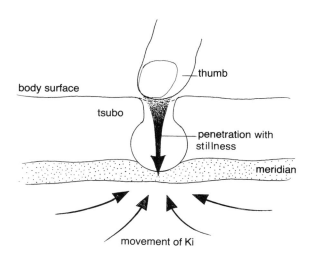

Fig. 14.1 *Tonifying touch.*

attract it, techniques such as stretches and rotations are not, strictly speaking, compatible with the tonification of Kyo areas. The stretch positions for the meridians are an exception, since they are a tonification method in themselves, However, it may be that a Kyo area has become physically stiff and stagnant from Deficiency. In such a case, a minimum of stretches and rotations can be performed after the area has been tonified by touch and penetration, if they are done slowly and sensitively.

Dispersing touch and techniques

Dispersing is often referred to as "sedation". This can be a misleading term, since it implies calming and stilling and some qualities of Jitsu need to be restored to natural active flow by dispersing compacted or stagnant Ki. The principles for dispersing are mostly the exact opposite to those of tonification but with one exception; whereas tonification touch is calm and non-invasive, dispersing touch is not agitated and aggressive! The giver remains focused and centred in the Hara and imparts only enough Yang control to her touch as is necessary to disperse the Ki.

A Jitsu area is signalled by an increase in reactivity of the Ki in the meridian, and often by an increased compactness and elasticity of the tissues. For this reason, you may need to be firmer in your penetration to the level of the meridian. Once you have reached the level of the meridian and its Ki flow, do not stay there but remove your thumb or elbow in order to penetrate once again. Your movement has the quality of physically moving the Ki along the channel of the meridian, away from where it has accumulated, like squeezing toothpaste along a tube.

This technique is not simply physical, however. Ki, even when it is dense and compacted, is best dispersed with Ki and awareness and it is important to identify and contact the individual quality of the Jitsu Ki in order to send it away, since Jitsu can have different qualities; for example, it may be agitated, or stuck, or resistant. (If you want to send someone away, it is more effective to single him out for the communication, rather than making general shooing noises.) Clarity and presence are required to make this contact without inviting the Jitsu Ki to linger and a steady focus is necessary to use your intention to disperse without force. It can help, as you "squeeze

the toothpaste along the tube", to visualize the Jitsu Ki being driven away from your thumb or elbow to a Kyo area or, if this is difficult, just to visualize it disappearing into the receiver's body space (Fig. 14.2).

On the whole, however, dispersing touch tends to be more physical, and also more Yang and moving, than tonification touch. When the majority of a body area is full of Excess Ki, causing congestion in the tissues around the meridians as well as the meridians themselves, massage techniques which combine pressure and movement, such as circular frictions or vibrations, may be used to encourage Ki and blood to move freely. These techniques are particularly successful when combined with tonification of any Kyo points discovered within the Jitsu area.

Kenbiki is a technique borrowed from Anma to deal with muscular tension in the back. The giver kneels facing the receiver's side and works down each side of the spine, pushing and pulling the longitudinal back

A An example of a jitsu condition in a meridian

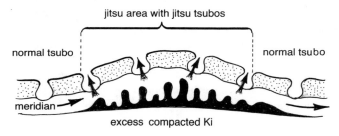

B Process of dispersal

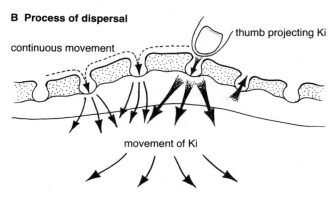

C Even flow re-established

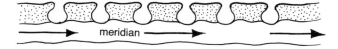

Fig. 14.2 *Dispersing touch.*

muscles "across the grain", using both hands side by side or one hand on top of the other. This should be done from the Hara and with a springy touch, so that the receiver's whole body undulates from side to side. Kenbiki is not suitable for receivers with weak backs or a Kyo condition in any of the back meridians.

On rare occasions, percussion techniques can be used to disperse large areas of compacted Ki. This should only be done by an experienced giver who is working with awareness of the receiver's Ki; indiscriminate slapping is not advisable. I have only seen this done once, by Pauline Sasaki on one of her students whose whole body appeared Jitsu with a build-up of Ki from unexpressed emotion. She firmly slapped down the length of the student's back and the receiver's body appeared to deflate instantly. The treatment profoundly altered the receiver's attitude and Ki.

Rotations are also useful dispersing techniques which help to move Ki in the joints. They should be performed with care, however, in order not to cause pain or overstretch contracted connective tissues. Stretches can also be used, but only after an area has been loosened with the dispersing techniques above.

Examples of tonification and dispersing touch in practice

Let us take two examples (opposite) of two receivers with a diagnosis of Lung Jitsu, Heart Protector Kyo, and imagine working the chest and arms in each case. With two meridians whose main area of activity is the Upper Burning Space, the chest and arms are likely to be significant in treatment, but the Ki may manifest in very different ways in different receivers.

The receiver's sensations during treatment

Pain

Although some degree of pain is often felt during a Shiatsu treatment, it is usually accompanied or closely

---

EXAMPLES

In receiver A, the Kyo Heart Protector is the deepest distortion in the chest area, with a noticeable concave area around CV 17, the Heart Protector Bo point, which is also the central point of the three branches of the Zen Shiatsu meridian in the chest. There is some Lung Jitsu apparent in the arms, however, as they look tight and are held in closely to the body. When treating this receiver, the Heart Protector in the chest would be generally treated with the even touch but with emphasis on tonifying the area around CV 17 and any other Kyo areas felt during treatment. The giver might then rest her mother hand gently and supportively on the CV 17 area in the centre of the sternum while her working hand disperses the Jitsu Lung meridian in the arms, allowing the Ki to flow up into the Kyo area in the chest.

In receiver B, the Lung Jitsu is the most noticeable in the chest, with a puffed-up area around Lu 1 which extends up into the shoulders. Both Lung and Heart Protector in the arms look weak and disconnected from the torso. In this case, after dispersing Lu 1 and the surrounding area, the giver could continue the dispersing by pushing gently down on the Lu 1 area with her mother hand while the working hand tonifies the most Kyo points in both Heart Protector and Lung in the arms, having discovered them by working down both meridians with the even touch. This will open up the flow of Ki from the Jitsu chest area down into the arms.

---

followed by sensations of pleasure or relief (one receiver called the sensation "grateful pain", another "grim satisfaction"!). However, since many Western receivers believe that pain is beneficial, some of them will endure an unnecessary degree of pain without complaint. It is important to be aware of this and to remain sensitive to any tension in the receiver's body. If pain is accompanied by relief, the receiver will remain relaxed; if not, he will tense up. Never ignore a receiver's pain. If you are working on an area which you know is Kyo and needs tonifying and the receiver's Ki is responding to your penetration but the receiver feels pain, you can:

- lighten your penetration to the minimum required to maintain contact with the receiver's Ki;

- increase the contact of the mother hand and its connection with the working hand;
- invite feedback from the receiver;
- encourage the receiver to breathe deeply into the painful area.

If the contact is still too painful, you may resort to gentle holding or off-the-body tonification, as described above.

If severe pain results from dispersing touch or techniques, you would be well advised to stop treating that particular area since the risks of causing damage to inflamed tissues and going beyond the receiver's tolerance outweigh the benefits of dispersing Ki.

Needing more

The receiver should be encouraged to contribute to the Shiatsu through feedback on what he feels or needs. If he requests extra attention to a point or area which has already been worked, it means that the tonification or dispersal process is not complete. However, in my own experience as a receiver, such points or areas require very little attention the second time around and it is wasting time to expend a great deal of effort on pleasing the receiver, when all that is required is a slight final nudge to the Ki.

Bodily processes

Since Shiatsu releases blocks and speeds elimination, it is quite common for receivers during treatment to experience:

- increased peristalsis, with stomach gurgling (stomach gurgles often but not always signal release of impeded Ki);
- flatulence;
- nasal discharge;
- slightly increased menstrual flow (if the Shiatsu treatment causes flooding, the treatment was excessive or inappropriate, unless the receiver was subject to this problem already).

Some receivers may feel tense or uncomfortable about these manifestations and should be reassured that they are normal signs of the effectiveness of the treatment.

Sexual arousal

This is also one the transitory states which may result from the energetic shifts occurring during a Shiatsu session. Although it probably occurs as frequently in women as in men, the effect is more obvious in men. If neither giver nor receiver pays undue attention to this change, it can pass without causing a problem. If the giver finds herself troubled by this manifestation in a receiver, she may need to talk to her Shiatsu teacher or another experienced practitioner. If the receiver deliberately focuses attention on his or her state, or if it happens frequently, the giver is justified in discontinuing treatment.

Avoidance

Avoidance tactics are not, strictly speaking, a sensation but the attempt to avoid experiencing sensation at a level which might induce change. The most common avoidance tactic is continual talking during the Shiatsu process. Although a funereal silence is not a necessary condition for the success of a Shiatsu treatment, you need a tranquil atmosphere in order to focus and the receiver should be told this. Another avoidance tactic is to sleep deeply throughout the session; if a receiver continually does this, consider changing your treatment mode to a more stimulating and challenging one.

Other reactions

It is fairly common for unexpressed grief to well up during treatment and to be released in tears. If this happens, pause in your treatment and wait in a position of comforting contact, check to see whether the receiver needs to talk and resume the treatment as appropriate.

Shiatsu produces many changes and receivers may report different sensations, from sudden hunger to seeing colours or even astral travelling. Most of these are unique to the receiver and their main importance is that the receiver may wish to talk about them and their relevance to his condition or the treatment process. While remaining open to the possible significance of such experiences, it is beneficial to view them as another transitory effect of the change in the receiver's Ki and encourage him not to become fixated upon them.

The timing of a treatment

It is important to keep the time of a treatment session to the minimum, for the following reasons:

- it saves the giver's energy;
- it sharpens the giver's focus and stops her drifting through a routine;
- it ensures that the receiver does not become tired from being overworked.

Within the normal 1-hour slot allowed for a session in a clinic, therefore, the actual Shiatsu need not exceed 45 minutes and may be as little as half an hour. While different givers have different natural time periods within which they feel comfortable and unhurried, it is important to keep treatment time short. It is often a sign of lack of confidence to take a long time treating. A shorter treatment will do the job as well, if not better, for the reasons given above.

It is also important, however, that the receiver feels properly cared for and is left with a feeling of completion and relaxation. You can accomplish this through:

- focusing the treatment on the areas you know are most significant;
- paying attention to the areas which the receiver feels are significant;
- proficiency and sensitivity with the even touch;
- an unhurried attitude during tonification techniques, making sure that relevant points are penetrated to the correct level and for the necessary length of time;
- being relaxed yourself;
- being familiar with the habits you fall into if tired, tense or hurried. (Most givers in this state will do one of two things; press too hard or not press hard enough.)
- going back to the basic "crawling" technique when you feel pressured. It deeply relaxes both receiver and giver.

Concluding the treatment

If possible, end the treatment with a concluding contact similar to the preliminary contact (the Hara or feet are good places to do this). This may be done before or after the final Hara diagnosis and rechecking the leg length. Both of these, and the final looking diagnosis, will provide information which should be written down in the case notes. The last part of the session is covered in the next chapter.

Incorporating points into a Shiatsu treatment

If the points to be used have already been decided upon, and if they lie on near the meridians in the Hara diagnosis, they can be incorporated into the Shiatsu treatment; otherwise, it may be less distracting for both giver and receiver if the points are treated separately after the work on the meridians.

The anatomical locations of major points are given in Section Three, but in order to locate points precisely, it can be helpful to stroke the surface of the skin all over the immediate vicinity of the point until you find a very slight hollow. Since tsubos have a lower electrical resistance than the surrounding area, you may also feel a characteristic sensation which indicates the presence of Ki. If locating all the points before you go into treatment mode to press them, you may need a fine felt-tipped pen to mark each of them with a dot.

The mother hand is not necessary when treating points but, unless you are pressing the point with one thumb on top of the other, it is comforting for the receiver if your other hand is resting on or supporting an adjacent body area. Sensation is important for the effective use of points and you should spend as much time as is necessary angling your pressure until the receiver feels a strong sensation, which may radiate outwards or towards another part of the body; it is desirable to obtain a sensation which radiates towards the area of the receiver's problem.

If the point is to disperse an Excess such as Dampness or Cold, you can use the dispersing touch; if it is to tonify Ki, Blood, Yin or Yang or an organ function, use the tonifying touch (remember to disperse Excess before tonifying Deficiency). In practice, deep pressure to the level where you sense the Ki, combined with the intention to disperse or tonify, is all that is needed. Adjust the strength of your pressure and intention to the condition of the receiver. It can help greatly if the receiver focuses on breathing into the Hara in order to increase his basic Ki.

Each point should be dispersed or tonified for a minimum of 1 minute, up to a maximum of 5 minutes; 2–3 minutes are usually enough to obtain the desired effect. Release the point every 20 seconds or so and start again, in order to maintain the receiver's sensations.

Magnets

Magnets, obtainable from acupuncture suppliers, can be used on points both during and after the Shiatsu treatment, in order to emphasize and prolong its effects. The stronger magnets (2500 gauss) should only be used for the treatment duration and replaced with weaker (800 gauss) magnets which may be left on. The North face of the magnet (the face which comes out of the packet first; it is a good idea to mark it for future reference) is more suitable for dispersing Jitsu or Excess conditions, the South face for tonifying Kyo or Deficient ones. The magnets can be used on points of local pain, tension or weakness, as appropriate, or they can be used on acupuncture points appropriate to the condition being treated (for example, Ki 3 for lower back pain associated with weak Kidney function). Different teachers suggest different ways of working with magnets*
and it appears that this method repays individual experimentation. Within my own limited experience of working with magnets, I have found them very effective in redirecting Ki flow.

Moxa

Moxa is one of the most effective ways of tonifying Ki and Yang Deficiency and of moving Cold, Damp and Stagnation. It is, however, used much more

extensively in Japan and China than in the West; perhaps one of its disadvantages for Westerners is its pronounced smoky smell when burned. However, this disadvantage is far outweighed by its usefulness, particularly in cold, damp climates. It is probably best used after the main Shiatsu treatment.

Moxa is the dried, powdered leaf of artemisia or mugwort. It comes in two forms: the loose powder or "punk" which can be the rough, dark Chinese variety or the ultrafine blonde Japanese fluff; and the moxa stick, which is the powder rolled in a paper cylinder, like an 8-inch cigarette.

The loose punk can be formed into cones of varying sizes which are burned on acupuncture points and usually removed before they burn down to the skin. This method, though effective, is best learned in a class situation, since it is easier to demonstrate than to describe.

The use of the moxa stick is almost equally effective and easier to learn and practise. The outer paper covering having been removed or peeled back to an appropriate level, the stick is lit, which takes a little time and a lighter rather than a match. Blowing on the lit end will reduce the time before it is ready to use, which is when the whole end is glowing red-hot. Have an ashtray handy, as ash quickly collects and must be tapped off constantly.

The stick can be used over points or over large areas.

Points

The glowing end of the stick is held above the point, which should first be marked with a fine felt-tip pen, close enough for the receiver to feel its warmth.

If the point is being used to disperse Cold or Damp, the stick can be moved up and down towards the point, like a bird pecking, while you visualize the Excess factor dispersing.

If it is being used to tonify Ki, Blood or Yang the stick can be held still above the point while you visualize Ki being drawn to the area; the point is likely to become uncomfortably hot and you can then take the stick away for a short time before recommencing.

When using either method, continue for 3–5 minutes, unless the receiver is uncomfortable. The skin should be faintly pink around the point.

---

*The most notable exponent of the use of magnets in the West is Kiiko Matsumoto, whose workshops on magnets, moxa and Hara treatment are highly recommended.

Local areas

Moxa can be used over large areas which are affected by Cold, Dampness (but not Damp-Heat) or stagnation. Examples of conditions which could benefit are:

- lower back pain, better with movement, worse in cold weather;
- severe menstrual pain; dark, clotted blood and a bluish-purple tongue; better with a hot water bottle;
- abdominal pain with loose stools, worse after cold food or drink; thick white, tongue coating
- sudden shoulder pain after sitting in a cold draught;
- bloating in the lower abdomen, with white vaginal discharge.

In such conditions, the glowing moxa stick is held as close as is comfortable over the affected area and moved back and forth to heat the area up. If you are centred in the Hara and have a mother hand somewhere on the receiver's body, you may find that the space above the area seems deficient in certain spots and dense and stagnant in others. If this is the case, you can employ the tonifying and dispersing methods mentioned above. Giving moxa in this way can be as enjoyable a method of interacting with Ki as giving Shiatsu. Continue for 10 minutes or so.

When the moxa treatment is over, the stick will need to be extinguished. Special moxa snuffers can be bought from acupuncture suppliers, but a bowl full of earth or sand will do as well. If all else fails, use scissors to cut the glowing end off the stick into a basin and run water over it.

The strong smell of moxa smoke will soon disappear if windows and doors are left open for half an hour.

15

After the treatment

The treatment has now been concluded and the final checks made on the Hara, the leg length and the Ki picture of the receiver. Ideally, the receiver should be covered with a blanket, if he is not already, and allowed to rest for a few minutes. The giver can use this time for writing up the relevant details on the treatment and its results in the case notes. While the information is still fresh, it may be helpful to jot down any ideas for the next treatment at this stage. Some practitioners offer a cup of herbal tea at this point but it is best not to commit yourself to the degree that one practitioner did when first starting out; after the treatment session, she would offer the receiver a hot bath and a cheese sandwich!

To talk or not to talk?

Many receivers will want to unburden themselves of emotional difficulties during the course of treatment, which is in many cases beneficial. The receiver needs someone to hear him and some time should be set aside to give him full attention. If the receiver is not truly communicating a problem, but obsessively pursuing the same topic every time, allowing time for listening becomes less of a priority.

Although at the time of writing there is a vogue for "psychological" Shiatsu, in which the giver acts as a kind of counsellor, the idea of considering body and mind as separate and treating the one with Shiatsu, the other with counselling, is foreign to the concepts of Oriental medicine. For the Oriental practitioner, the emotions are not distinct from physical symptoms and it is difficult to apply counselling based on

Western concepts of emotional affect within a system which regards emotion as a form of the universal Ki. Shiatsu in itself, the restoring of balance to the Ki in the meridians, is designed to heal the emotions as well as the body, especially when combined with the comfort of physical touch and an understanding and receptive listener when needed.

In cases where a receiver is already in a counselling situation with a qualified psychotherapist, Shiatsu can be a useful parallel treatment, since the emotional effect of the Shiatsu can be brought into consciousness and discussed in the counselling sessions. It is not appropriate, however, for a Shiatsu giver to offer advice or counselling unless properly trained.

Recommendations

To repeat a point made earlier, Shiatsu treatment does not involve the manipulation of a passive receiver by an active therapist. Although the procedures involved may give such an impression, the experience of Shiatsu can be very different, especially if the giver avoids controlling the receiver's Ki and, instead, encourages it to find its own balance through focused but non-invasive touch and intention. Your aim is to allow the receiver to participate as fully as possible in the healing process and to this end you can make recommendations which will help the receiver to do something for himself between treatment sessions.

There are two types of recommendation: one type is specifically connected to the meridians and points used in the treatment and consists of exercises to stretch and tonify the meridians, and points to press or moxa; the other type involves changes in the receiver's lifestyle which may eliminate or reduce the cause of the condition.

Type 1 recommendations: points and meridian exercises

Points

If the receiver has a recognizable TCM syndrome (a pattern, such as Blood Deficiency or Cold Phlegm in the Lungs) there will be certain points (as indicated in Chapter 5 and the individual chapters in Section Three) which will be beneficial, first to disperse any external or internal pathogenic factor and second, to tonify any weakness of the organs.

If there is no Heat present and moxa is suitable, you can teach the receiver to moxa the points himself and suggest that he does it every day or every other day.

If moxa is not suitable, then the receiver can press the points once or twice a day (getting up and going to bed are good times to introduce a new routine). Mark the points for him and show him how to obtain a sensation, focus his Ki and breathe into the point. Pressing points is an excellent way of introducing receivers to the experience of focusing on their own healing. If no point seems particularly relevant, then the source point of a meridian which seems chronically Kyo would be a good choice and St 36 is usually beneficial.

Meridian exercises: the Makko-Ho

This series of exercises will be familiar to most Shiatsu students, since they almost always accompany introductory classes. However, for the student who does not know them, they are included here as helpful recommendations. When recommending a Makko-Ho exercise, suggest one for the meridian that is Kyo; not only will it tonify the meridian through emphasizing the fascial connections, but it will also focus the receiver on an aspect of the cycle of Ki which he is neglecting in his life. It is, in addition, likely to be easier to do than the exercise for the Jitsu

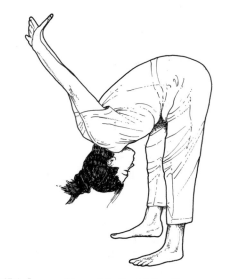

Fig. 15.1 *Lung and Large Intestine Makko-Ho.*

meridian. When teaching the exercise, stress that it is to be done slowly, without effort and always moving on the outbreath, as these concepts are usually unfamiliar to Western receivers.

Lung and Large Intestine

Stand with your feet shoulders width apart, knees "soft" (not locked) and link your thumbs behind your back. Breathe deeply into your Hara. Stretch your fingers out and imagine your body filling with Ki to the fingertips. Now breathe out and, as you do so, bend forward into the position shown in Figure 15.1, keeping your fingers stretched out and relaxing as much as you can.

Still in the position shown, breathe deeply again into the Hara and, as you breathe out, concentrate on letting go all tension and all thought. Feel your body relax. Breathe in once more, imagining yourself taking in new Ki, and breathe out again, relaxing and letting go still more. Breathe in deeply once more and, as you breathe out, come slowly to an upright position. The exercise can be repeated with the thumbs linked the other way around.

Stomach and Spleen

This exercise is usually taught as three stages, but in my experience only the most limber can accomplish

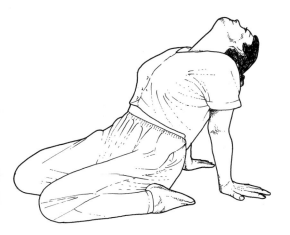

Fig. 15.2A *Stomach and Spleen Makko-Ho – Stage 1.*

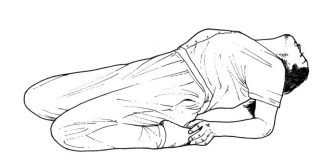

Fig. 15.2B *Stomach and Spleen Makko-Ho – Stage 2.*

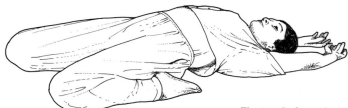

Fig. 15.2C *Stomach and Spleen Makko-Ho – Stage 3.*

the third stage and even the second stage may be a strain. Teach only the stages which are possible for your receiver and emphasize that he should not go beyond what is comfortable.

Stage 1. Kneel on a padded surface such as a thick carpet or futon; sit between your heels if possible, sit on your heels if you cannot sit between them and sit on a cushion placed between your ankles if you can do neither. Breathe deeply into your Hara. As you breathe out, rest your hands facing backward on the floor behind you and lean your torso backwards. Relax your neck and let your head fall back (Fig. 15.2A). Look behind you, rolling your eyes upward. Repeat for two cycles of breath. This stage of the exercise stretches the upper part of the Stomach and Spleen meridians in the chest, throat and face and the lower part in the knees, shins and feet.

If this stage is as much as the receiver can manage he can come back upright on the fourth outbreath. If he could use slightly more of a stretch, encourage

him to lift his pelvis up and forwards if he comfortably can, to stretch some of the rest of the meridian, while breathing out.

Stage 2. On the next outbreath, lean back further on to your elbows. Continue to keep your head relaxed backwards. Stay in this position for two cycles of breath. This position stretches the meridians down to the groin (Fig. 15.2B).

Stage 3. On the next outbreath, if you can, lay your body back on to the floor, with your arms stretched above your head. Relax for two cycles of breath. This final stage stretches the front of the hips and thighs and increases the stretch to the rest of the body. The stretch is increased the more your knees are drawn together (Fig. 15.2C).

When coming up from this position, do so slowly in stages and on the outbreath, rather than scrambling up anyhow. Your head should be the last part to come upright.

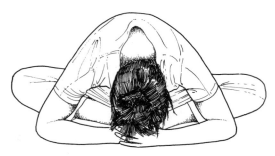

Fig. 15.3 *Bladder and Kidney Makko-Ho.*

Heart and Small Intestine

Sit on the floor with the soles of your feet touching, your legs relaxed outwards and your back upright. Breathe in deeply and clasp your toes. As you breathe out, relax your head, neck and torso forward between your knees, allowing your elbows to relax towards the floor (Fig. 15.3). Stay in the position for two cycles of breath, allowing yourself to relax into it more on each outbreath, and come up on the fourth outbreath.

Although this exercise is hard on the hips and thighs at first, with practice your legs will relax outwards, allowing your torso to curl downwards more and focusing your Ki in the centre of your chest. As this happens, your elbows will reach further towards the floor, stretching the Small Intestine meridian in the shoulders and arms.

Kidneys and Bladder

This exercise is a slightly modified version of the Yoga forward bend; the modifications are important, however, since they add forward impetus to the stretch.

Sit with your legs straight out in front of you, but relaxed outwards. Breathe in and, as you do so, stretch your whole spine upwards and stretch your arms above your head, palms facing out. Breathe out and, as you do, lean forwards, flexing at the hips but with a straight back and straight legs. Breathe in again into your Hara and, as you breathe out, reach as far forward between your feet as you can (Fig. 15.4). Imagine the motive force propelling you forward from your sacrum.

Breathe in again and, on the outbreath, allow your body to relax down towards your legs and rest.

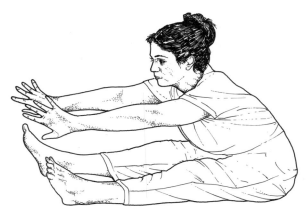

Fig. 15.4 *Heart Protector and Triple Heater Makko-Ho.*

Breathe in again and, on the outbreath, uncurl your body, vertebra by vertebra, bringing your head up last.

Heart Protector and Triple Heater

Sit cross-legged, with your back straight. Cross your arms and place your hands on your knees, with the outside arm on the same side as the outside or uppermost leg. Breathe in deeply and, on the outbreath, relax your body downwards towards the floor. Allow your hips to spread and settle if you do not feel enough of a stretch, or "walk" your hands further apart on your knees (Fig. 15.5).

Hold the position for two cycles of breath and, on the fourth outbreath, come back to the upright position. Repeat, crossing your legs and arms the other way around.

Liver and Gall Bladder

Sit on the floor with your legs as far apart as you can while keeping your spine upright. Link your fingers and stretch your arms above your head, palms up. Breathe in deeply and turn to look at your right foot. Breathe out and lean your body sideways towards your left, stretching your arms out towards your left foot. You should be facing your right foot still and not your left knee! Hold the position and relax into it for two cycles of breath, then come up on the fourth outbreath and repeat the sequence to the other side (Fig. 15.6).

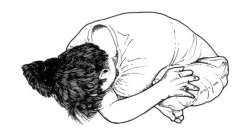

Fig. 15.5 *Heart and Small Intestine Makko-Ho.*

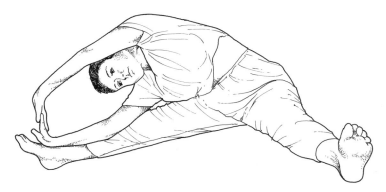

Fig. 15.6 *Gall Bladder and Liver Makko-Ho.*

If you are quite "stretchy", you can complete the sequence by stretching your palms forward in front of you on the next outbreath, leaning forward from the hip joints with a straight back, relaxing into the position for two cycles of breath and coming up on the fourth outbreath.

Type 2 recommendations: lifestyle changes

The field of recommendations is as wide as your experience and if you have other areas of expertise such as physiotherapy, herbs or nutritional supplements, you will obviously be able to make appropriate recommendations from your own specialist viewpoint. The giver who has no such special skills, however, can take heart from the knowledge that if the "yuan" (see p. 9) between

herself and the receiver is good, simply recommending a glass of hot water and lemon every day before breakfast will have a strong healing effect.

General considerations

However enthusiastic you may be about, for example, meditation or jogging, it is essential to give the receiver a recommendation which is in line with his general tastes and outlook. When teaching on one occasion, I observed a giver, who was a Yoga teacher, counselling a down-to-earth receiver with a Stomach diagnosis about breathing and relaxation. As the giver warmed to her subject, I saw the receiver's expression settle into one of controlled derision and stopped the exercise, pointing out to the giver that she was wasting her time, since the receiver had preconceptions about the value of her recommendation. In this case, the receiver had problems with the area of acceptance (Stomach), as well as a dislike of anything appearing hippy or New Age, and needed an extra careful approach.

It is also a mistake to give too many recommendations. In my experience, most receivers find it hard to encompass the changes, even minor changes, which recommendations demand of their lifestyle. One appropriate recommendation, communicated with intention and clarity, can see the receiver through to the next session. Two may underline your concern for the receiver's well-being, but are unlikely to be carried out fully. More than two begin to seem like a chore.

Giving up habits

There are two situations in which you may need to support a receiver in giving up a habit: the first is when the receiver comes for treatment specifically with the intention of giving the habit up; the second is when you, as giver, see that some habit is contributing to the receiver's condition.

1. It sometimes happens that a receiver will come for Shiatsu for help in giving up smoking, drinking or drug taking. This is a specialist subject and not within the scope of this book to discuss at length, but you should be clear, both with yourself and the receiver, that the success of the Shiatsu is ancillary to the genuineness and strength of the receiver's resolve. A more realistic aim for treatment would be to minimize symptoms and reduce stress associated with the habit, without expecting the receiver to abandon it.
2. Far more frequently, it transpires that the receiver's lifestyle incorporates habits which are directly affecting the outcome of treatment. When the habit has some element of addiction attached to it, such as cigarette smoking or excessive drinking of alcohol, the problem is often compounded by guilt on the receiver's part, induced by social disapproval of his habit. It is important, in such a case, to avoid adding to this guilt and to help the receiver to resolve his conflict with himself. It would be unrealistic to expect him to give up smoking or drinking altogether, but he can be encouraged to cut down by various means and, above all, to have awareness of the situations which

drive him to indulge. As treatment progresses, his increased health and balance can greatly ease the compulsion of the habit and perhaps, with time, allow it to drop away altogether.

It is my personal opinion that addictions such as smoking or drinking are tied in to a primary weakness in the organ or organs affected by the drug and that the habit arises as an instinctual attempt to protect a vulnerable organ or stimulate a sluggish one, but one which subsequently causes more damage. So, for example, a receiver who smokes and has a Lung imbalance may well have had it *before* he began to smoke, although he will have made it worse over time. Relinquishing the habit is therefore likely to be even harder and a gradual reduction to a reasonable level, with encouragement and support, is often all that can be expected in the long term.

It is, however, part of the giver's responsibility to let the receiver know that the habit is contributing to his condition, rather than to ignore it. Many receivers want to hear this as a confirmation of what they already suspect and as a form of authority and support in cutting down. This information only has value, however, if it is expressed matter-of-factly and without condemnation.

Knowledge of anatomy, physiology and pathology is especially useful when recommending changes in lifestyle, since most receivers are more receptive to information when it is communicated in a form they can understand, rather than in the unfamiliar terms of Oriental medicine and "energy". A little help with bridging the gap is all that is required and a receiver will often find it easier to accept, for example, that drinking a lot of black coffee is bad for his sciatica (manifesting as Bladder Jitsu) if "overstimulation of the lower spinal nerves" is mentioned.

Recommending other therapies

Other therapies can often be a useful adjunct to Shiatsu treatment and also, for the receiver who feels Shiatsu is not for him, a replacement. Since different therapies suit different types of receiver, I have made some suggestions below. Since there are far more therapies in existence than the ones mentioned here, the reader is invited to contribute his or her own.

Suggested recommendations for each meridian pair

Lung and Large Intestine

Breathing exercises are very beneficial for both. If you know any breathing techniques, you can choose from among them, but simple Hara breathing works very well; for the Lungs, the inbreath is the focus, for the Large Intestine, attention is directed to the outbreath and release. The receiver will require support and encouragement, however, since the taking in and letting go represented by the breathing process are problematic for him; the Lungs receiver may feel unequal to the task and the Large Intestine receiver may suffer from low motivation.

Physical exercise is another way of encouraging a Metal receiver to breathe deeply. For the Large Intestine receiver a more vigorous type of exercise may be suitable (as long as lower back pain is not a symptom) and social sports such as tennis or squash may help him to overcome the isolation which tends to be a factor in a Metal imbalance. The Lungs receiver may not have enough Ki to exercise vigorously and will benefit from Tai Chi, Qi Gong or Yoga, all of which encourage the flow of Ki as well as improving the breathing.

Entertainment is important for providing new experiences for the Metal receiver, who may otherwise sit at home feeling depressed. The best form of entertainment is one which will help to remind the receiver of the significance and beauty of life – music, art, theatre, dance; reading is less helpful, since the receiver needs the stimulation of a different environment. For someone who has trouble with letting go and expressing grief, listening to wistful music or watching a sad film in the home environment may allow the floodgates to open.

Although many Metal receivers love the pungent taste of spicy, hot foods, because it moves the Ki, too much hot food is not advised since the pungent taste also disperses Ki which, particularly in a Lungs receiver, may be Deficient and should not be dispersed. If an underlying Spleen imbalance is causing Dampness and Phlegm in the Lungs, the dietary recommendations for the Spleen (below) maybe helpful.

Smoking is likely to be a problem with the Lungs receiver and he should be encouraged to cut down. Useful methods are to practise Hara breathing when the desire for a cigarette arises and to try to be aware each time of whether the cigarette is really wanted, is desired to suppress an unwelcome emotion, or is a routine mechanical habit.

If a Lungs or Large Intestine receiver has chronic respiratory problems, such as chronic bronchitis or sinusitis, steam inhalations with essential oils can be helpful. Books on aromatherapy will suggest oils to use. Try and choose a book which details whether oils are warming and drying or moistening, in order to fit them as closely as possible to the receiver's TCM syndrome. Essential oils are generally good for the receiver to use, for example in the bath, to activate the corporeal soul via the sense of smell; they can also be helpful for skin problems.

Other therapies. Aromatherapy is a good choice, for the reasons given above. Bereavement counselling may be needed for the receiver who is mourning a death or loss. Homoeopathy is often very effective for Lung problems when Shiatsu is not appropriate and herbs can be helpful for bowel problems. Acupuncture, Chinese herbs and homoeopathy all have good track records for skin conditions.

Stomach and Spleen

Advice on food is likely to be very important for the Earth receiver.

Eating too fast, overeating and constant nibbling are habits which damage the Stomach and Spleen but which will also improve with treatment of the Stomach and Spleen meridians. It is doubtful whether advising a receiver with a weight problem to diet or substantially to change his eating habits will help, since he is already oppressed by social disapproval, but any initiative on his part should be warmly welcomed and supported.

Not eating breakfast and eating too late at night are habits which carry less emotional charge and the Earth receiver will be happy to know that food consumed in the morning is burned off faster than food consumed at night. The receiver's digestion and energy will improve greatly with modification of these habits. If Stomach Yin Deficiency is a suspected TCM syndrome, the receiver may well be eating irregularly and under stressed conditions and should be guided towards regular and peaceful mealtimes.

Overconsumption of fruit, salads and other raw and cold food is a modern fetish which damages the Spleen Yang. Since the average overweight receiver is already Spleen Yang Deficient, he will lose weight and feel better if he saves salads for very hot weather and has lightly steamed or stir-fried vegetables or a warming vegetable soup at other times. Iced drinks are also to be avoided and ice-cream is (almost) taboo!

Foods which cause Dampness are sugar, dairy products, peanuts, bananas, fatty foods and alcohol. All these are contraindicated for the Spleen and Stomach receiver, but in my experience such dietary changes can be quite difficult for the receiver to maintain.

If the receiver has a noticeably Hot or Cold condition where diet is likely to be a factor, the table of Hot and Cold foods on p. 76 may be useful. (If the cause is primarily emotional, which is particularly likely in the case of Heat, then dietary recommendations will not be so helpful.)

Meditation is often recommended for Stomach and Spleen receivers in order to counteract the problem of "overthinking", but this may be too confrontational an approach. Because Earth's major source of cognitive security is the thinking mind, meditation styles which aim to diminish its activity often create anxiety and resistance rather than increasing calm. The Stomach and Spleen receiver is likely to be better off with a form of moving meditation such as Tai Chi, which increases his physical grounding while allowing mental activity to quieten naturally. Since he has a sequence of movements to memorize, his mind has a task to distract it while the meditative state creeps up unawares through the slow harmony of the movements. Yoga has the same kind of effect. For the resolutely sceptical Western receiver, the Pilates system of exercise is a good alternative. Slow, controlled movements, performed with attention to the breath and working from the stomach (the Hara centre), often to an accompaniment of classical music in a tranquil atmosphere, make this system the Western equivalent to Yoga.

Learning Shiatsu is also a good recommendation for the receiver with a problem in Stomach or Spleen. Giving Shiatsu is not only a moving meditation in a similar way to Tai Chi but also offers an opportunity to create a balance between giving and receiving, which is often a problem for the Earth Element. The grounding in the Hara which is a part of Shiatsu training from the beginning, the use of bodily sensing rather than conceptual thought and the recognition that he is both giving and receiving something of real value combine to stabilize and nourish the energies of Stomach and Spleen.

Physical exercise is extremely important for the Stomach and Spleen receiver; Earth controls the muscles and these may become underactive while the brain works overtime. Often, too, an Earth imbalance will manifest with symptoms in the "child" Element, Metal, such as shortness of breath and bowel problems, which are improved by exercise. Since Stomach and Spleen need enjoyment, the type of exercise taken should be carefully chosen to fit the receiver's tastes. Anything he enjoys, from regular walks in the park to Scottish dancing, will nourish as well as exercise him. He should take it easy at first, however, since his feet and knees are vulnerable.

Nourishment and enjoyment are key factors for the Earth receiver but often his way of enjoying himself will be exacerbating his condition. Reading, for example, taxes the thinking mind far more than listening to music, which is a non-conceptual activity; simply suggesting more music to a Stomach Jitsu speed-reader may help to relax him by resting his overactive mind. It is also important for Earth receivers to find a balance between enjoying the company of others and being alone. They tend not to have the same problems with isolation as Metal individuals (although this is not always the case) and often need to spend time by themselves, attending to their own needs. For those with a spiritual bent, retreats are ideal; for others, just an hour to devote to themselves every day can make a difference.

Other therapies. Herbs can be very helpful in cases of severe digestive problems. If a receiver seems severely Blood Deficient, Chinese herbs will be necessary and nutritional advice or supplements will also help.

Heart and Small Intestine

Meditation is the recommendation of choice for a consistent Heart and Small Intestine diagnosis. The Shen is likely to be agitated or Deficient as a result of emotional stress and needs to be stabilized and strengthened; meditation, which calms the emotions, creates a tranquil space in the Heart where the Shen can peacefully reside. Meditation should be taught by a qualified and competent teacher, however; inappropriate techniques may take the imbalance worse, since the Shen is already too volatile. This applies particularly to techniques which focus the attention in a particular area of the body. Watching the breath, a Zen technique, is a safe one to advise if the receiver is willing to try meditation but does not have a method.

For the receiver who views meditation with suspicion for whatever reason, relaxation tapes are now widely available and provide a calming effect. If an older, more traditionally minded receiver finds the concept of relaxation slightly offbeat, crafts or hobbies which absorb the attention without straining the concentration can perform something of the same function; carving or painting, knitting or crocheting can all relax and calm.

Singing, in a choir or with a society, can be a wonderful opener for the Heart/Small Intestine receiver who has difficulty communicating or perhaps even for someone with a speech impediment. The discipline of the form, the support of other voices and the internal resonance of the different notes all combine to give the experience of joy sometimes associated with "singing one's heart out". For the more adventurous receiver, there are many experiential voice therapy groups in large cities, which work with the voice in a specific way to release emotional blocks. It would be advisable to do some research on the individual group and teacher before recommending this type of work.

Other therapies. Psychotherapy or counselling may be helpful in many cases where emotional problems have affected the Heart or where the Small Intestine is blocking off areas of feeling from the receiver's awareness. Voice therapy, as mentioned above, can also be helpful. Healing, if you personally know a healer with skills in this area, can help to stabilize scattered Shen, if you feel it is beyond your capacity.

Bladder and Kidneys

Rest and moderation is one of the most useful recommendations for the Bladder or Kidneys receiver.

It is a difficult one to make, however, since the lives of such receivers are usually inextricably tied to the factors that are exhausting them: a business which is failing, three children to bring up without help, and so on. The Shiatsu will already provide at least an hour when the receiver can relax and if the suggestion to take more time for rest is made, persistently but gently and with understanding of the receiver's real problems in this area, it may eventually have effect.

Water receivers, if they have nothing else to overstretch and tax them, often overexercise. In my experience, counselling moderate exercise rather than marathon running has little effect, but it is worth trying.

Herbs can be helpful over a long period of time to revive and balance an exhausted nervous system. Ginseng is readily available and can be helpful in cases of Kidney Yang Deficiency if there are no signs of Heat, in which case it is contraindicated. The receiver should be told not to take ginseng when suffering from a cold, flu or other acute condition. Royal Jelly can be taken for not longer than 2 months at a time for Kidney Yin Deficiency. Herbs for relaxation are available in tablet form and may help some receivers. Diuretic herbs are better than chemical diuretics in cases of water retention, since they replace lost potassium. Unless you have some training in the use of herbs, however, it is better to leave prescribing to a professional.

Diet. Coffee and tea are favourite means for the Water receiver to draw extra energy from his Source Ki. In my experience, a Kidney diagnosis frequently goes with coffee, while a Bladder type of receiver characteristically drinks pints of tea. Sometimes they can be successfully weaned in easy stages on to decaffeinated coffee or herb tea for 80% of their intake, saving the caffeine hit for the lowest time of day (often mid- to late afternoon). Since fear is the prevailing emotion of these receivers, a gentle warning of the effect of stimulants on their condition will go a long way.

Alcohol will also over time affect the Water Element to some extent. White wine in particular may affect the Bladder type of receiver, perhaps because of the extra acidity. Cigarettes, because of their drying effect, may injure Kidney Yin, via the Lung Yin. Most recreational drugs, whether stimulants or narcotics, injure the Kidneys, Source Ki and Bladder; those in common use which particularly do so are cocaine, cannabis, amphetamines and amphetamine derivatives such as Ecstasy.

Other therapies. Autogenic training and biofeedback can be useful aids to relaxation for a Water type of receiver, since he is likely to want to control the process and may not abandon himself completely to Shiatsu. Herbal treatment is also helpful to restore the nervous system and to revitalize depleted tissues. Chinese herbs are the treatment of choice for Kidney Yin Deficiency.

Triple Heater and Heart Protector

In general, *reconnecting* on one level or another is essential for the receiver with a consistent diagnosis in these meridians, although it is difficult to make recommendations of this nature for the receiver whose boundaries are overprotected. He needs first to re-establish connections within himself on either a physical or psychological level before connecting outwards, with other people, social groups and the environment.

Disciplines involving awareness of his own internal Ki connections, such as Qi Gong, can be very helpful in reconnecting such a receiver. The Pilates system of exercise described above is also an excellent "connector", since it involves muscle groups and fascial connections throughout the body and the deep breathing and attention to the abdomen encourages the Triple Heater/Hara connection. Awareness takes time to manifest, however, and the receiver may need to spend some time with either of these disciplines before feeling the subtler benefits. Yoga can also be mentioned here, although it is possible to do Yoga for years as an advanced form of muscle stretching without enjoying the sensations of Ki or prana, unless it is well taught.

Expressive dance can establish a link between the emotional core and the physical body. Any kind of dancing will help to some extent, but there are many classes and workshops in specific types of dance and movement designed to foster awareness of emotions and energy. Circle dancing will also help to link the receiver's Ki with that of a group.

Certain breathing and meditational techniques

have the effect of distributing awareness throughout the body. These should, however, be taught by a properly qualified and experienced teacher. You should be well informed about the method and the teacher and preferably have experienced it yourself before recommending it. Examples are Qi Gong forms which involve "breathing" Ki around the body in certain cycles; Vipassana meditation; Yogic or Tibetan Buddhist forms of breathing which enable the receiver to gain control over the different "locks" dividing the Three Burning Spaces; meditations connecting the chakras.

Once the receiver is in touch with his own core and the connections throughout his body, he can begin to extend himself outwards. Giving massage or Shiatsu would be an ideal beginning, since the contact involved is limited by the boundaries of the session. Amateur dramatics might encourage both communication and a sense of group identity in a safe form.

On the physical level, circulation is likely to be a problem for receivers with either meridian consistently appearing in the diagnosis. Since the problem stems from the centre, circulatory stimulants alone are unlikely to suffice; however, they may be useful adjuncts. The Heart Protector receiver needs to be warned to change his working posture frequently. Spicy foods with chillies and cayenne will help the circulation, although the Triple Heater receiver may have a sensitive digestion; ginger is milder. Skin-brushing and salt-rubs will stimulate the surface, although the Triple Heater receiver may have sensitive skin. Saunas and Turkish baths may place too much strain on the circulation for these receivers.

The Triple Heater receiver, particularly, is likely to be both sensitive to the environment and vulnerable to infection. Food allergies may be a problem and persistent colds, skin problems, fluid retention or digestive troubles should be investigated with this in mind. (The commonest allergens are dairy products, wheat products, citrus fruits, corn and chocolate.) Antibiotics should be avoided as much as possible and instead, precautions against external pathogenic factors should be taken, by keeping warm and covered as much as possible and avoiding air conditioning and draughts. Ionizers and essential oil diffusers purify the domestic atmosphere in different ways and chemicals should be kept to a minimum in the home environment.

Other therapies. Bioenergetics and Feldenkrais (Awareness through Movement) strengthen energetic connections in the body with the receiver's conscious awareness. Craniosacral therapy (sometimes called cranial osteopathy) works through linking all the fascial connections with the pulse of the cerebrospinal fluid and, while very similar in effect to Shiatsu, may be a gentler method for extremely sensitive receivers. A nutritionist may be needed to check for food allergies. Homoeopathy can also be helpful for stubborn allergies of all kinds.

Liver and Gall Bladder

While the central issue for the receiver with these two meridians in the diagnosis may be to do with life choices and decisions, this issue will be addressed by the Shiatsu treatment itself. Recommendations will be directed towards evening out the receiver's use of his energy and resources, detoxifying and relaxing.

Overconcentration on work is often a problem with the goal-oriented Liver and Gall Bladder receiver and he should be encouraged not necessarily to rest, but to balance work with play. Creativity is to be encouraged – the Wood meridians give the energy for new beginnings and the receiver needs to express his individuality. Any creative talent or preference, such as painting, music-making or writing, which enables him to find his authentic voice will both relax and focus him.

Outdoor pursuits are very beneficial for the Liver or Gall Bladder type of receiver and they are often good at gardening. Receivers with a lot of robust but stagnated energy may thrive on vigorous mowing of lawns!

Physical exercise can often be quite vigorous (unless the receiver is Blood or Ki Deficient) in order to release stagnation, but competitive sports such as tennis carry the risk of extending the Wood receiver's habitual aggression or timidity into the area of play, so that for complete relaxation non-competitive activities, such as swimming, aerobics or long walks, are preferable. Martial arts training, if taught by an experienced teacher, is often an exception, especially for the timid type of receiver, since in the best forms non-aggression is emphasized. Dancing is also good, although Liver and Gall Bladder receivers often combine dancing with situations of overindulgence.

For the localized joint pain often experienced by Wood receivers, a blend of essential oils may be helpful, either as a rub or in the bath.

Diet. Coffee and hot or spicy food are other factors which affect the Liver by stagnating Ki after an initial fast dispersal. Fatty foods may cause a build-up of Heat or Dampness in the Liver and Gall Bladder. In cases of mild Liver Blood Deficiency, proprietary herbal blood tonics are often a helpful supplement to the Shiatsu treatment.

Check what medication a receiver of this type is taking, since many prescribed drugs, in particular anti-inflammatories, tranquillizers, the contraceptive pill and hormone replacement therapy, may have a strong effect on the Liver energy. Some recreational drugs, particularly opium, cannabis and heroin, also affect the Liver and Gall Bladder.

Alcohol intake may need to be controlled if it is affecting the Wood meridians and the receiver should be encouraged to find other forms of enjoyment. It should be remembered that the alcohol may not be a primary factor in the imbalance but an attempt to deaden emotional pain or frustration and the receiver needs other rewards before he can relinquish it.

Other therapies. Psychotherapy can be helpful for the receiver under emotional stress, particularly forms which encourage active expression, such as Gestalt. Art therapy may also be helpful. For the timid receiver, assertiveness traning may be an option. Family therapy or couples therapy may help to resolve self-perpetuating conflicts. Receivers who are in serious difficulties with alcohol or drugs should be referred to a support group which specializes in such problems. Chinese herbs may be necessary in cases of serious Liver Blood Deficiency or Blood stagnation.

After the recommendations

If the receiver is coming for the first time or if you feel that there has been a particularly strong change during the treatment, you may like to suggest that he can telephone you for advice or reassurance. It is rarely a good move to mention that he may experience reactions to treatment, since you may encourage him to imagine some.

Treatment reactions

It is not common, but it does happen that receivers experience reactions to Shiatsu treatment. The most frequent reaction is extreme fatigue, occasioned by the redistribution of the receiver's Ki away from its accustomed pattern. This should last for no longer than a day and a half, however, after which the receiver should feel his normal energy, or slightly better, as he acquires new awareness of his Ki system. If the extreme fatigue lasts, it means that you have overtaxed him with too long or too focused a treatment.

Other common treatment reactions may occur in the form of discharge, such as a snuffly cold, diarrhoea or, very occasionally, a skin rash. There may also be some muscular discomfort if you made postural adjustments to the back during treatment; this should not last, however. If a pain appears in the receiver's back where there was no pain before and does not disappear within a couple of days, it is likely that you made a mistake during treatment, such as dispersing a tense area which was compensating for a weak one, without tonifying the weak area.

Other symptoms which appear after a treatment should be considered very carefully as a possible worsening of the receiver's condition, a possibly unconnected factor (such as food poisoning), or as the result of a mistake you made. Do not automatically assume that they are all signs of improvement. While making this assessment, however, do not be too hard on yourself, since most wrong Shiatsu treatment does not have lasting results. In general, a treatment can be considered to be successful if the receiver reports increased well-being, even if other symptoms appear during the changes which are part of the process of recovery.

Suggesting further treatments

It will help both you and the receiver if you put the first treatment in context. If he is consulting you about the treatment of a disorder, rather than trying Shiatsu for relaxation purposes, he will want to know your opinion of his condition and prognosis. If you feel that you can help, give him an idea of the time it may take and suggest a trial period of the minimum time you think will be required for improvement to show. Be encouraging without being enthusiastic. Your sincerity will be an extension of your Shiatsu.

Appendices

Appendix One: An example of diagnosis and treatment in practice

A woman of 29 came for treatment following an episode of manic behaviour for which she had been hospitalized and sedated. She had weathered the illness well and during it had partially remembered two traumatic incidents from her childhood which she had previously repressed, one of sexual abuse at the age of 3, the second of an incident in her childhood in the tropics, when a snake wound itself around her throat. She felt that remembering these events was part of a process of cure for an illness of which this episode was the third manifestation.

Symptoms

Her illness had left her feeling frail, vulnerable and emotionally exhausted by any social contact. She had a pain down the centre of her epigastrium from her chest. She slept badly, though not every night, and suffered drenching night sweats. Immediately following her release from hospital she caught a cold and lost her voice.

Medication

She was taking a mixture of ginseng and Royal Jelly, also vitamin B complex, and valerian at night.

Personality

She appeared quiet and reserved, with a sweet, "singing" voice and a shy smile. It transpired that her manic episodes were characterized by extreme outspokenness, in contrast to her normal behaviour, in which she rarely expressed negative emotions.

Although attractive, she had difficulty in forming intimate relationships and found intercourse physically painful. She was highly intelligent and enjoyed literature, music and art.

Looking diagnosis

She was red in the face. Her tongue was swollen, pale, moist, quivering and had teethmarks around the edge: it was red at the tip, with red spots and had no coating. When she lay down, there seemed to be a noticeable absence of Ki in her throat area, but there was an Excess in the front of her thighs.

Hara diagnosis

There was general tightness and congestion in the upper Hara and coldness and emptiness in the lower Hara. The Bladder was particularly Kyo and reacted with the Stomach, which was Jitsu.

Interpretation of diagnosis

The receiver is in a state of exhaustion (Bladder Kyo); her nervous system (Bladder) has been oversedated by medication after the hyperexcitement of the manic phase, which must in itself have cost her considerable energy. The Bladder may also reflect the fear contained in her newly unearthed childhood memories. The memories are also embodied in the emptiness in the lower Hara, possibly relating to the abuse and her sexual difficulties, and the lack of Ki in the throat area (the snake around her throat), which is probably also related to her recent loss of voice. The

Stomach Jitsu relates on the physical level to the pain in her epigastrium. It also reflects a long-standing imbalance in the receiver's Earth Element, possibly dating from her childhood when she was sent away to boarding school; her need (Stomach) for nurturing has never been fulfilled and she compensates with her intellect (Stomach) and refined aesthetic sense. (She mentioned that during her breakdown "her brain was functioning overtime".) The gap in the throat area may also indicate that she is used to functioning with her intellect, which is reluctant to connect with the traumatic memories contained in her body.

The TCM interpretation of her symptoms and tongue corroborates the diagnosis. The pale, wet, quivering tongue with teethmarks indicates Ki Deficiency stemming from lack of Spleen and Kidney Yang, hence her exhaustion. The long term Spleen Yang Deficiency which her tongue indicates stems from the same causes as the Stomach Jitsu.

She has a slight Yin Deficiency, which is giving her insomnia and night sweats. It may be the result of the hospital medication combined with her emotional state or it may be the Deficiency of Kidney Yin which ensues from long term depletion of Kidney Yang. It has not yet manifested significantly in her tongue.

The red tip of the tongue with red spots derives from Heat in the Heart, of emotional origin. Her face is also red, indicating a Heat condition in addition to her slight Yin Deficiency, and to which the ginseng is probably contributing.

The imbalance uppermost is that of the Hara diagnosis, Earth and Water, but the Heart needs some attention as the seat of consciousness and there are symptoms of Heat and Yin Deficiency to be addressed.

Treatment method

Treatment was kept short, because of her exhaustion, and focused on specific areas.

Starting in the supine position, the Stomach Jitsu in the thighs was dispersed, allowing the Ki to flow up to the mother hand on the Bladder diagnostic area of the Hara. Bladder and Kidney were both tonified in the feet and special attention was paid to Ki 1, 3 and 6, which all tonify the Yin and were all Kyo. Kidney was then tonified in the chest, with some attention to Heart where it felt Kyo. Stomach was dispersed in the upper chest. The arms were ignored,

to keep the treatment short, since they showed no significant Ki imbalance in the looking diagnosis. Occipital balancing concentrated on Bl 10, as well as local points, and was a focal point of the treatment, with the aim of filling the Ki gap in the throat area.

The prone position followed and the Bladder meridian was worked throughout. Its upper part felt Kyo but inflamed and oversensitive, so only the Heart Yu point was tonified. The middle back felt congested (like the upper Hara, whose energy it mirrors) and was dispersed. The lower back, corresponding to the sexual areas and the uterus, as well as the Bladder and Kidney diagnostic areas, was very Kyo and was a focal point for tonification. Working down the back of the legs, more Ki was felt in the Bladder meridian but is was reluctant to connect with the back and needed considerable encouragement.

Result

Looking diagnosis revealed more flow throughout, but there was still a gap in the throat area. Occipital balancing had not been enough to connect the Ki of the head with that of the body. Kidney in the throat was therefore deeply tonified and Stomach and Spleen dispersed. On rechecking with the looking diagnosis, the throat gap was still there, but only just. She looked less red.

The final Hara diagnosis was Gall Bladder Jitsu, Lung Kyo, with an underlying continuing Spleen Jitsu. Her body energies were now focused on detoxification and finding a path; there was an underlying sadness and sense of loss still to be addressed and a continued need for nurturing.

Recommendations

I suggested the points HP 6 and Ht 7 for self-treatment and recommended that she do some work on connecting her Ki by chakra breathing, holding each chakra in turn and breathing into it. This would help to connect the empty throat and Hara with the rest of the body. The ginseng was too heating and I suggested Royal Jelly alone. Melissa tea (said to "comfort the heart" and a tonic for the nervous system) was suggested as a regular drink.

As she was already receiving psychotherapy and Ki healing, the next appointment was scheduled for nearly a month away, in order not to overload her.

Appendix Two: The Governing and Conception Vessels

The Governing and Conception (or Directing) Vessels are not used as meridian pathways in Shiatsu, since the first runs down the centre of the spine and the second descends the midline of the Hara and is replaced by the diagnostic areas. There are, however, some important points which lie on these meridians. The Governing Vessel is the "Sea of Yang" and the points on it stimulate the Yang, the Source Ki and the Defensive Ki and clear the mind. They have a tendency to support and raise Ki. The Conception Vessel is the "Sea of Yin" and the points on it nourish the Yin, Blood and Essence. They have a tendency to stabilize and descend Ki.

Here are the locations and actions of the points on the Governing Vessel and Conception Vessel, mentioned in Chapter 5.

The Governing Vessel

Governing Vessel 4

Ming-Men, Gate of Vitality. Between the spinous processes of the second and third lumbar vertebrae.

Actions

- Tonifies Source Ki
- Benefits Essence
- Benefits Kidney Yang and the Gate of Vitality
- Expels Cold

MOXA SHOULD NOT BE USED ON THIS POINT IF THERE IS HEAT ANYWHERE IN THE BODY, AS IT WILL MAKE IT WORSE.

Governing Vessel 14

Between the spinous processes of the seventh cervical and first thoracic vertebrae.

Actions

- Expels Wind and releases the Exterior
- Tonifies Yang generally (especially with moxa)
- Clears Exterior and Interior Heat
- Clears the mind

Governing Vessel 20

On the crown of the head, at the midpoint of a line drawn between the tips of the ears.

Actions

- Tonifies Yang
- Strengthens the ascending function of the Spleen
- Eliminates Interior Wind
- Clears the mind
- A resuscitation point

The Conception Vessel

Conception Vessel 3

On the midline of the abdomen, one thumb's width above the upper border of the pubic bone.

Actions

- Bo point of the Bladder
- Clears Heat and Damp-Heat
- Benefits Bladder function

Conception Vessel 4

On the midline of the abdomen, one palm's width below the centre of the umbilicus.

Actions

- Bo point of the Small Intestine
- Benefits the Source Ki
- Benefits the Lower Burning Space
- Roots the ethereal soul
- Nourishes Blood and Yin (without moxa)
- Strengthens Yang (with moxa)
- Tonifies the Kidneys and regulates the uterus
- Anchors Ki in the Hara and clears the mind

Conception Vessel 5

On the midline of the abdomen, three fingers' width below the centre of the umbilicus.

Actions

- Bo point of the Triple Heater
- Tonifies Source Ki
- Promotes transformation and excretion of fluids in the Lower Burning Space and opens the water passages

Conception Vessel 6

On the midline of the abdomen, two fingers' width below the centre of the umbilicus.

Actions

- Tonifies Source Ki
- Tonifies Ki and Yang
- Regulates Ki
- Resolves Dampness

Conception Vessel 9

On the midline of the abdomen, one thumb's width above the centre of the umbilicus.

Actions

- Promotes the transformation, transportation and excretion of fluids throughout the body
- Resolves Dampness and Phlegm
- Controls the Water passages

Conception Vessel 12

On the midline of the abdomen, one palm's width above the centre of the umbilicus.

Actions

- Bo point of the Stomach
- Resolves Dampness
- Tonifies and regulates Stomach and Spleen
- Benefits the Middle Burning Space

Conception Vessel 17

On the midline of the sternum, between the nipples.

Actions

- Bo point of the Heart Protector
- Tonifies and regulates Ki
- Benefits the Upper Burning Space
- Clears the chest and Lungs
- Resolves Phlegm
- Benefits the diaphragm and breasts

Appendix Three: Bibliography

The Book Of Shiatsu, Paul Lundberg, Gaia Books, 1992

Chinese Acupuncture and Moxibustion, Foreign Languages Press, Beijing, 1987

Chinese Medicine from the Classics: The Heart, The Lung, The Kidneys, Spleen and Stomach, Heart Master Triple Heater, Claude Larre and Elisabeth Rochat de la Vallee, Monkey Press, 1989–91

Five Elements and Ten Stems, Kiiko Matsumoto and Stephen Birch, Paradigm Publications, 1983

The Foundations of Chinese Medicine, Giovanni Maciocia, Churchill Livingstone, 1989

Hara Diagnosis: Reflections on the Sea, Kiiko Matsumoto and Stephen Birch, Paradigm Publications, 1988

The Joy of Feeling, Iona Marsaa Teeguarden, Japan Publications, 1987

Nan Ching, The Classic of Difficult Issues, translated and annotated by Paul U. Unschuld, University of California Press, 1986

Shiatsu: The Complete Guide, Chris Jarmey and Gabriel Mojay, Thorsons, 1991

Tongue Diagnosis in Chinese Medicine, Giovanni Maciocia, Eastland Press, 1987

The Yellow Emperor's Classic of Internal Medicine, translated by Ilza Veith, University of California Press, 1972

Zen Imagery Exercises, Shizuto Masunaga, Japan Publications, 1987

Zen Shiatsu, Shizuto Masunaga, Japan Publications, 1977

Suggested further reading

Acupuncture Energetics, Mark Seem, Healing Arts Press, 1991

Acupuncture in the Treatment of Children, Julian Scott, Eastland Press, 1991

Barefoot Shiatsu, Shizuko Yamamoto, Japan Publications, 1979

Classical Moxibustion Skills in Contemporary Clinical Practice, Sung Baek, Blue Poppy Press, 1990

The Complete Book of Shiatsu Therapy, Toru Namikoshi, Japan Publications, 1981

Medicines, Peter Parish, Penguin Books, 1976

The Natural Family Doctor, edited by Dr Andrew Stanway, Promotional Reprint Company, 1993

Natural Medicine for Children, Julian Scott, Unwin Hyman, 1990

Oriental Diagnosis, Michio Kushi, Sunwheel Publications, 1978

Prince Wen Hui's Cook, Bob Flaws and Honora Lee Wolfe, Paradigm Publications, 1983

The Way of Energy, Master Lam Kam Chuen, Gaia, 1991

Appendix Four:
Useful addresses

UK

The Shiatsu Society,
5 Foxcote,
Wokingham,
Berks RG11 3PG

USA

American Oriental Bodywork Therapy Association,
50 Maple Place,
Manhasset,
New York 11030

Australia

Shiatsu Therapy Association of Australia,
P O Box 1,
Balaclava,
Victoria 3183

Austria

Dachverband fuer Shiatsu Oesterreich,
Mariatrosterstr. 113,
A-8043 Graz

Belgium

Internationale Macrobiotiche Shiatsuverenigung,
Zwartezustersstraat 39,
B 9000 Gent

Germany

Gesellschaft fuer Shiatsu in Deutschland,
Wilhelmsallee 11,
10997 Berlin 31

Italy

Federazione Italiana Shiatsu,
Via P. Custodi 14,
20136 Milano
(This body also acts as the secretariat for the
European Shiatsu Federation)

Spain

Instituto Internacional de Shiatsu,
Mare de Deu Del Coll 25,
08023 Barcelona

Switzerland

Shiatsugesellschaft (Schweiz),
Munzachstr. 14,
4410 Liestal

Index

Page numbers in bold refer to illustrations and tables